ESSENTIAL
EMERGENCY
TRAUMA

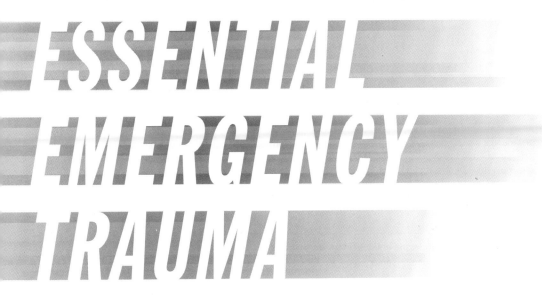

ESSENTIAL EMERGENCY TRAUMA

Editor-in-Chief

Kaushal Shah, MD, FACEP
Residency Site Director
Department of Emergency Medicine
Elmhurst Hospital
Mt. Sinai School of Medicine
New York, New York

Editors

Daniel Egan, MD
Associate Residency Director
Department of Emergency Medicine
St. Luke's-Roosevelt Hospital Center
New York, New York

Joshua Quaas, MD
Director of Trauma Services
Department of Emergency Medicine
St. Luke's-Roosevelt Hospital Center
New York, New York

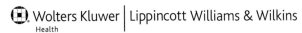

Wolters Kluwer | Lippincott Williams & Wilkins
Health

Philadelphia · Baltimore · New York · London
Buenos Aires · Hong Kong · Sydney · Tokyo

Acquisitions Editor: Frances DeStefano
Product Manager: Julia Seto
Production Manager: Alicia Jackson
Senior Manufacturing Manager: Benjamin Rivera
Senior Marketing Manager: Angela Panetta
Design Coordinator: Holly McLaughlin
Production Service: Aptara, Inc.

Library of Congress Cataloging-in-Publication Data

Essential emergency trauma / senior editor, Kaushal Shah; editors, Daniel Egan, Joshua Quaas.
    p. ; cm.
  Includes bibliographical references and index.
  ISBN 978-1-60831-894-0 (alk. paper)
  1. Traumatology–Handbooks, manuals, etc. 2. Emergency medicine–Handbooks, manuals, etc. 3. Wounds and injuries–Treatment–Handbooks, manuals, etc. I. Shah, Kaushal. II. Egan, Daniel, MD. III. Quaas, Joshua.
  [DNLM: 1. Emergencies–Handbooks. 2. Emergency Medicine–methods–Handbooks. 3. Wounds and Injuries–Handbooks.   WB 39 E7695 2010]
  RD93.E75 2010
  617.1–dc22

                                                                                              2010011840

Care has been taken to confirm the accuracy of the information presented and to describe generally accepted practices. However, the authors, editors, and publisher are not responsible for errors or omissions or for any consequences from application of the information in this book and make no warranty, expressed or implied, with respect to the currency, completeness, or accuracy of the contents of the publication. Application of the information in a particular situation remains the professional responsibility of the practitioner.

The authors, editors, and publisher have exerted every effort to ensure that drug selection and dosage set forth in this text are in accordance with current recommendations and practice at the time of publication. However, in view of ongoing research, changes in government regulations, and the constant flow of information relating to drug therapy and drug reactions, the reader is urged to check the package insert for each drug for any change in indications and dosage and for added warnings and precautions. This is particularly important when the recommended agent is a new or infrequently employed drug.

Some drugs and medical devices presented in the publication have Food and Drug Administration (FDA) clearance for limited use in restricted research settings. It is the responsibility of the health care provider to ascertain the FDA status of each drug or device planned for use in their clinical practice.

To purchase additional copies of this book, call our customer service department at (800) 638-3030 or fax orders to (301) 223-2320. International customers should call (301) 223-2300.

Visit Lippincott Williams & Wilkins on the Internet: at LWW.com. Lippincott Williams & Wilkins customer service representatives are available from 8:30 am to 6 pm, EST.

10 9 8 7 6 5 4 3 2 1

Dedication

Kaushal Shah

I dedicate this book to the emergency medicine residents of St. Luke's-Roosevelt Hospital (NYC) from 2003-2010 because they have been my inspiration. It's with a heavy heart that we all move on from the places we grow to love.

I also dedicate this book to my wife, Vanisha Gilja Shah. Without her support, none of this would be possible.

Daniel Egan

To my family: your continuous support, encouragement, and love have gotten me where I am today.

To the SLR EM residents: your quest for knowledge and growth over time are what give me the drive to keep teaching and learning. You make me a better physician and educator each shift I work with you and I thank you.

Joshua Quaas

I dedicate my portion of this book to my parents, my wife, and my children for their love and support. I also dedicate this to my patients, who continue to teach me about medicine and life.

Contributors

Sarah Battistich, MD
Resident
Department of Emergency Medicine
Harbor-UCLA Medical Center
Torrance, California

Suzanne K. Bentley, MD
Chief Resident
Department of Emergency Medicine
The Mount Sinai School of Medicine;
Chief Resident
Department of Emergency Medicine
The Mount Sinai Hospital
New York, New York

Russell E. Berger, MD
Resident
Beth Israel Deaconess Medical Center
Harvard Affiliated Emergency Medicine Residency
Boston, Massachusetts

Kriti Bhatia, MD
Clinical Instructor
Harvard Medical School;
Associate Residency Director
Department of Emergency Medicine
Brigham and Women's Hospital
Boston, Massachusetts

Jesse Borke, MD
Resident Physician
Department of Emergency Medicine
University of Illinois at Chicago, Illinois;
Resident Physician
Department of Emergency Medicine
Advocate Christ Medical Center
Oak Lawn, Illinois

Casey Buitenhuys, MD
Clinical Instructor
Department of Emergency Medicine
University of California, Los Angeles;
Pediatric Emergency Medicine Fellow
Department of Emergency Medicine
Harbor-UCLA Medical Center
Torrance, California

Erica Cavallo, MD
Department of Emergency Medicine
St. Luke's-Roosevelt Hospital Center;
Attending
Department of Emergency Medicine
Albert Einstein-Weiler Hospital
Bronx, New York

Amit Chandra, MD, MSc
Attending Physician
Department of Emergency Medicine
New York Hospital Queens
Flushing, New York

Christopher H. Cheng, MD
Resident Physician
Department of Emergency Medicine
St. Francis Memorial Hospital/
St. Luke's Hospital
San Francisco, California

Elizabeth Cho, MD
Emergency Medicine Resident
Department of Emergency Medicine
Mount Sinai School of Medicine;
Emergency Medicine Resident
Department of Emergency Medicine
The Mount Sinai Hospital
New York, New York

Clinton J. Coil, MD, MPH
Assistant Clinical Professor of Medicine
Department of Emergency Medicine
David Geffen School of Medicine at ULCA
Los Angeles, California;
Patient Safety Officer
Harbor-UCLA Medical Center
Torrance, California

Matthew Constantine, MD
Senior Resident
Mt. Sinai School of Medicine
New York, New York

Herbert C. Duber, MD, MPH
Assistant Professor
Department of Emergency Medicine
Tufts University School of Medicine
Boston, Massachusetts;
Attending Physician
Department of Emergency Medicine
Baystate Medical Center
Springfield, Massachusetts

Andrea F. Dugas, MD
Department of Emergency Medicine
Beth Israel Deaconess Medical Center
Boston, Massachusetts

Sayon Dutta, MD
Clinical Research Fellow
Department of Emergency Medicine
Harvard Medical School;
Department of Emergency Medicine
Massachusetts General Hospital
Boston, Massachusetts

Daniel J. Egan, MD
Associate Residency Director
Department of Emergency Medicine
St. Luke's-Roosevelt Hospital Center
New York, New York

Mary P. Eldridge, MD
Resident Physician
Department of Emergency Medicine
Mount Sinai School of Medicine;
Resident Physician
Department of Emergency Medicine
The Mount Sinai Medical Center
New York, New York

Robert P. Favelukas, MD
Resident Physician
Department of Emergency Medicine
St. Luke's-Roosevelt Hospital Center
New York, New York

Megan L. Fix, MD
Assistant Professor
Department of Emergency Medicine
Tufts University School of Medicine
Boston, Massachusetts;
Director of Medicine Student Education
Department of Emergency Medicine
Maine Medical Center
Portland, Maine

Jennifer L. Galjour, MD, MPH
Resident
Department of Emergency Medicine
The Mt. Sinai School of Medicine
New York, New York

Nicholas Genes, MD, PhD
Informatics Fellow
Department of Emergency Medicine
Mount Sinai School of Medicine;
Clinical Instructor
Department of Emergency Medicine
Mount Sinai Medical Center
New York, New York

Jonathan St. George, MD
Instructor in Medicine
Emergency Department
Weill-Cornell Medical College, Cornell University;
Attending Physician
Emergency Department
New York Presbyterian Hospital
New York, New York

Darin Geracimos, MD
Attending Physician
Emergency Department
New York Downtown Hospital
New York, New York

Samuel Jeffrey Gerson, MD
Resident
Department of Emergency Medicine
New York Presbyterian Hospital
New York, New York

Hina Zafar Ghory, MD
Chief Resident
Department of Emergency Medicine
NewYork-Presbyterian Hospital
New York, New York

Brandon J. Godbout MD
Emergency Medicine Resident
Department of Emergency Medicine
St. Luke's-Roosevelt Hospital
New York, New York

Elisabeth Gomes, MD
Resident Physician
New York Presbyterian Hospital
New York, New York

Jeffrey P. Green, MD
Attending Physician
New York Hospital Queens
Flushing, New York

Sanjey Gupta, MD
Clinical Assistant Professor
Department of Emergency Medicine
Weill Cornell College of Medicine
Attending Physician
Department of Emergency Medicine
New York Hospital Medical Center of Queens
Flushing, New York

Joseph Habboushe, MD, MBA
Physician
Department of Emergency Medicine
New York Hospital – Queens of Cornell
University
Queens, New York

Azita G. Hamedani, MD, MPH
Division Chief
Department of Emergency Medicine
University of Wisconsin, School of Medicine &
Public Health;
Medical Director, Director of Quality
Department of Emergency Medicine
University of Wisconsin, Hospital & Clinics
Madison, Wisconsin

Jessica Hernandez, MD
Senior Resident
Department of Emergency Medicine
St. Luke's-Roosevelt Hospital
Columbia College of Physicians & Surgeons
New York, New York

Timothy Horeczko, MD
Clinical Instructor
Department of Emergency Medicine
David Geffen School of Medicine at the
University of California,
Los Angeles;
Clinical Instructor
Department of Emergency Medicine
Harbor-UCLA Medical Center
Torrance, California

Erin R. Horn, MD
Resident
Department of Emergency Medicine
Harvard Affiliated Emergency Medicine
Residency;
Beth Israel Deaconess Medical Center
Boston, Massachusetts

Ula Hwang, MD, MPH
Assistant Professor
Department of Emergency Medicine & the
Brookdale Department of Geriatrics and Adult
Development
Mount Sinai School of Medicine
New York, New York

Jonathan Ilgen, MD
Assistant Professor
Division of Emergency Medicine
University of Washington;
Assistant Professor
Division of Emergency Medicine
Harborview Medical Center &
University of Washington Medical Center
Seattle, Washington

Jason Imperato, MD, MBA
Assistant Professor
Department of Medicine
Harvard Medical School
Boston, Massachusetts;
Director of Operations
Department of Emergency Medicine
Mount Auburn Hospital
Cambridge, Massachusetts

Daniel J. Irving MD
Chief Resident
Department of Emergency Medicine
New York Hospital Queens
Flushing, New York

Lisa Jacobson, MD
Chief Resident
Department of Emergency Medicine
Mt. Sinai School of Medicine;
Department of Emergency Medicine
The Mount Sinai Hospital
New York, New York

Amy H. Kaji, MD, PhD
Assistant Clinical Professor
Department of Emergency Medicine
David Geffen School of Medicine at UCLA;
Faculty Attending
Department of Emergency Medicine
Harbor-UCLA Medical Center
Torrance, California

Fahad R. Khan, MD
Attending Physician
Department of Emergency Medicine
Lutheran Medical Center
Brooklyn, New York

Anupam Kharbanda, MD, MSc
Assistant Professor of Clinical Pediatrics
Department of Pediatrics
Columbia University;
NewYork-Presbyterian Morgan Stanley
Children's Hospital
Division of Pediatric Emergency Medicine
New York, New York

Barbara Kilian, MD
Attending Physician
Department of Emergency Medicine
Columbia University
St. Luke's-Roosevelt Hospital Center
New York, New York

Jonathan Kirshner, MD
Assistant Professor of Clinical Emergency
Medicine
Department of Emergency Medicine
Indiana University;
Attending Physician
Department of Emergency Medicine
Methodist Hospital
Indianapolis, Indiana

Andreana Kwon, MD
Attending Physician
Department of Emergency Medicine
Bronx Lebanon Hospital
Bronx, New York

Zuleika Ladha, MD
Attending Physician
Department of Emergency Medicine
Long Island College Hospital
Brooklyn, New York

Alden M. Landry, MD
Clinical Instructor
Department of Emergency Medicine
Harvard Medical School;
Clinical Instructor
Department of Emergency Medicine
Beth Israel Deaconess Medical Center
Boston, Massachusetts

Sarah J. Lannum, MD
Attending Physician
Department of Emergency Medicine
Kaiser Permanente
Walnut Creek, California

Jarone Lee, MD, MPH
Chief Resident
Department of Emergency Medicine
St. Luke's-Roosevelt Hospital Center
New York, New York

Patricia Van Leer, MD
Resident
Department of Emergency Medicine
St. Luke's-Roosevelt Hospital
New York, New York

Penelope Chun Lema, MD
Assistant Professor
Department of Emergency Medicine
New York Hospital Queens/Weill Cornell
Medical College;
Attending Physician
Department of Emergency Medicine
New York Hospital Queens/Weill Cornell
Medical College
Flushing, New York

Jay Lemery, MD, FACEP
Assistant Professor
Department of Emergency Medicine
Weill Cornell Medical College;
Attending Physician
Department of Emergency Medicine
NewYork-Presbyterian Hospital
New York, New York

Elan Levy, MD
Resident Physician
Department of Emergency Medicine
Columbia University;
Department of Emergency Medicine
St. Luke's-Roosevelt Hospital
New York, New York

Resa Lewiss, MD
Assistant Clinical Professor of Medicine
Columbia University College of Physicians and
Surgeons;
Attending Faculty
Department of Emergency Medicine
St. Luke's-Roosevelt Hospital
New York, New York

May H. Li, MD
Columbia University;
Resident
Department of Emergency Medicine
St. Luke's-Roosevelt Hospital
New York, New York

Ari M. Lipsky, MD, PhD
Senior Researcher
National Center for Trauma & Emergency
Medicine Research
The Gertner Institute for Health Policy &
Epidemiology
Tel Hashomer, Israel;
Attending Physician
Department of Emergency Medicine
Santa Monica-UCLA Medical Center and
Orthopaedic Hospital
Santa Monica, California

Mirtha Macri, MD
Senior Resident
St.Luke's-Roosevelt Hospital
New York, New York

Chilembwe M. Mason, MD
Attending Physician
Department of Emergency Medicine
Bronx-Lebanon Hospital Center
Bronx, New York

Ryan P. McCormack, MD
Clinical Assistant Professor
Department of Emergency Medicine
New York University School of Medicine;
Department of Emergency Medicine
Bellevue Hospital Center
New York, New York

Mariah McNamara, MD, MPH
Assistant Professor
Department of Emergency Medicine
University of Massachusetts Medical School;
Attending Physician
Department of Emergency Medicine
UMass Memorial Medical Center
Worcester, Massachusetts

Jamie Meade, MD
Resident Physician
Department of Emergency Medicine
University Medical Center
Las Vagas, Nevada

Kamal Medlej, MD
Resident
Department of Emergency Medicine
St. Luke's-Roosevelt Hospital Center
New York, New York

Bret P. Nelson, MD, RDMS, FACEP
Assistant Professor
Department of Emergency Medicine
Mount Sinai School of Medicine;
Associate Director
Emergency Medicine Residency Program
Department of Emergency Medicine
Mount Sinai Hospital
New York, New York

Sara W. Nelson, MD
Clinical Instructor
Department of Emergency Medicine
Maine Medical Center/Tufts University
School of Medicine;
Attending Physician
Department of Emergency Medicine
Maine Medical Center
Portland, ME

Maria Nemethy, MD
Fellow, Wilderness Medicine/EMS
Division of Emergency Medicine
University of Utah School of Medicine;
Visiting Instructor
Department of Surgery
University of Utah School of Medicine
Salt Lake City, Utah

Marisa L. Oishi, MD, MPH
Resident
Department of Emergency Medicine
Mount Sinai School of Medicine;
Resident
Department of Emergency Medicine
The Mount Sinai Hospital
New York, New York

Francis O'Connell, MD

Neil Patel, MD
Assistant Clinical Professor
Department of Medicine
David Geffen School of Medicine, UCLA;
Attending Physician
Division of Emergency Medicine
West Los Angeles VA Medical Center
Los Angeles, California

Ronak B. Patel, MD, MPH
Clinical Instructor
Department of Emergency Medicine
Harvard Medical School;
Attending Physician
Department of Emergency Medicine
Brigham and Women's Hospital
Boston, Massachusetts

Armin Perham Poordabbagh, MD
Resident Physician
Department of Emergency Medicine
North Shore University Hospital
Manhasset, New York

Joshua W. Quaas, MD
Director of Trauma Services
Department of Emegency Medicine
St.Luke's-Roosevelt Hospital Center
New York, New York

Jeffrey S. Rabrich, DO
Medical Director of Emergency Services
Department of Emergency Medicine
St. Luke's-Roosevelt Hospital Center
New York, New York

Oscar Rago, MD, MBA
Attending Physician
Department of Emergency Medicine
Sunrise Hospital
Las Vegas, Nevada

Prakash Ramsinghani, MD
Resident
Department of Emergency Medicine
Columbia University;
Resident
Department of Emergency Medicine
St. Luke's-Roosevelt Hospital
New York, New York

Anthony Ratanaproeksa, MD
Department of Emergency Medicine
Harbor-UCLA Medical Center
Torrance, California
Providence Portland Medical Center
Portland, Oregon

David C. Riley, MD, MS, RDMS
Assistant Clinical Professor of Medicine
Department of Emergency Medicine
Columbia University Medical Center;
Ultrasound Research Director
Department of Emergency Medicine
Columbia University Medical Center
New York, New York

Lindsay S. Roberts, MD
Resident Physician
Department of Emergency Medicine
Beth Israel Deaconess Medical Center
Boston, Massachusetts

Michael Rosselli, MD, MPH
Sports Medicine Fellow
North Shore University Hospital
Manhasset, New York

Dana Sacco, MD
Resident
Department of Emergency Medicine
New York Presbyterian Hospital
New York, New York

Dana R. Sajed, MD
Clinical Assistant Instructor
Department of Emergency Medicine
SUNY Downstate
Brooklyn, New York;
Department of Emergency Medicine
Kings County Hospital Center/University
Hospital of Brooklyn
Brooklyn, New York

Leon D. Sanchez, MD, MPH
Assistant Professor
Department of Medicine
Harvard Medical School;
Director of Clinical Operations
Department of Emergency Medicine
Beth Israel Deaconess Medical Center
Boston, Massachusetts

Turandot Saul, MD, RDMS
Assistant Clinical Professor
Department of Emergency Medicine
Columbia University;
Ultrasound Fellowship Director
Department of Emergency Medicine
St. Luke's-Roosevelt Hospital
New York, New York

Sonya Seccurro, MD, MS
Chief Resident
Department of Emergency Medicine
St. Luke's-Roosevelt Roosevelt/
Columbia University
New York, New York

Todd A. Seigel, MD
Assistant Professor
Department of Emergency Medicine
Brown University
Providence, Rhode Island

Monique I. Sellas, MD
Instructor
Department of Surgery
Harvard Medical School;
Attending Physician
Department of Emergency Medicine
Massachusetts General Hospital
Boston, Massachusetts

Emily Senecal, MD
Clinical Instructor
Department of Emergency Medicine
Harvard Medical School;
Attending Physician and Associate
Clerkship Director
Department of Emergency Medicine
Massachusetts General Hospital
Boston, Massachusetts

Kaushal Shah, MD, FACEP
Residency Site Director
Department of Emergency Medicine
Elmhurst Hospital
Mt. Sinai School of Medicine
New York, New York

Pranav Shetty, MD
Resident Physician
Department of Emergency Medicine
Harbor-ULCA Medical Center
Torrance, California

Sanjay Shewakramani, MD
Assistant Professor
Department of Emergency Medicine
Georgetown University Hospital
Washington, DC

Steven Shuchat, MD
Attending Physician
Department of Emergency Medicine
Phoenixville Hospital
Phoenixville, Pennsylvania

Daniel J. Singer, MD
Senior Resident
Department of Emergency Medicine
Mount Sinai School of Medicine;
Department of Emergency Medicine
The Mount Sinai Medical Center
New York, New York

Aparajita Sohoni, MD
Clinical Faculty/Fellow
Department of Emergency Medicine
Alameda County Medical Center – Highland
Hospital
Oakland, California

Dean Jared Straff, MD
Instructor in Medicine
Department of Emergency Medicine
Weill Cornell Medical College;
Attending Physician
Department of Emergency Medicine
NewYork-Presbyterian Hospital
New York, New York

Alison E. Suarez, MD
Clinical Instructor
Department of Emergency Medicine
Weill Cornell Medical College;
Assistant Program Director
Department of Emergency Medicine
New York Hospital Queens
Flushing, New York

Darrell Sutijono, MD
Clinical Instructor
Department of Emergency Medicine
SUNY Downstate;
Resident
Department of Emergency Medicine
Kings County Hospital Center/University
Hospital of Brooklyn New Haven, Connecticut
Brooklyn, New York

Christopher Tainter, MD
Resident Physician
Department of Emergency Medicine
The Mount Sinai Hospital
Resident Physician
Department of Emergency Medicine
The Mount Sinai Hospital
New York, New York

Jennifer M. Teng, MD
Attending Physician
Emergency Department
Kaiser Permanente
Hayward, California

Jose Dionisio Torres, Jr., MD
Clinical Instructor
Department of Emergency Medicine
Weill Cornell Medical College;
Attending Physician
Department of Emergency Medicine
New York Hospital Queens
Flushing, New York

Ann Vorhaben, M.D
Resident
Department of Emergency Medicine
St. Lukes- Roosevelt Hospital
New York, New York

Graham Walker, MD
Visiting Clinical Fellow
Columbia University College of Physicians
and Surgeons;
Chief Resident
Department of Emergency Medicine
St. Luke's-Roosevelt Hospital Center
New York, New York

Joseph H. Walline, MD
Instructor
Surgery-Emergency Medicine Division
Saint Louis University;
Attending Physician
Surgery-Emergency Medicine Division
Saint Louis University Hospital
Saint Louis, Missouri

Jonathan Wassermann, MD
Attending Physician
Department of Emergency Medicine
St. Luke's-Roosevelt Hospital Center
New York, New York

Raymond V. Wedderburn, MD, FACS
Chief, Trauma and Critical Care
Associate Director,
Surgical Residency Program
St. Luke's-Roosevelt Hospital Center
New York, New York

Benjamin A. White, MD
Instructor
Department of Surgery
Harvard Medical School;
Staff Physician
Department of Emergency Medicine
Massachusetts General Hospital
Boston, Massachusetts

Lucy Willis, MD
Attending Physician
Department of Emergency Department
New York Downtown Hospital
New York, New York

Kathleen A. Wittels, MD
Clinical Instructor
Department of Medicine (Emergency Medicine)
Harvard Medical School;
Associate Director of Student Programs
Department of Emergency Medicine
Brigham and Women's Hospital
Boston, Massachusetts

Steven S. Wright, MD, FACEP, MS
Instructor in Emergency Medicine in
Clinical Medicine
Department of Emergency Medicine
Cornell University;
Director of Undergraduate Education
Department of Emergency Medicine
New York Hospital Queens
New York

Brian Wright, MD

Jean F. Yang, MD
Resident
Department of Emergency Medicine
St. Luke's-Roosevelt Hospital Center
New York, New York

Jeffrey Yao, MD
Assistant Professor
Department of Orthopedic Surgery
Stanford University Medical Center
Palo Alto, California;
Medical Director of Emergency Services
Emergency Department
St. Luke's-Roosevelt Hospital Center
New York, New York

Preface

Trauma management is one of the major foundations of emergency medicine and frontline medical care. It ranges from the simple evaluation of elbow injuries for occult radial head fractures to complex decisions about whether a major motor vehicle collision patient should go to the computed tomography (CT) scanner, operating room, IR suite or be transferred to another institution. These decisions we make every day matter a great deal—emergency physicians need to feel comfortable and confident making them.

There is no doubt that trauma management can be both "cookbook" and complex. Emergency physicians and surgeons need to have a much deeper understanding of trauma than ATLS training provides. Some of that comes from experience but much of it comes from knowing the essentials of emergency trauma. To that end, we have developed a textbook of trauma that emphasizes the first 15 minutes and provides a framework for decision making. The information is presented in bullet points with heavy reliance on tables and images in hopes of high-yield knowledge transfer.

Practicing emergency physicians will appreciate the up-to-date review and the focus on "best evidence" at the end of every chapter. Residents will benefit from studying the algorithms and understanding the injury patterns that are laid out as (a) pathophysiology, (b) diagnosis, (c) evaluation, and (d) management. Medical students should absolutely read/study a book such as this one before a trauma or emergency medicine rotation. It will allow a much deeper appreciation for trauma care that often occurs quickly and furiously with little discussion.

Those caring for severely injured trauma patients do not always have the luxury of time. Knowing the medicine in advance benefits both the physicians and the patients.

Kaushal Shah, MD, FACEP
Residency Site Director
Department of Emergency Medicine
Elmhurst Hospital
Mt. Sinai School of Medicine

The more we sweat in peace, the less we bleed in war.
—Vijaya Lakshmi Pandit (1900–1990)

Acknowledgments

We acknowledge all the editors (Frances DeStefano, Julia Seto, and Sarah Granlund) for believing in us and making the process smooth and (relatively) painless. Thank you, Fran, Julia, and Sarah.

Contents

Section Editor: Jeffrey Rabrich

1

General Trauma: The First 15 Minutes, Algorithm, and Decision Making

Jeffrey Rabrich

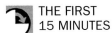 THE FIRST
15 MINUTES

Prehospital Phase
- Obtain as much information as possible from emergency medical service (EMS).
- Mobilize resources before the patient arrives. If you are at a facility with an organized trauma team, they should be activated. Even more importantly, in the nontrauma center, the physician should consider alerting the surgeon on call if there is a potential need for his or her services.
- Additional resources to mobilize prior to arrival include the respiratory therapist, radiology technician, and any other service the physician feels may be needed on the basis of the preliminary information.

Patient Arrival
- Initial observations of the patient as he or she is being wheeled in by EMS.
  - Patient intubated? Or assisted with BVM?
  - Is there adequate intravenous (IV) access?
  - Does the patient appear awake?
- Get "the bullet" (brief synopsis of what happened) from EMS.
  - Remember that the EMS providers actually saw the scene of the trauma and can provide details (such as amount of damage, external blood loss) that cannot be obtained from any other source.
  - Remember to ask about prehospital vitals as several recent studies indicate that prehospital hypotension may predict need for operative intervention, as well as worse prognosis.

Primary Survey
Immediate goal of simultaneous assessment and treatment of life-threatening injuries.

- Airway must be evaluated with c-spine precautions.
  - Look in the mouth for potential obstructions such as blood, vomitus, and loose or broken teeth.
  - If there is any concern for the patient's ability to maintain his or her airway, the physician should have a low threshold for intubation with manual in-line stabilization.
- Assess the breathing.
  - Evaluate chest wall motion, lung sounds, respiratory rate, and oxygen saturation.

- Consider early intubation for poor respiratory effort, inadequate oxygenation or Glasgow Coma Scale (GCS) score of 8 or less.
- Assess the circulation.
  - Examine for life-threatening hemorrhage by looking externally; however, some experts have suggested that this would include looking for internal hemorrhage as well and advocate the FAST examination being done during "C," whereas others feel that this should be done after the primary survey.
  - Two large-bore IVs should be established if not already done.
- Disability or neurologic assessment.
  - Must include an assessment of the GCS score as well as pupil examination. Pitfalls here include not documenting an initial GCS score as well as being falsely reassured by a rapidly improving mental status that may actually represent a "lucid interval" of a serious head injury.
- Expose fully.
  - Look for any other injuries that may not be readily apparent.
  - Hypothermia is a major concern in the trauma patient. It has been well documented in the literature that trauma patients who are allowed to become hypothermic have worse outcomes. The clinician must be cognizant of the fact that the patient is naked in a large trauma room that is often cold, as well as receiving blood and or crystalloid that is cold. Every effort must be made to maintain body temperature, as well as giving warmed IV fluids and blood.

Imaging Studies

- "Trauma Series"
  - Once the primary survey has been completed an initial "trauma series" should be obtained. Traditionally, this has included a chest x-ray (CXR), AP pelvis, and lateral c-spine.
  - More recently, the lateral c-spine has been abandoned for the faster and more accurate computed tomographic scan of the cervical spine.
- FAST or e-FAST
  - If not performed during the primary survey, the FAST examination should be performed to evaluate for intraperitoneal blood.
  - Recently, the e-FAST or extended-FAST examination has been advocated to assess for pneumothorax and hemothorax as well.

Tubes

- Foley
  - A Foley catheter should be placed for evaluation for hematuria as well as monitoring urine output.
- Rectal examination
  - Traditional teaching is that a rectal examination must be done prior to placement to evaluate for signs of urethral injury such as high-riding prostate as well as blood at the urethral meatus.
  - Recently, at least one study has questioned this practice, but until more data are available to dispute the need for a rectal examination, the classic dogma should be followed.

The Secondary Assessment

- Once the primary survey has been completed and life-threatening concerns addressed, an organized, head-to-toe assessment must be undertaken. This examination should proceed in an organized fashion and evaluate each area for injury or abnormality.

- Some pitfalls in the secondary assessment include not looking in recesses or difficult to see areas such as the axillae and perineum. These sites can hide evidence of injury such as exit wounds and stab wounds.
- SAMPLE (**S**igns/**S**ymptoms, **A**llergies, **M**edications, **P**ast medical history, **L**ast meal, **E**vents) history should be obtained if the patient is alert. If unable to obtain from the patient, often details such as medical history or allergies can be obtained from family or EMS.

Platinum 10 Minutes

All of the previously described assessments should be obtainable in the first 10–15 minutes. By this time, the initial resuscitation and stabilization of most patients should be completed, and the patient should be ready to leave the trauma bay. The patient should be on his or her way to (a) the operating room (**OR**) if immediate surgery is indicated, (b) **the imaging suite** if he or she is stable, (c) the intensive care unit if observation is the planned course of action, or (d) a regular gurney/stretcher in the emergency department for observation before discharge home.

DECISION MAKING

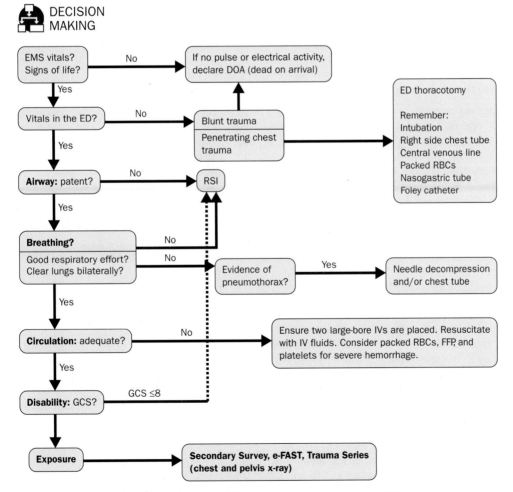

General trauma: Decision making algorithm. EMS, emergency medical services; DOA, dead on arrival; ED, emergency department; RBCs, red blood cells; RSI, rapid sequence intubation; IVs, intravenous lines; FFP, fresh frozen plasma; GCS, Glasgow Coma Scale.

2 Emergency Medical Services

Kamal Medlej

Introduction

Emergency medical services (EMS) is an extension of emergency medical care into the community. They were created and designed to shorten the time of delivery of essential care and to optimize the transport of patients from their site of injury/illness to the most appropriate hospital or care center. There is no one single EMS system, rather, like most health care systems in this country there are a patchwork of local systems defined by geographic and political variables.

The importance of EMS stems from the fact that the survival rate of certain medical conditions is significantly improved when these are recognized on-site, and their treatment initiated rapidly, before transport to the hospital. Such conditions include cardiac arrests secondary to the "shockable rhythms" of pulseless ventricular tachycardia (V-tach) and ventricular fibrillation (V-fib) in which it was found that decreasing the time from arrest to electrical defibrillation significantly improved outcome. Multiple emergent conditions benefit from rapid on-site intervention: acute trauma, hypoglycemia, severe anaphylactic reactions, narcotic overdoses, and so forth.

Another important role of an EMS system is to recognize the need of certain patients for specially equipped and staffed facilities such as a trauma center, burn center, or a cardiac catheterization laboratory. Depending of their accessibility and the patient's condition, the ambulance crew can be directed to these facilities, bypassing closer hospitals that are not appropriately equipped to deal with specific patient pathology. The goal is to optimize the patient's transport and care to the most appropriate facility and to decrease the resources used for subsequent transfer of these patients once their initial resuscitation and stabilization is achieved.

Training

Four main levels of certification exist at the federal level as established by the Department of Transportation. Their recognition at the state level varies from state to state but is generally along the following lines.

First Responder: Basic Life Support

It represents the first person at the scene, usually from the fire or police department. They are responsible for the initial scene and patient assessment, as well as the initiation of basic airway management (bag-valve mask ventilation) and cardiopulmonary resuscitation. Once the initial life-saving measures are under way, they can provide hemorrhage control by direct pressure over the injury as well as spinal immobilization. First responders should be trained in the use of the automated external defibrillator.

Emergency Medical Technician—Basic (EMT-B): Basic Life Support

This level of certification is the minimum required to staff a basic life support ambulance. The EMT-B possesses all the skills and training of the first responder but receives further formation in triage, detailed patient assessment, and patient transportation.

4

Emergency Medical Technician—Intermediate (EMT-I): Basic or Advanced Life Support
This certification level sees a wide variation nationwide in terms of the level of training it receives. It offers a compromise between the EMT-B and EMT-P in that it allows for the delivery of more advanced care at a lesser cost of training. EMT-I is usually allowed to start intravenous lines and to manually defibrillate. They may also use blind-insertion airway devices and certain medications. Their designation as Basic Life Support (BLS) or Advanced Life Support (ALS) varies from state to state.

Emergency Medical Technician—Paramedic (EMT-P): Advanced Life Support
The EMT-P is the most advanced prehospital provider and performs a number of procedures such as endotracheal intubation, needle decompression of tension pneumothorax, needle or surgical cricothyrotomy, and transthoracic cardiac pacing. They are also trained in cardiac rhythm recognition and in the use of a wider number of medications.

Transportation

Ground Transport
An EMS system is based on the concept of mobility and efficiency. The EMS personnel must be able to reach their site of intervention quickly in a vehicle that is designed to carry all the equipment they might need and to provide safe transport for the patient(s). Each system is designed with local setting and community needs: urban/rural, geography (mountains, ocean, etc.), regional hospital distances, regional hospital types, and so forth.

Ambulances have evolved from horse-drawn carriages, to stripped-down motorized vans, to the sophisticated vehicles in use today. Indeed, they are equipped with lighting, power outlets, communications devices, and suction and oxygen delivery systems. The ambulance interior is set up to securely transport up to two patients. It is also designed so that the ambulance crew can have easy access to patients to manage them in terms of airway and ventilatory support during transportation.

Ambulance crews can be combined in different ways but are most commonly organized into BLS crews and ALS crews. The ambulances are also labeled as ALS and BLS ambulances and will vary in how they are equipped.

Air Medical Transport (AMT)
The concept of air medical evacuation goes back to the first air transport of wounded soldiers in World War I by fixed-winged airplanes. It was revolutionized by the introduction of the helicopter during World War II and matured into a large-scale means of evacuating the injured during the Korean and Vietnam wars. This mode of transportation greatly improved the outcome of traumatic casualties by accelerating their transfer to field hospitals located behind the front lines.

This once mostly military application proved its usefulness and resulted in the development of civilian AMT programs. The helicopter remained the most used carrier given its ability to vertically take off and land and to forego the need of a long runway. This also allowed the helicopters to land in the immediate vicinity of the hospitals and decreased the delay a transfer from an airplane to an ambulance would involve. Fix-winged aircraft remains in use, however, for transport of critically ill individuals over longer distances, as well as interfacility transport and repatriations.

The makeup of the air medical crew differs from the ground transport crew in that it is composed of a registered nurse and a paramedic in the majority of cases. The flight nurses are generally experienced in intensive care units or emergency department care and may be specialized to care for adults, children, or neonates. Respiratory therapists are sometimes also included as part of the AMT crew to provide expertise in airway and ventilator management.

Certain limitations affect AMT and are usually related to cost, weather, and the difficulty of managing critical patients in this particular setting. As in other modes of transportation, AMT operates only in circumstances that do not jeopardize the safety of its crew. Certain environmental, situational, and geographic requirements must be met before the dispatch of an AMT unit can be allowed. Weather requirements in terms of wind speed, temperature, and visibility are established by the local authorities and are usually similar to those imposed on civilians. The site of intervention itself must also be safe and appropriate for helicopter landing and takeoff. Given the cost of AMT compared with ground transport, certain criteria must be met relating to the condition of the patient, the distance from an appropriate hospital facility, and the benefit of his air transport in terms of time saved and care given.

The effect of AMT on trauma patients compared with ground transport remains another area of controversy. Although some studies have shown that the overall mortality in patients transported by helicopter is reduced, this benefit pertains to only moderately to severely injured patients. Critical patients or those in posttraumatic cardiac arrest did not benefit from these dispositions.

Protocols

There is a clear consensus that patients with traumatic arrests need to be transported to the nearest hospital, regardless of its designation as a level I trauma center. The EMS prehospital treatment protocols are clear on this matter and Advanced Trauma Life Support (ATLS) is usually started on route to the extent possible.

The management of unstable trauma patients, however, remains controversial, with some favoring a rapid transport to the nearest trauma center without delay, whereas others opt for an initial attempt at patient stabilization on-site with endotracheal intubation and fluid boluses. While evidence favors a rapid transport to the nearest facility after airway management, fluid boluses as a mean to restoring blood pressure are falling out of favor as evidence suggests that they do not improve outcomes and prolong the time spent on-site. "Permissive hypotension" in cases of penetrating trauma to the chest/torso is a theory practiced in many trauma centers, further arguing that patient transport should not be delayed except for obvious medical circumstances.

Ambulance crew provide the hospital of destination with an early notification of their impending arrival with a seriously ill or unstable patient whenever possible. The two-person crew has to deal with operating the vehicle and managing their patient and will sometimes not be able to contact the hospital directly. They might rely on a dispatcher such as a trained EMS dispatcher to whom they can provide some information on the situation, or a police officer who was present at the scene. The notification allows for the emergency department staff to set up the trauma/resuscitation room and be prepared for the patient's arrival and expedite care. Level I trauma centers have designated trauma teams that are usually composed of EM physicians, EM nurses, and surgeons. The team is activated by the notification and will be present at the bedside for quick resuscitation and assessment of the patient and to transport to the operating room if need be. Table 2.1 lists the procedures that—given the circumstances and the composition of the EMS team (BLS vs. ALS)—could already have been performed on-site or en route. Indications that a patient should be transported to the nearest hospital instead of the nearest trauma center are listed in Table 2.2.

TABLE 2.1: Possible on-site or en route procedures performed on traumatic arrests

Advanced airway management[a]

Needle decompression (if a tension pneumothorax was suspected)[a,b]

Defibrillation in nonpenetrating chest trauma (V-fib or pulseless V-tach on ECG)[b]

Rapid infusion of normal saline or Ringer's Lactate via one or two large bore IVs[a,c]

Rigid cervical collar placement

Patient placed on a long spinal board

Deformed joints immobilized in the position found[b]

[a]These procedures are performed only by ALS crews.
[b]These steps are performed en route in unstable or traumatic arrests.
[c]Controversial step, still included in certain EMS protocols.

V-fib, ventricular fibrillation; V-tach, ventricular tachycardia; ECG, electrocardiogram; IVs, intravenous lines; ALS, Advanced Life Support; EMS, emergency medical services.

Transfer of Care

The transfer of care occurs between the EMS crew and the trauma team in the presence of the physician running the trauma survey. The EMS team provides the receiving team with all the information it needs to start assessing and treating the patient, including the mechanism and time of injury, initial vital signs, and progression of physiological status, as well as what was performed in terms or procedures and treatment on-site or en route. The receiving physician should prompt the EMS team for any other information that could have been gathered from surveying the scene (i.e., presence of alcohol bottles, mechanism of injury, field Glasgow Coma Scale score).

It is the receiving physician's responsibility to confirm the placement and functioning of airway adjuncts and vascular access equipment. It is also very important to do so given that endotracheal tubes and intravenous access can easily be dislodged during the patient's transfer.

TABLE 2.2: Indications for transporting major trauma patients to the nearest hospital rather than the nearest trauma center

The patient is in cardiac arrest (medical or traumatic)

The patient has an unmanageable airway (failure of both basic and advanced airways)

An on-line medical control physician so directs

Definition

Shock

On a global level, shock is the failure of the circulatory system to maintain adequate blood flow. At a cellular level, shock is impaired metabolism due to inadequate oxygen delivery. Acute hemorrhage is the main cause of shock and hypovolemia in the trauma patient requiring fluid resuscitation. Other causes include neurogenic shock (from spinal cord trauma), burns (including chemical and electrical) and dehydration. Although rare, cardiogenic shock may occur because of trauma to the heart, and septic shock may occur in patients with underlying illness or who are slow to arrive to a higher level of care.

Pathophysiology

In hemorrhagic shock, decreased circulating blood volume is detected by cardiac stretch and aortic baroreceptors, which then increase sympathetic tone to restore intravascular volume and maintain perfusion. Sympathetic activation leads to vasoconstriction, increased heart rate, and increased myocardial contractility. The renin-angiotensin system is also activated by the kidneys leading to more vasoconstriction from angiotensin II.

At some point, however (see shock classes below), the degree of hemorrhage exceeds the body's ability to compensate, causing decreased perfusion which leads to lactic acidosis of nonvital tissues, hypotension, and shock.

Diagnosis/Evaluation

Hemorrhage may be occult in trauma, but all sources must be considered as patients may have multiple bleeding diatheses.

All trauma patients should ideally have two peripheral large bore intravenous line (IVs) (16G or larger) placed on or prior to arrival, and the patient should be immediately placed on a cardiac monitor to obtain a full set of initial vital signs. The vital signs will provide a framework for the level of hemorrhage based on the degree of shock (Table 3.1). If a patient is tachycardic, assume that it is due to hemorrhage and not simply pain or anxiety. If mental status is altered, consider severe hemorrhage or head injury as opposed to intoxication. Also recall that vital signs may be masked by patient factors or medications, for example, beta-blockers that prevent tachycardia.

Consider that patient factors may affect parameters:

- Young, healthy patients have increased cardiac reserve and may be able to tolerate greater hemorrhage but may deteriorate rapidly once compensatory mechanisms are exhausted.
- Athletes, who may have resting heart rates in the 40s and 50s, may be relatively tachycardic with heart rates in the 80s and 90s.
- The elderly may not respond to hemorrhage with tachycardia because of heart disease or medications (typically chronotropes, such as beta-blockers, digoxin).

TABLE 3.1: Shock classes[a]

Parameter	Class I	Class II	Class III	Class IV
Blood loss in mL	≤750 mL	750–1500 mL	1500–2000 mL	≥2000 mL
Blood loss as percent total blood volume	≤15%	15–30%	30–40%	≥40%
Pulse	Often <100	>100	>120	≥140
Blood pressure	Normal	Normal	Decreased	Decreased
Pulse pressure	Normal or increased	Decreased	Decreased	Decreased
Capillary refill	Normal	Delayed	Delayed	Delayed
Respirations	14–20	20–30	30–40	>35
Urine output	≥30 mL/hr	20–30 mL/hr	5–10 mL/hr	Minimal
Mental status	Slightly anxious	Mildly anxious	Anxious/confused	Confused and lethargic

[a]Assumes a normal blood volume: 7% of the of the 70 kg patient = 5 L of blood (3 L plasma, 2 L red blood cells)

- Pregnant patients, especially in the third trimester, may have a more pronounced response to minor hemorrhage, given poor venous return from a gravid uterus, and also have a significantly increased circulating volume.
- Those with heart transplants will not respond sufficiently to hemorrhage or shock.
- Nonhemorrhagic causes of hypotension are listed in Table 3.2.

Although urine output is an important measure to guide resuscitation efforts, in the initial assessment of the trauma patient it is not useful.

Although few blood tests have any benefit in the evaluation of the acute trauma patient, consider ordering the following trauma panel: complete blood count, basic metabolic panel, coagulation profile, toxicologic screen (including alcohol level), lactate, type and screen, and pregnancy test. Arterial blood gas may be helpful in major trauma.

- The initial hematocrit is usually normal even in the setting of significant hemorrhage, though serial hematocrits can be useful to guide resuscitative efforts and help characterize injury.
- A lactate level above 2 mmol/L has been correlated with intensive care unit admission and length of stay, signifying that tissues are using anaerobic metabolism due to poor perfusion.

TABLE 3.2: Nonhemorrhagic causes of hypotension in the trauma patient

Cardiac tamponade
Tension pneumothorax
Spinal cord injury (neurogenic shock)
Toxic ingestions
Primary cardiac dysfunction

- A base deficit of less than −4 indicates inadequate resuscitation due to lactic acidosis.
- A basic metabolic panel may be useful in the evaluation of a patient's renal function.
- A coagulation panel will provide coagulation status (especially useful if the patient is on warfarin [Coumadin]).

Although rarely done emergently in the emergency department, for further evaluation of fluid status, a central venous oxygen saturation catheter may be inserted. If the mixed central venous saturation is low, this suggests inadequate resuscitation.

Management

Follow the ABCs and ATLS guidelines. The patient should be placed on 100% oxygen and a cardiac monitor. A full set of vital signs should be immediately obtained while procuring IV access (Table 3.3).

If peripheral access is difficult, central venous catheterization may be necessary. Often the femoral vein is most accessible and fastest to procure during a trauma resuscitation. If there is concern for hemorrhage below the diaphragm (i.e., penetrating vascular injury to the abdomen or lower chest), cannulation of the subclavian or internal jugular veins is preferred.

A Cordis central catheter will allow for more rapid infusion of IV fluids than a triple lumen catheter. Remembering Poiseuille's law, flow of liquid is inversely related to the length of the tube and directly related to the radius of the tube to the fourth power.

If there are abnormal vitals or a mechanism concerning for potential hemorrhage, begin fluid resuscitation with a 2 L crystalloid bolus (normal saline or lactated ringer's) in the adult patient and a 20 mL/kg crystalloid bolus in the pediatric patient. Consideration may be given to allow so-called "permissive hypotension" in the patient with penetrating trauma, as returning the patient to a normal blood pressure will only accelerate the extravasation of blood (see Best Evidence, below). This is currently very controversial and not yet standard of care at most institutions.

When crystalloid is infused, only approximately 30% stays intravascular; thus, a 3:1 rule is used to approximate the crystalloid volume necessary for resuscitation. (For example, if 1 L of blood is lost, it will take 3 L of crystalloid to replace this intravascular volume.)

Blood products may be required for significant hemorrhage or continued abnormal vital signs despite fluid resuscitation. Standard practice is to give 2 units of packed red blood cells (RBCs) if hypotension persists despite 2–3 L of crystalloid, hematocrit is <20 (or <25 in cardiac patients), or sooner if cardiovascular collapse is impending or there is obvious devastating hemorrhage. While typed and matched blood is preferable, when time does not permit, type O blood should be given; O+ is preferred for everyone other than

TABLE 3.3: Ideal venous access in trauma resuscitation

Two large peripheral IVs
Cordis catheter
Triple lumen catheter
Intraosseous needle

TABLE 3.4: Indications for packed red blood cells

Hypotension persists despite 2–3 L of crystalloid
Hematocrit <20 (or <25 in cardiac patients)
Impending cardiovascular collapse
Obvious devastating hemorrhage

women of childbearing age who should be given O– to prevent Rh sensitization. Each unit of packed RBCs should raise the hematocrit approximately three points (Table 3.4).

Platelets and coagulation factors drop because of consumption and dilution from resuscitative fluids. Acidosis and hypothermia also interfere with the normal functioning of the coagulation cascade. Trauma patients are especially prone to these conditions. In the patient, IV fluids and blood products should be warmed when possible (Table 3.5).

While there is no consensus on when to transfuse blood products (other than packed RBCs), most experts recommend rechecking coagulation factors (including fibrinogen) after a patient has received 5–7 units of packed RBCs. If values exceed 1.5× normal, patients should receive 2 units of fresh frozen plasma (FFP). Each unit of FFP will increase clotting factor levels by 10%. If fibrinogen levels are significantly low (<100 mg/dL), cryoprecipitate may be given. Platelet counts are also reduced through hemodilution, such that 10–12 units of blood can reduce the platelet concentration by 50%; after 10–20 units of packed RBCs, most physicians agree on giving a standard 6 units of platelets to increase the platelet count by 30,000–60,000, depending on patient characteristics.

Simple IV replacement categorization:

- Crystalloid sufficient for Shock Classes I and II
- Crystalloid and blood for Shock Classes III and IV

Note: other colloids besides blood (starches, albumin, etc.) have not shown any benefit over standard crystalloid for resuscitation.

Special Considerations

Vasopressors in trauma patients are generally discouraged. If they are utilized because of persistent hypotension, it should occur only after very aggressive fluid and blood resuscitation and a thorough evaluation for hemorrhage. In a hypovolemic patient, pressors without adequate fluid resuscitation will lead only to further peripheral vasoconstriction and tissue hypoxia. One exception to the rule is in cases of neurogenic shock; vasopressors (dopamine alone or with other agents) along with IV fluids may be used to improve blood pressure, since this hypotension is due to loss of sympathetic tone, and *not* blood loss. However, the initial management of neurogenic shock is the same: fluid resuscitation, *then* vasopressor therapy.

Shock does **not** occur from isolated brain injuries. Do not make the mistake of attributing a patient's hypotension to a head injury!

TABLE 3.5: "Lethal triangle" of trauma

Coagulopathy
Acidosis
Hypothermia

Best Evidence/Clinical Decision Rules

Permissive Hypotension

ATLS recommends initiating intravenous fluid therapy with 2 L of a balanced salt solution with the goal of a normal blood pressure in cases of hypotension from traumatic hemorrhage. Multiple animal studies have demonstrated that this leads to *increased* bleeding (due to increased pressure, dilution of clotting factors, and decrease in blood viscosity) and decreased tissue oxygen delivery. "Permissive hypotension" is the practice of allowing patients of penetrating trauma to the torso to remain hypotensive until reaching the operative room where the source of bleeding can be definitely addressed. In theory, avoiding aggressive fluid hydration will prevent "popping the clot" and increased hemorrhage.

The first large randomized study of permissive hypotension was performed in the early 1990s in Houston, Texas (Bickell et al., 1994). It was demonstrated that those with delayed fluid resuscitation had a 70% survival to discharge from the hospital versus 62% survival for those with immediate fluid resuscitation in the field by emergency medical services ($p < 0.04$). An attempt to repeat the study of permissive hypotension at Maryland's Shock Trauma (Dutton et al., 2002) proved to be futile with 92.7% survival in both arms of the study, those titrated to a systolic blood pressure (SBP) of 100 (aggressive fluid resuscitation arm) and those titrated to a SBP of 70 (permissive hypotension arm).

Although there is no clear correct method of resuscitation, it is a mistake to practice "permissive hypotension" on all trauma patients. It has been studied only on patients with penetrating trauma to the torso. **Patients with traumatic brain injury should never be allowed to remain hypotensive as this second insult has clearly been demonstrated to be harmful.**

Transfusion Protocols

In anticipated massive transfusion (requiring more than 10 units of packed RBCs), recent observational data from the US military hospitals in Iraq and Afghanistan suggest that these patients should be transfused in a RBC:FFP:platelet ratio of 1:1:1, as many of these patients are either coagulopathic on arrival or rapidly become coagulopathic from hemorrhage and hemodilution.

Tourniquets

After high rates of amputation and neurovascular compromise from tourniquet use in the Vietnam War, tourniquets fell out of favor but are again being investigated because of their use in the Iraq and Afghanistan wars. While most bleeding should be controlled with direct pressure, if direct pressure is not adequate, limited and prudent tourniquet use should be considered. Certainly, a patient should not die from extremity hemorrhage when a tourniquet could potentially be life-saving.

Suggested Readings

Bickell WH, Wall MJ Jr, Pepe PE, et al. Immediate versus delayed fluid resuscitation for hypotensive patients with penetrating torso injuries. *N Engl J Med*. 1994;331(17):1105–1109.

Borgman MA, Spinella PC, Perkins JG, et al. The ratio of blood products transfused affects mortality in patients receiving massive transfusions at a combat support hospital. *J Trauma*. 2007;63(4):805–813.

Dutton RP, Mackenzie CF, Scalea TM. Hypotensive resuscitation during active hemorrhage: impact on in-hospital mortality. *J Trauma*. 2002;52(6):1141–1146.

Fraga GP, Bansal V, Coimbra R. Transfusion of blood products in trauma: an update [published online ahead of print April 1, 2009]. *J Emerg Med*.

4

Trauma Airway

Darin Geracimos

Airway Evaluation
- Airway evaluation occurs simultaneously with obtaining of vitals signs and placement of an intravenous line, oxygen and monitor on the patient.
- Initial evaluation of the trauma airway: LOOK, LISTEN, FEEL.

LOOK
- Is patient in c-spine immobilization? If yes, intubation will be more difficult and require a second person to hold in-line stabilization. If no and mechanism warrants a c-collar, place one immediately.
- Is there trauma to the head? Head trauma can cause rise in Intracranial pressure (ICP). You may consider using pretreatment agents to blunt the rise in ICP that occurs with endotracheal intubation.
- Is there direct trauma to the upper airway (maxillofacial, larynx, trachea)? The traumatized airway may have distorted anatomy complicating intubation. Have rescue airway equipment available and consider deferring to the more experienced intubator given the circumstances. Rapid sequence oral intubation often is still the best method of securing the airway.
- Is there trauma to the chest? Evaluate for bilateral chest rise. Is there a pneumothorax, hemothorax, or flail chest causing ventilation or oxygenation problems? If so, they must be dealt with simultaneously with securing an airway.
- Is there trauma to Zone II of the neck? If yes, worsening injury and anatomical distortion are possible. Early intubation should be strongly considered.

LISTEN
- Ask the patient to speak. This gives you quick assessment of airway patency and neurological status. If the patient is hoarse, be concerned about airway compromise and consider intubation in the right clinical setting.
- Listen to the neck for stridor. Stridor in the trauma patient is a sign of impending airway compromise and should prompt consideration for aggressive, early intubation.
- Listen to bilateral lung fields.

FEEL
- Palpate the neck for crepitus. Subcutaneous air is suggestive of a pneumothorax. Remember that the application of positive pressure into the lungs can convert a simple pneumothorax into a tension pneumothorax.
- Feel the neck for hematomas. An expanding hematoma indicates vascular injury that will likely require exploratory surgery for definitive management. Intubate these patients immediately as the airway can become compromised in minutes.
- Locate the cricoid membrane in the event you need to perform a cricothyrotomy.

Special Considerations

Airway Patency
- Injury to maxillofacial area, larynx, or trachea can distort normal anatomy leading to a progressively more difficult intubation and possibly airway obstruction. Strongly consider early intubation and be prepared for a surgical airway.
- Airway edema caused by smoke inhalation or caustic ingestion can also compromise airway patency.
- Always have difficult airway tools available (e.g., gum-elastic bougie, laryngeal mask airway, video laryngoscope, fiberoptic scope). But, in cases of lost airway patency, surgical cricothyrotomy may be the only option.
- Some patients may have an injured airway that requires urgent but not emergent intubation. If you anticipate a "cannot intubate–cannot ventilate" scenario, consider an awake intubation (sedation without paralysis) via nasal or fiberoptic airway. These patients may be better managed in the controlled setting of the operating room where a tracheostomy can be performed, if necessary.
- A fractured larynx is a contraindication to a surgical cricothyrotomy. These patients need an emergent surgical tracheostomy in the operating room.

Chest Injury
- Pneumothorax, hemothorax, flail chest, and pulmonary contusion are all possible complications of chest trauma that can cause problems with ventilation and oxygenation and must always be addressed.
- Positive pressure ventilation can exacerbate a pneumothorax. If you intubate a patient with a moderate or large size pneumothorax, most sources advocate needle decompression prior to intubation, followed by tube thoracostomy. Some advocate that a tube thoracostomy can be avoided if the patient is monitored closely (e.g., intensive care unit setting) for progression to a tension pneumothorax, especially in cases of small pneumothoraces.

Head/C-Spine Injury
- When the Glasgow Coma Scale score is ≤8, it is standard practice to immediately intubate for airway protection.
- Although controversial, consider using pretreatment medications to ameliorate the rise in ICP that can accompany intubation. Note that atropine and a defasciculating agent are no longer recommended in the third edition of Ron Wall's *Manual of Emergency Airway Management.*
  - **L**idocaine 1.5 mg/kg IV
  - **O**pioid (fentanyl 3 mcg/kg IV)
  - **A**tropine 0.02 mg/kg in children younger than 10 years only to prevent bradycardia
  - **D**efasciculating agent (rocuronium 0.06 mg/kg IV or vecuronium 0.01 mg/kg IV)
- Always maintain c-spine immobilization; a second person should be responsible for immobilization of spine during intubation.
- In cases of head injury, etomidate is usually the preferred induction agent due to its favorable hemodynamic effects [decreases ICP and maintains cerebral perfusion pressure (CPP)].
- Avoid hypotension and hypoxia. A single episode of hypotension (systolic blood pressure <90 mm Hg) or hypoxia (PO_2 <60) has been shown to dramatically increase mortality of traumatic brain injury patients.

Hemodynamically Unstable Patient
- Use etomidate or ketamine for induction/sedation as they have the best hemodynamic profiles; until recently, it was recommended that ketamine be

avoided in patients with closed head injuries but recent evidence suggests there is no association with increased ICP.
- It is important to be aware of the factors that can cause a drop in blood pressure as a result of rapid sequence intubation.
  - Induction/sedation agents
  - Decreased catecholamine release
  - Vagal stimulus from laryngoscopy
  - Positive pressure ventilation

Considerations in Cricothyrotomy
- Reserved for patients who you are unable to intubate or ventilate.
- Surgical cricothyrotomy is generally contraindicated in age <12 years. Needle cricothyrotomy is the surgical airway of choice in this age group.
- Contraindicated when the larynx is fractured.
- Can be difficult in penetrating neck trauma, tracheal tears, and expanding neck hematomas. Consider fiberoptic intubation in these patients, if available and feasible.

Combative Patient
- There are many causes of combativeness in the trauma patient, such as alcohol and drug intoxication, hypoxia, anxiety, and traumatic brain injury.
- The decision to sedate with haloperidol or benzodiazepines or use rapid sequence intubation needs to be made taking into account the extent of injury, the plan for further evaluation, and the safety of the patient.
- Proper and thorough evaluation of the trauma patient is paramount. If temporary sedation and intubation are required to obtain the necessary tests, these should be initiated without delay.

For specific technique of rapid sequence intubation, see the Procedures section in Chapter 96, Rapid Sequence Intubation and Gum-Elastic Bougie.

5 Trauma Center Referrals

Jonathan Kirschner

Trauma Systems

The regionalization of trauma care is based on the premise that patients presenting to nontertiary care emergency departments are stabilized and rapidly transferred to a trauma center for specialized multidisciplinary care.

Trauma centers must meet specific criteria mandated by the state and typically require specific personnel, facilities, resources, patient volume, quality control measures, and trauma administration. Trauma centers vary in their capabilities and are designated by level. A Level 1 center is generally a tertiary teaching center capable of all treatment with 24-hour multispecialty services on call (trauma surgery, neurosurgery, orthopedics, anesthesia, critical care, etc.). Level 2 hospitals have most of the same capability and level of resource, whereas Level 3 centers have less. The American College of Surgeons maintains the standard of trauma care and helps confirm and maintain an individual hospital's ability to meet this standard.

In rural settings, direct transfer to a trauma center from the scene is not practical and stabilization at nontrauma hospitals is often necessary.

Trauma care can be very expensive and, as such, there have been many trauma center closings in the past 10 years. Many states have no Level 1 trauma centers (Table 5.1).

Decision to Transfer

The decision to transfer a patient to a trauma center should be made in coordination with the receiving facility and should be based on clinical factors, resource availability, and patient need.

The goals of the provider in the nontertiary center should be prompt evaluation, stabilization, and rapid transfer if necessary. **Nonessential diagnostic testing should be avoided and identifying associated minor injuries prior to transfer is not required.** In the unstable patient with life-threatening injuries, the only acceptable reason for transfer is lack of resources or qualified personnel.

Transfer Process

Communication between receiving and transferring facility and providers is crucial. Copies of essential imaging and laboratory testing should be sent with the patient. Do not delay transfer for nonessential studies.

Decompensation during transport should be anticipated. The high level of care and monitoring established in the emergency department (ED) should be maintained throughout the transfer process, requiring qualified personnel as well as resuscitation equipment and medications.

TABLE 5.1: Essential elements of trauma systems

Presence of a lead agency with legal authority to designate trauma centers

Use of a formal process for designation of trauma centers

Use of American College of Surgeons (or similar) standards for verification of trauma centers

Use of an out-of-state survey team for designation of trauma centers

Mechanism to limit the number of designated trauma centers in a community on the basis of community need

Written triage criteria that form the basis for bypassing nondesignated centers

Presence of continuous monitoring systems for quality assurance

Statewide availability of trauma centers

Nathens AB, Brunet FP, Maier RV. Development of trauma systems and effect on outcome after injury. *Lancet.* 2004;422:17–22.

The mode of transport is dependent on regional factors such as resource availability and distance between hospitals. Most studies show no mortality benefit between ground and air transportation. Since air transport often takes longer to initialize, time to arrival at a trauma center is often faster via ground transportation for short to moderate distances.

The patient transfer process is expedited when established protocols for transfer are in place. Utilization of transfer coordinators at the transferring or receiving centers can facilitate a rapid and smooth transfer (Table 5.2).

Outcomes of Trauma Center Transfer

Multiple studies have confirmed that trauma centers improve mortality in the urban setting, though this benefit is not clear in the rural setting. In one study, the risk of death in transferred patients was 60% greater than in patients admitted to a trauma center directly from the scene; however, these transfer patients likely represent a sicker population.

Trauma systems with protocols for initial management at nontertiary centers were associated with lower mortality, and instituting transfer protocols increased survival in rural areas. In mild to moderately injured patients, functional outcomes (i.e., independence, ability to feed self, mobility) have been shown to be only slightly improved for patients treated at trauma centers compared with outside hospitals.

These outcome studies are inherently flawed as scoring systems for injury severity are anatomically rather than physiologically based and study populations are typically quite different.

TABLE 5.2: Ideal trauma transfer process

Follow established protocols for decision to transfer

Physician-to-physician communication

Appropriate level of emergency medical services transfer care

Copies of notes and laboratory/imaging tests accompany patient

In the nontertiary setting, the decision to transfer an injured patient should be based on the judgment of the experienced clinician as well as the availability of resources and qualified personnel.

Best Evidence/Clinical Decision Rules

Relying on the mechanism of injury to determine the need for transfer results in over-triage of injured patients. Are there clinical criteria that may aid in predicting which patients will need trauma center referral?

Newgard et al. identified five clinical criteria to detect high-need patients presenting to nontertiary centers: emergent airway intervention (prehospital or ED), initial ED Glasgow Coma Scale score of <11, ED blood transfusion, initial ED systolic blood pressure (SBP) <100 or >220 mm Hg, and initial ED respiratory rate <10 or >32. The presence of one or more criteria portends a positive likelihood ratio (+LR) of 3.5 for early mortality/early resource need, two or more increased the +LR to 9.1, and three or more increased to 16.2. These criteria have not been validated but may provide a useful tool in identifying trauma patients who may benefit from early transfer.

Suggested Readings

Harrington DT, Connolly M, Biffl WL, et al. Transfer times to definitive care facilities are too long: a consequence of an immature trauma system. *Ann Surg.* 2005;241:961–966.

MacKenzie EJ, Rivara FP, Jurkovich G, et al. A national evaluation of the effect of trauma center care on mortality. *New Engl J Med.* 2006;354:366–378.

Newgard CD, Hedges JR, Adams A, et al. Secondary triage: early identification of high-risk trauma patients presenting to non-tertiary hospitals. *Prehosp Emerg Care.* 2007;11:154–163.

Newgard CD, McConnell KJ, Hedges JR. Variability of trauma transfer practices among non-tertiary care hospital emergency departments. *Acad Emerg Med.* 2006;13:746–754.

Newgard CD, McConnell KJ, Hedges JR, et al. The benefit of higher level of care transfer of injured patients from nontertiary hospital emergency departments. *J Trauma.* 2007;63:965–971.

Nirula R, Brasel K. Do trauma centers improve functional outcomes: a national trauma databank analysis? *J Trauma.* 2006;61:268–271.

Rivara FP, Koepsell TD, Wang J, et al. Outcomes of trauma patients after transfer to a level I trauma center. *J Trauma.* 2008;64:1594–1599.

Utter GH, Maier RV, Rivara FP, et al. Inclusive trauma systems: do they improve triage or outcomes of the severely injured? *J Trauma.* 2006;60:529–535.

Section Editor: Daniel Egan

6

Head Trauma: The First 15 Minutes, Algorithm, and Decision Making

Daniel Egan

 THE FIRST
15 MINUTES

ABCs
- Follow Advanced Trauma Life Support (ATLS) guidelines and the Head Trauma Algorithm.
- When securing the patient's airway, the use of rapid sequence intubation is evidence-based and the safest for the patient. Protective premedication with lidocaine, a defasciculating agent (e.g., vecuronium), and an opiate may be considered.

Glasgow Coma Scale
- Calculation of the Glasgow Coma Scale (GCS) score will allow you to follow a patient's neurologic status over the course of his or her time under your care.
- This is a valuable tool for communication with trauma and neurosurgical colleagues.
- Decorticate posturing is the involuntary flexion of the muscle groups in the extremities.
- Decerebrate posturing is the involuntary extension of the muscle groups in the extremities.

Physical Examination
- Palpate the skull to identify any obvious skull fractures, depressions, and step-offs.
- Clinical findings of a basilar skull fracture: raccoon eyes, Battle's signs, and hemotympanum.
- Examine the ear canal and nose for evidence of cerebrospinal fluid (CSF) leak, characterized by clear fluid drainage. This can also be tested for a glucose level, which is typically in the range of two-third the serum glucose value.
- **Cranial nerve examination**
  - Close examination and documentation of the baseline pupillary examination is critical as the examination may be one of the first to change with herniation.
- **Neurologic examination**
  - Motor and sensory function in all extremities.
  - Reflexes, including Babinski.
- Keep in mind that the mechanism of injury may also put the patient at risk for spinal cord injury, making spinal immobilization critical during the evaluation.
- Vital signs (Table 6.1).

TABLE 6.1: Cushing's triad—associated with increased ICP

Elevated blood pressure
Bradycardia
Respiratory irregularity

Emergency Interventions
- Maintain normotension and avoid hypoxia.
- Provide rapid evaluation and assessment for other potentially life-threatening injuries.
- Arrange for rapid neuroimaging when indicated.
- Involve neurosurgical consultants early when clinical suspicion warrants.
- Provide hyperventilation after intubation for patients with clinical evidence of herniation only.

Memorable Pearls
- Up to 20% of the general population will have anisocoria.
- Hypotension is not typically associated with isolated head trauma and should prompt further evaluation for other injury.
- Patients with a GCS score of 8 or less should have their airway secured with the use of rapid sequence intubation (Table 6.2).

Essential Considerations
- Given the fact that most computed tomographic (CT) scanners are not in the emergency department, the emergency physician must ensure patient safety and airway security before patient transport.
- Consideration of neuroimaging (CT scan) for patients with minor head trauma is less clear. The Canadian Head CT Rules and New Orleans criteria may help guide this decision and are discussed in the "Minor Head Injury" chapter.

TABLE 6.2: Glasgow Coma Scale

Category	Response	Score
Eye opening	Spontaneous	4
	To voice	3
	To pain	2
	None	1
Verbal response	Oriented	5
	Confused	4
	Inappropriate words	3
	Incomprehensible	2
	None	1
Motor response	Normal	6
	Localizes pain	5
	Withdraws to pain	4
	Decorticate posturing	3
	Decerebrate posturing	2
	None	1

Consultations

- Neurosurgical consultation is indicated for most head trauma including skull fractures and intracranial injuries.
- Neurologic consultation may be indicated for patients with concussion and ongoing neurologic impairment.

 DECISION
MAKING

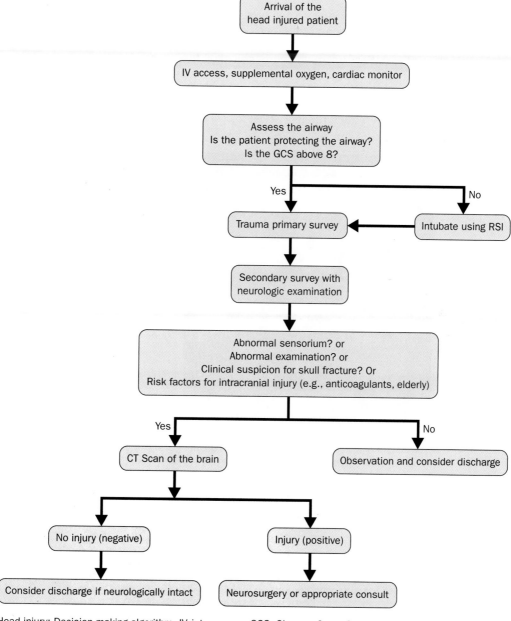

Head injury: Decision making algorithm. IV, intravenous; GCS, Glasgow Coma Scale; RSI, rapid sequence intubation; CT, computed tomography.

7

Skull Fracture

Megan Fix

Definition

- Skull fractures are divided into two types: those of the cranial vault and those of the skull base (basilar), and then each of those is further classified (Table 7.1).
- Most skull fractures are simple linear fractures of the vault and do not require surgical intervention; however, depressed skull fractures and basilar skull fractures are separate entities and may require surgical intervention.
  - Approximately 20% of skull fractures are basilar skull fractures.
  - Most depressed skull fractures are in the frontoparietal region and 75–90% of them are open fractures (Fig. 7.1).

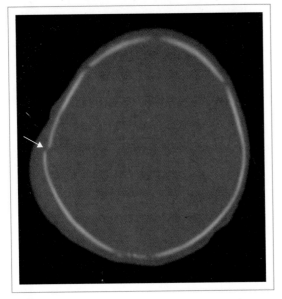

FIGURE 7.1: Computed tomographic image demonstrating a slightly displaced right-sided skull fracture with overlying soft tissue swelling. (Courtesy of Daniel Kloda, MD, Maine Medical Center.)

TABLE 7.1: Classification of skull fractures

Vault fractures	Skull base fractures
Linear or stellate	With or without CSF leak
Depressed or nondepressed	With or without CN VII palsy
Open or closed	

CSF, cerebrospinal fluid; CN, cranial nerve.

Pathophysiology
- Skull fractures are caused by either blunt or penetrating trauma to the calvarium.
- **The accumulation of blood from a basilar skull fracture may lead to classic signs such as raccoon eyes (periorbital ecchymosis), Battle's sign (retroauricular ecchymosis), and cerebrospinal fluid (CSF) rhinorrhea or otorrhea.**
- Linear skull fractures may run through vascular channels or venous sinus grooves and lead to epidural hematomas or venous sinus thrombosis.
- Basilar skull fractures through the temporal bone may run through the facial nerve canal, the inner ear, or the vestibulocochlear apparatus leading to facial nerve palsies, hearing loss, or disturbances in equilibrium.

Diagnosis
- Skull fractures can be suspected on physical examination in any trauma patient with hematomas, laceration, or penetrating trauma. Basilar skull fracture should be suspected with any of the following: raccoon eyes (periorbital ecchymosis), Battle's sign (retroauricular ecchymosis), and CSF rhinorrhea or otorrhea.
  - The "ring sign" showing a halo around a drop of blood from the nose/ear on tissue paper suggests CSF leakage.
- Vault skull fractures can be diagnosed on plain x-ray film but definitive diagnosis for other types of skull fractures requires noncontrast computed tomographic (CT) imaging of the skull and CT scan is now considered the gold standard.
  - If a basilar skull fracture is identified and it traverses the carotid canals, consider computed tomography angiography or cerebral arteriography.
  - Temporal bone fractures are best identified using thin cuts (1 mm) through the skull base with sagittal reconstruction (Fig. 7.2).

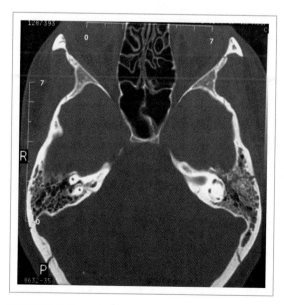

FIGURE 7.2: Computed tomographic scan demonstrating a basilar skull fracture of the left temporal bone. (Courtesy of Daniel Kloda, MD, Maine Medical Center, Portland, Maine.)

Evaluation
- Facilitate rapid CT scan to identify skull fracture and any underlying intracranial pathology.

- Evaluation should focus on identifying associated injuries, including cervical spine injury, underlying intracranial hematomas, and, in the case of basilar skull fractures, carotid injury (dissection, pseudoaneurysm, or thrombosis) or nerve injury.
  - Identify signs of altered mental status or weakness that may signal carotid injury.
  - Identify signs of facial paralysis, hearing loss, nystagmus, or ataxia that may signal seventh and eighth nerve damage.
  - Fractures of the occipital condyles are rare and very serious. They are associated with cervical spine injuries and damage to cranial nerves IX, X, and XI.
- Special consideration should be given to pediatric patients with skull fracture. Always complete a thorough history and physical to identify any suspicion for nonaccidental trauma.

Management

- Appropriate wound care and tetanus booster should be administered in patients who have associated lacerations, unless the wound is grossly contaminated and warrants operative repair. Consider antibiotics for grossly contaminated wounds.
- Adults with simple linear skull fractures that are neurologically intact with no complications (e.g., epidural hematoma) may have their wounds repaired and be safely discharged home.
- Children and infants with skull fractures should be admitted for observation and neurosurgical consultation.
- Depressed skull fractures require neurosurgical consultation. Many of these will be treated expectantly; the guidelines for surgical intervention are outlined in Table 7.2.
  - Seizure prophylaxis should be considered, especially if the patient had loss of consciousness or any neurologic compromise.
- Occipital condylar fractures require neurosurgical consultation for possible operative intervention or halo traction. All are kept in strict cervical spine immobilization.
- Adults with basilar skull fractures should have consultation with a specialist, but most often they are treated conservatively, without antibiotics.
  - Any patient with signs of facial nerve palsy, hearing loss, or tympanic membrane rupture requires ENT referral. Most times the tympanic membrane heals on its own.
  - Delayed nerve palsies (secondary to neuropraxia) may occur and are treated with corticosteroids.

Special Considerations

- Current management of CSF leak includes head elevation, bed rest, stool softeners, avoidance of nose blowing/sneezing and other forms of straining, and, in selected patients, placement of a lumbar drain or intermittent spinal taps.
- When considering CT scans in children and young adults, consider the impact of radiation. There are guidelines for CT scans, including those referenced below in the articles by Kuppermann et al. and Schutzman et al.

TABLE 7.2: Indications for surgical intervention of depressed skull fracture

Depressed fragment >5 mm below inner table of adjacent bone
Gross contamination
Dural tear with pneumocephalus
Underlying hematoma

Best Evidence/Clinical Decision Rules

Should I start my patients empirically on antibiotics if they have a basilar skull fracture?

A recent 2006 Cochrane review reports that current evidence shows no difference in the incidence of meningitis in those with basilar skull fractures who have received prophylactic antibiotics after basilar skull fracture. Its recommendation does not support routine use of antibiotics in basilar skull fractures, regardless of evidence of CSF leakage.

Suggested Readings

Heegaard WG, Biros MH. Head injuries. In: Marx JA. *Rosen's Emergency Medicine: Concepts and Clinical Practice*, 6th ed. Philadelphia, PA: Mosby, 2006:349–382.

Johnson F, Semaan MT, Megerian CA. Temporal bone fracture: evaluation and management in the modern era. *Otolaryngol Clin North Am*. 2008;41(3):597–618.

Kuppermann N, Holmes JF, Dayan PS, et al. Identifying children at very low risk of clinically-important traumatic brain injuries after blunt head trauma. *Lancet*. 2009;374:1160–1170.

Legros B, Fournier P, Chiaroni P, et al. Basal fracture of the skull and lower (IX, X, XI, XII) cranial nerves palsy: four case reports including two fractures of the occipital condyle—a literature review. *J Trauma*. 2000;48(2):342–348.

Qureshi NH. Skull fracture. emedicine.medscape.com. Updated February 1, 2008.

Ratilal BO, Costa J, Sampaio C. Antibiotic prophylaxis for preventing meningitis in patients with basilar skull fractures. *Cochrane Database Syst Rev*. 2006 Jan 25;(1):CD004884.

Schutzman SA, Barnes P, Duhaime AC, Greenes D, Homer C, Jaffe D, Lewis RJ, Luerssen TG, Schunk J. Evaluation and management of children younger than two years old with apparently minor head trauma: proposed guidelines. *Pediatrics*. 2001;107(5):983–993.

8

Minor Head Trauma and Concussion

Jonathan Ilgen

Definition

- Minor head injury, also known as concussion or minor traumatic brain injury (TBI), is defined as blunt trauma to the head, with a history of loss of consciousness, amnesia, or disorientation, and with normal or minimally altered mental status upon presentation (Glasgow Coma Scale [GCS] score of 13–15).
- To be classified as a minor head injury, patients cannot have lost consciousness for more than 15 minutes or have posttraumatic amnesia for more than 1 hour.

Pathophysiology

- Based on animal data, concussions may cause cellular injury as a result of decreased cerebrovascular blood flow in the setting of increased cellular glucose needs.
- Loss of consciousness after a blunt head injury is thought to result from disruption of the reticular activating system. This is a product of rotational forces centered at the thalamus and upper midbrain.
- The mechanism whereby blunt injury induces amnesia is unknown.

Diagnosis

- Minor head injury rarely results in intracranial complications (6–21%), though a minority of these are potentially life-threatening and necessitate neurosurgical intervention (0.4–1.0%).
- The diagnosis of intracranial complications after minor head injury can be rapidly facilitated by computed tomography (CT).
- Concussions will typically have normal neuroimaging studies. Symptoms of concussions are listed in Table 8.1. The severity of concussions is determined by the type, duration, and severity of symptoms.

Evaluation

- Minor head injuries are common, and while complications are rare, they can be potentially life-threatening. To avoid subjecting all patients to the ionizing radiation and costs inherent to CT, the challenge is deciding which patients need imaging.
- Two clinical decision rules with high sensitivities, the New Orleans Criteria (NOC) and the Canadian CT Head Rule (CCHR), may guide the decision to forgo a head CT (Tables 8.2 and 8.3).

Management

- Neurosurgical consultation and management will be dictated by the presence and type of injuries seen on CT.

TABLE 8.1: Acute signs and symptoms suggestive of minor head injury

Cognitive	Somatic	Affective
Confusion	Headache	Emotional liability
Posttraumatic amnesia	Fatigue	Irritability
Retrograde amnesia	Disequilibrium	
Loss of consciousness	Dizziness	
Disorientation	Nausea/vomiting	
Vacant state	Photophobia	
Delayed verbal and motor responses	Blurred/double vision	
Slurred or incoherent speech	Phonophobia	
Excessive drowsiness		

Adapted from Concussion (mild traumatic brain injury) and the team physician: a consensus statement. *Med Sci Sports Exerc.* 2006;38(2):395–399.

- Patients with a normal neurologic examination can be safely discharged into the care of a responsible person after 2 hours of observation. These patients should receive written instructions regarding signs and symptoms for which they should return to the hospital.
- There are no class I studies to guide the treatment of concussions or to determine whether athletes are safe to return to play after these injuries.
- The postconcussive syndrome can follow minor head injuries and last for days to weeks. Symptoms include headache, dizziness, disequilibrium, and difficulty concentrating. Therapy focuses on patient education and though not evidence-based, may include mild analgesics, meclizine, antiemetics, and vestibular exercises.

Special Considerations

- A CT scan should be performed in most anticoagulated patients with minor head injury because therapeutic anticoagulation increases the likelihood of severe TBIs and overall mortality.

TABLE 8.2: The New Orleans Criteria

Glasgow Coma Scale score of 15, without:
    Headache
    Vomiting
    Age >60
    Alcohol or drug intoxication
    Persistent anterograde amnesia
    Evidence of traumatic soft tissue or bone injury above the clavicles
    Seizure

Adapted from Haydel MJ, Preston CA, Mills TJ, Luber S, Blaudeau E, DeBlieux PM. Indications for computed tomography in patients with minor head injury. *N Engl J Med.* 2000;343(2):100–105.

TABLE 8.3: The Canadian CT Head Rule

Glasgow Coma Scale scores of 13–15, age >16 years, and without:
  High risk of neurosurgical intervention
  Glasgow Coma Scale score of <15 within 2 hours after injury
  Suspected open or depressed skull fracture
  Any sign of basilar skull fracture
  Two or more episodes of vomiting
  Age >65
  Moderate risk of brain injury detected by computed tomography
  Retrograde amnesia for >30 minutes
  Dangerous mechanism, defined as:
  Pedestrian struck by motor vehicle
  Ejected from motor vehicle
  Fall from >3 ft or >5 stairs

Adapted from Stiell IG, Wells GA, Vandemheen K, et al. The Canadian CT Head Rule for patients with minor head injury. *Lancet.* 2001;357(9266):1391–1396.

- Management of pediatric minor head injury continues to be a clinical challenge. The most recent American Academy of Pediatrics guidelines from 1999 state that, in the absence of neurologic abnormalities, both observation and initial CT imaging are acceptable management options. Observation should last for 24 hours and can be performed in the emergency department, hospital, clinic, or home.
  - Important factors identifying children who are at low risk for TBI are listed in Table 8.4.

TABLE 8.4: Children at low risk for traumatic brain injury

Absence of:
  Abnormal mental status
  Signs of skull fracture
  History of vomiting
  Scalp hematoma (in children <2 years)
  Headache

Best Evidence/Clinical Decision Rules

When should I perform a CT scan in patients with minor head injury?

In 2005, Stiell et al. compared the NOC (Table 8.2) and the CCHR (Table 8.3).

- Both the NOC and the CCHR had sensitivity of 100% for predicting the need for neurosurgical intervention and detecting clinically important brain injury.
- The CCHR, however, was significantly more specific than the NOC for the same predictions.

Suggested Readings

Cassidy JD, Carroll LJ, Peloso PM, et al. Incidence, risk factors and prevention of mild traumatic brain injury: results of the WHO Collaborating Centre Task Force on Mild Traumatic Brain Injury. *J Rehabil Med.* 2004;43 (suppl):28–60.

Cohen DB, Rinker C, Wilberger JE. Traumatic brain injury in anticoagulated patients. *J Trauma.* 2006;60(3):553–557.

Concussion (mild traumatic brain injury) and the team physician: a consensus statement. *Med Sci Sports Exerc.* 2006;38(2):395–399.

Haydel MJ, Preston CA, Mills TJ, Luber S, Blaudeau E, DeBlieux PM. Indications for computed tomography in patients with minor head injury. *N Engl J Med.* 2000;343(2):100–105.

Palchak MJ, Holmes JF, Vance CW, et al. A decision rule for identifying children at low risk for brain injuries after blunt head trauma. *Ann Emerg Med.* 2003;42(4): 492–506.

Pieracci FM, Eachempati SR, Shou J, Hydo LJ, Barie PS. Degree of anticoagulation, but not warfarin use itself, predicts adverse outcomes after traumatic brain injury in elderly trauma patients. *J Trauma.* 2007;63(3):525–530.

Ropper AH, Gorson KC. Clinical practice: concussion. *N Engl J Med.* 2007;356(2): 166–172.

Stiell IG, Clement CM, Rowe BH, et al. Comparison of the Canadian CT Head Rule and the New Orleans Criteria in patients with minor head injury. *JAMA.* 2005;294(12):1511–1518.

Stiell IG, Wells GA, Vandemheen K, et al. The Canadian CT Head Rule for patients with minor head injury. *Lancet.* 2001;357(9266):1391–1396.

The management of minor closed head injury in children. Committee on Quality Improvement, American Academy of Pediatrics. Commission on Clinical Policies and Research, American Academy of Family Physicians. *Pediatrics.* 1999;104(6):1407–1415.

9 Subarachnoid Hemorrhage

Daniel Egan

Definition

- Subarachnoid hemorrhage (SAH) is defined as bleeding within the subarachnoid space, between the pia mater and the arachnoid layer of the meninges.
- Traumatic SAH (tSAH) appears to be a distinct entity from aneurysmal SAH (aSAH), with different mechanism, treatment, and outcome.

Pathophysiology

- tSAH is poorly understood. It is thought that tSAH comes from bleeding cortical arteries or diffusion from brain contusions rather than bleeding from bridging veins or ruptured aneurysms.
- The accumulation of blood in the subarachnoid space may lead to intracranial hypertension and hydrocephalus. Vasospasm of the cerebral vasculature can lead to parenchymal ischemia.
- Morbidity and mortality of tSAH is correlated with hypoxia, hypotension, and intracranial hypertension.
- tSAH is frequently associated with traumatic brain injury (up to 60%). Early tSAH is frequently an indicator of other evolving traumatic brain lesion(s).

Diagnosis

- tSAH can be suspected on physical examination in any trauma patient with altered mental status or depressed Glasgow Coma Scale (GCS) score, though normal mental status does not rule out tSAH.
- Definitive diagnosis requires noncontrast computed tomographic (CT) imaging of the brain.
  - On CT imaging, blood may be seen within the ventricles, along the sulci, and/or following the distribution of the falx and tentorium.
  - CT imaging of the brain immediately after injury is highly sensitive for tSAH (Fig. 9.1).

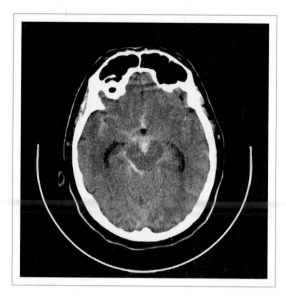

FIGURE 9.1: Subarachnoid hemorrhage. Hyperdensity within the subarachnoid space most visible in the sulci or cerebral peduncles. (Reprinted with permission from Mick N, Peters JR, Egan D, et al. *Blueprints Emergency Medicine*, 2nd ed. Philadelphia: Lippincott Williams & Wilkins, 2005.)

Evaluation

- Facilitate rapid CT scan to identify injury.
- Evaluation should focus on identifying associated injuries (especially c-spine injury).
- Special consideration should be given to early intubation. **Immediately intubate any patient who is actively decompensating or presents with a GCS score of ≤8.** Agitated patients with head injury usually require intubation to facilitate CT, prevent exacerbation of injury, and to protect against future decompensation.
- Identify signs of elevated ICP:
  - Cushings's triad: Bradycardia, hypertension, irregular respirations.
  - Uncal herniation: fixed pupil(s), flexion (decorticate), or extension (decerebrate) posturing.

Management

- Neurosurgical consultation is mandated when tSAH is identified. Consider early involvement of neurosurgery and trauma surgery teams when index of suspicion is high.
- **The goal of management of patients with head trauma is to minimize further brain injury from secondary insults:**
  - Hypotension: treat aggressively with intravenous (IV) fluids.
  - Seizure prophylaxis is controversial. In the emergency department, this usually is done with loading of phenytoin 15–20 mg/kg IV over 20 minutes to 1 hour.
  - Ischemia secondary to vasospasm: Calcium channel blockers may be associated with decreased morbidity and long-term sequelae of tSAH.
- Increased ICP needs aggressive management:
  - Sedation: benzodiazepines or propofol are first-line agents to prevent agitation.

- Osmotherapy: hypertonic saline and mannitol have both shown effectiveness in lowering ICP. These therapies are usually used for small volume hemorrhage or as a bridge to more invasive management.
- Cerebrospinal fluid drainage: external drain placement and cerebral perfusion pressure (CPP) measurement are most effective in managing significant intracranial hypertension.
- Decompressive craniectomy is a consideration for severe head injury with elevated ICP.
- Maintenance of pCO2 in a range of 30–35 preserves vascular tone.
  - Identify and correct coagulopathy.

Special Considerations

- Minor tSAH in stable patients with clear sensorium can be followed with repeat CT scans. These patients are often amenable to discharge 24 hours later with close follow-up.
- Patients with significant tSAH and/or other traumatic lesions should be managed in a neurologic or surgical intensive care unit.

Best Evidence/Clinical Decision Rules

Should I start my patients empirically on IV calcium channel blocker therapy when tSAH is diagnosed?

A recent 2007 Cochrane review reports that there is mixed evidence on the routine prophylactic use of calcium channel blocker therapy in aneurysmal SAH. It is not recommended routinely. However, if blood pressure management is necessary, calcium channel blocker therapy is prudent given the added benefit of decreased vasospasm.

Suggested Readings

Armin SS, Colohan AR, Zhang JH. Traumatic subarachnoid hemorrhage: our current understanding and its evolution over the past half century. *Neurol Res.* 2006;28:445–452.

Dorhout Mees SM, Rinkel GJ, Feigin VL, et al. Calcium antagonists for aneurysmal subarachnoid hemorrhage. *Cochrane Database Syst Rev.* 2007;3:CD000277.

10 Subdural Hematoma

Kriti Bhatia

Definition

- Subdural hematoma (SDH) refers to a collection of blood in the space between dural and arachnoid membranes, surrounding the brain.
- It is the most common type of traumatic intracranial hemorrhage.
- SDH can be acute (<24 hours old), subacute (24 hours to 2 weeks old), or chronic (>2 weeks old).

Pathophysiology

- There are three main mechanisms that are known to cause SDH: venous injury, arterial damage, and intracranial hypotension.
- **Typically, SDH formation occurs from tearing of the bridging veins between the cortex and the venous sinuses.**
- High-risk groups for SDH are outlined in Table 10.1.
- SDH resulting from arterial injury is most often seen in the temporoparietal regions.
- Low cerebrospinal fluid (CSF) pressure is usually caused by a spontaneous or iatrogenic CSF leak. Reduced CSF pressure causes traction of the supporting structures, including the bridging veins, making them susceptible to shearing.
- Small asymptomatic SDHs usually resolve spontaneously and are gradually resorbed over weeks.

Diagnosis

- Presentations of patients with SDHs vary greatly.
- Signs and symptoms may be fluctuating depending on location of the lesion and rate of development of the collection.
- Headache and confusion are the most common presenting complaints.
- Patients may report focal weakness, seizures, and incontinence.
- Increased intracranial pressure or mass effect may result in cerebral hypoperfusion with resultant cerebral infarction.

TABLE 10.1: High-risk groups

Patients with brain atrophy
Alcoholics
Prior brain injury
Elderly
Infants—have not yet developed adhesions in the subdural space
Anticoagulated patients

- Subacute and chronic SDHs can be difficult to diagnose.
    - They can present insidiously, making an antecedent traumatic event difficult to identify.
    - Symptoms may not only be prolonged but also develop days to weeks after the inciting incident.
    - Patients may present with progressive symptoms such as unexplained, lingering headache; changes in personality and appetite; uncharacteristic lethargy; apathy; lightheadedness.

Evaluation

- Imaging is the mainstay of diagnosis.
- Computed tomographic (CT) scan of the head is the most widely used imaging modality given its relative simplicity, easy availability, and speed of test completion.
- Acute SDHs.
    - **Appear as a high-density crescent-shaped collection that is concave toward the brain and unrestricted by suture lines (Fig. 10.1).**
    - The most common location is over the cerebral convexity in the parietal region followed by the area above the tentorium cerebelli.

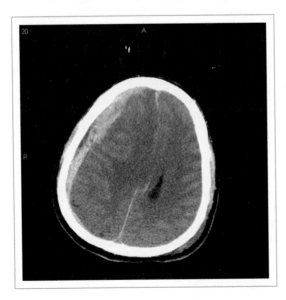

FIGURE 10.1: Right subdural hematoma appears concave as it tracks below the dural membrane. (Reprinted with permission from Wolfson AB, Hendey GW, Ling LJ, et al. *Harwood-Nuss' Clinical Practice of Emergency Medicine,* 5th ed. Philadelphia: Lippincott Williams & Wilkins, 2009.)

- Subacute subdurals.
    - Typically, the subdural will have varying densities and layering.
    - May become lens-shaped and can be confused with epidural hematomas (Fig. 10.2).

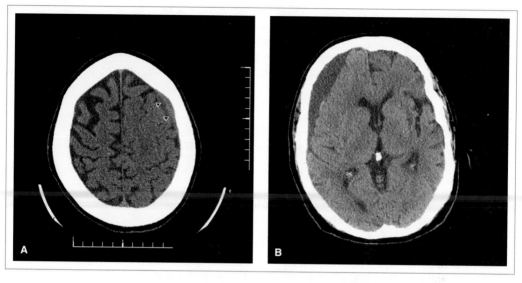

FIGURE 10.2: A: Subacute subdural hematoma. The arrows outline the isodense collection of blood in the subdural space. Blood becomes isodense on CT scan 1 to 2 weeks after injury. This finding is easily missed if the CT scan is not carefully inspected. B: Chronic subdural hemoatoma. The hypodensity in the right frontal region represents a chronic subdural hematoma. Blood becomes hypodense on CT scan 2 weeks after the injury. Note the small area of hyperdensity within the chronic subdural hematoma. This area represents acute hemorrhage within the chronic subdural hematoma. (Reprinted with permission from Wolfson AB, Hendey GW, Ling LJ, et al. *Harwood-Nuss' Clinical Practice of Emergency Medicine,* 5th ed. Philadelphia: Lippincott Williams & Wilkins, 2009.)

- ▪ Chronic SDHs.
  - ● May be difficult to detect.
  - ● Typically appear as isodense or hypodense crescent-shaped lesions.
- ▪ Moderate to large SDHs produce some degree of midline shift. Bilateral lesions may negate this finding (Fig. 10.3).

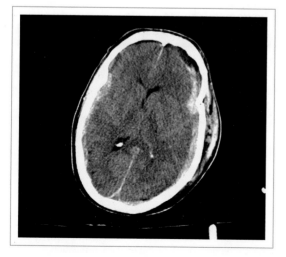

FIGURE 10.3: Subdural hematoma. Concave density adjacent to the skull that crosses suture lines. (Reprinted with permission from Mick N, Peters JR, Egan D, et al: *Blueprints Emergency Medicine,* 2nd ed. Philadelphia: Lippincott Williams & Wilkins, 2005.)

- Brain magnetic resonance imaging is more sensitive than head computed tomography but its use is limited in most emergency settings. CT imaging is the recommended modality for expeditious evaluation of brain hemorrhage in the acute setting.
- Lumbar puncture is contraindicated because of the risk of herniation.

Management
- The goals for management of acute SDH are:
  - prevention of secondary brain injury and death by hematoma expansion or herniation.
  - Identify and correct coagulopathy.
  - maintenance of appropriate intracranial pressure.
- The mainstay of treatment is the determination of whether surgical evaluation of the hematoma is indicated (see Best Evidence Section).
- Administration of an antiepileptic agent should be considered to prevent seizures.
- Steroids are not effective and should not be given.
- Patients managed nonoperatively may require:
  - close monitoring, often in an intensive care unit setting.
  - intracranial pressure monitoring.
  - serial brain imaging for any changes in neurological status.
- There are no guidelines for the management of chronic SDHs. Surgical management can be considered if there is potential for recovery and there has been neurological deterioration.

Special Considerations
- Very small, chronic SDHs.
  - These patients may be discharged home after neurosurgical evaluation.
  - Must be given explicit discharge instructions with criteria to return to the emergency department.
  - These patients must have a competent person to oversee them and evaluate them for changes in neurological status.
- SDHs in children can present differently than in adults.
  - Inflicted injury is a common etiology. This is especially true in pediatric patients younger than 2 years.
  - History is usually not consistent with the severity of injury.
    - Common presenting complaints include seizures, apnea, altered mental status, lethargy, and difficulty breathing.
    - Examine infants' fontanelles for bulging.
    - No clear criteria for operative management exist for pediatric patients.

TABLE 10.2: Indications for SDH surgery

The acute SDH is associated with a midline shift ≥5 mm
The hematoma exceeds 1 cm in thickness
The patient is comatose with an acute SDH <1 cm in thickness with a midline shift <5 mm if any one of the following criteria are met: If the GCS score decreases by 2 or more between the time of injury and hospital evaluation The patient presents with fixed and dilated pupils The ICP is >20 mm Hg

SDH, Subdural hematoma; GCS, Glasgow Coma Scale; ICP, intracranial pressure.

Best Evidence

- Indications for SDH surgery are outlined in Table 10.2.
- Mathew et al. reported that for all patients in their series with acute SDH initially treated nonoperatively who went on to require surgery, all had SDHs that were at least 10-mm thick on their initial head CTs.
- For those patients who meet criteria for surgical intervention, evidence suggests that surgery performed within 2–4 hours of neurological deterioration results in better outcome.
- Hyperglycemia.
  - Evidence suggests that hyperglycemia (defined as glucose ≥200 mg/dL) in patients with intracranial hemorrhage results in higher infection rates, mortality rates, as well as brain edema and perihematomal cell death.

Suggested Readings

Bullock MR, Chesnut R, Ghajar J, et al. Surgical management of acute subdural hematomas. *Neurosurgery*. 2006;58:S16.

Cenic A, Bhandari M, Reddy K. Management of chronic subdural hematoma: a national survey and literature review. *Can J Neurol Sci*. 2005;32(4):501–506.

Mathew P, Oluoch-Olunya DL, Condon BR, Bullock R. Acute subdural haematoma in the conscious patient: outcome with initial non-operative management. *Acta Neurochirn*. 1993;121(3–4):100–108.

Salim A, Hadjizacharia P, Dubose J, et al. Persistent hyperglycemia in severe trauma brain injury: an independent predictor of outcome. *Am Surg*. 2009;75(1):25–29.

Santarius T, Lawton R, Kirkpatrick PJ, Hutchinson PJ. The management of primary chronic subdural haematoma: a questionnaire survey of practice in the United Kingdom and the Republic of Ireland. *Br J Neurosurg*. 2008;22(4):529–534.

Song EC, Kon C, Sang-Wuk J, et al. Hyperglycemia exacerbates brain edema and perihematomal cell death after intracerebral hemorrhage. *Stroke*. 2003;34(9):2215–2220.

11

Epidural Hematoma

Ryan McCormack

Definition

Epidural hematoma (EDH) is the accumulation of blood and clot within the epidural space, between the skull and the dura mater.

Pathophysiology

- EDHs occur as the result of blunt head trauma, most commonly in the temporoparietal region with resultant disruption of the middle meningeal artery.
- The vast majority will have an associated skull fracture. The high pressure of the bleeding vessel rapidly dissects the dura away from the skull.
- In about 15% of patients, the bleeding is from one of the dural sinuses. In these cases, the hematoma and clinical findings develop more slowly.
- EDH is rarely seen in the elderly because the dura becomes increasingly adherent to the skull with advancing age.
- It is also rare in children younger than 2 years for similar anatomic reasons. Children are less likely to have the associated skull fractures because of the elasticity of the skull during childhood.

Diagnosis

- EDH should be considered in any patient with blunt head injury, particularly when associated with loss of consciousness, skull deformity, or any signs of clinical deterioration with serial examinations.
- The **classic presentation**, occurring in one-third of patients, is described as a transient loss of consciousness, followed by a lucid interval, and then rapid clinical deterioration. The lucid interval typically lasts hours but may last several days with venous bleeding.

Evaluation

- Airway protection and cervical spine precautions should always be considered.
- Facilitate prompt computed tomographic scan to identify the potential EDH.
- **On computed tomographic scan, EDH is hyperdense and the shape is biconvex (football shaped). The borders are well defined and usually do not extend beyond the dural attachments at the suture lines (Fig. 11.1).**
- Monitor the patient closely for signs of elevated ICP (headache, vomiting, decreasing level of consciousness, Cushing's triad) or herniation, typically uncal (Table 11.1).

TABLE 11.1: Clinical signs of herniation

Ipsilateral third nerve palsy (dilated, nonreactive pupil)
Contralateral hemiparesis
Contralateral increased deep tendon reflexes
Contralateral upgoing Babinski

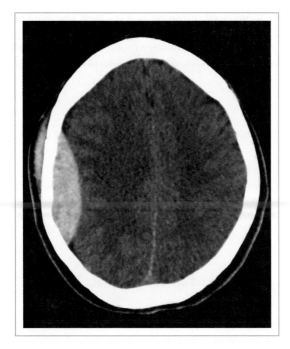

FIGURE 11.1: Right-sided epidural hematoma with characteristic biconvex shape and hyperdensity. (Reproduced with permission from Greenberg MI, Hendrickson RG, Silverberg M, et al. *Greenberg's Text-Atlas of Emergency Medicine.* Philadelphia: Lippincott Williams & Wilkins, 2005.)

- About 20% will have other intracranial lesions, usually subdural hematomas or contusions.
- Lumbar puncture is contraindicated in patients with EDH.

Management

- Prompt neurosurgical evaluation and intervention is essential. Without surgical intervention, EDH has a nearly 100% mortality.
  - Open craniotomy for evacuation of the clot and hemostasis is typically required.
- Patients with signs of herniation may need emergency decompression by trephination (burr holes).
  - This procedure should be considered in the emergency department if definitive neurosurgical care is not available.
- Identify and correct coagulopathy.
- Protect the brain from potential secondary insults:
  - Prevent hypotension with intravenous fluids as needed.
  - Seizure prophylaxis typically with phenytoin.
- Initiate nonsurgical interventions for elevated intracranial pressure (ICP) until definitive treatment. Options include hypertonic saline, mannitol, hyperventilation, and elevation of the head of the bed.

Special Considerations

- EDHs are often associated with lower-energy trauma and have less resultant primary brain injury. **If the hematoma is evacuated early, before neurologic**

deficit or signs of herniation, functional outcome is excellent and full recovery is often seen.
- Patients with EDH require immediate surgical intervention and frequent neurologic monitoring necessitating management in an intensive care unit.

Best Evidence/Clinical Decision Rules

The majority of EDHs attain their maximum size within minutes of injury. Borovich et al. showed that 9% continue to expand during the first 24 hours. Occasionally, the hematoma progression occurs more slowly and clinical deterioration occurs days after the injury.

EDH is rarely seen in the elderly because the dura becomes increasingly adherent to the skull with advancing age. Children are less likely to have the associated skull fractures because of the elasticity of the skull during childhood.

Suggested Readings

Borovich B, Braun J, Guilburd JN, et al. Delayed onset of traumatic extradural hematoma. *J Neurosurg.* 1985;63(1):30–34.

Dinh-Zarr TB, Goss CW, Heitman E, Roberts IG, DiGuiseppi C. Interventions for preventing injuries in problem drinkers. *Cochran Database Syst Rev.* 2004;(3):CD001857.

Heegaard WG, Biros MH. Systems injuries—head. In: Marx JA, John A, Hockberger Robert S, Walls Ron M, et al., eds. *Rosen's Emergency Medicine: Concepts and Clinical Practice*, 6th ed. Philadelphia: Mosby Inc, 2006:349–382.

12 Intraparenchymal Hemorrhage

Sanjay Shewakramani

Definition

- Traumatic intraparenchymal hemorrhage is defined by intra-axial intracranial bleeding (bleeding from the brain tissue itself), as opposed to extra-axial causes like subdural, epidural, and subarachnoid bleeding.
- The spectrum of disease ranges from small contusions to large hematomas.
- As opposed to extra-axial hemorrhage, intraparenchymal hemorrhage tends to be associated with worse outcomes, as it is more difficult to treat.

Pathophysiology

- **Intracranial contusions** are bruises on the surface of the brain, which form when the brain comes into contact with skull and thus are due to *direct* trauma.
  - Parenchymal blood vessels are damaged, and the resulting areas of petechial hemorrhage within the grey matter cause local edema.
  - Edema and progressive hemorrhage can lead to local mass effect.
  - Contusions can be classified as *coup* (in the area where direct trauma to the head occurred) or *contrecoup* (on the opposite side of the coup injury). These two entities can occur individually or together.
- **Intracerebral hematomas (ICHs)** occur deep within the brain tissue and occur when small arterioles are damaged because of shearing or tensile forces and thus are due to *indirect* trauma.
  - Small petechial hemorrhages coalesce to form larger ICHs.
  - These tend to occur in the more vascular, deeper areas of the brain.

Diagnosis

- Intraparenchymal bleeding should be considered in any trauma patient with a significant mechanism (either direct head injury or rapid acceleration/deceleration injury).
- Symptoms vary widely:
  - Patients may be asymptomatic.
  - Mild symptoms include headache, nausea/vomiting, and visual changes.
  - Moderate to severe injuries can cause focal neurological deficits, seizures, or coma.
- Computed tomographic (CT) imaging of the brain is the fastest and easiest method of diagnosis.
  - Nearly 85% of ICHs are found in the frontal and temporal lobes and are often found in patients with extra-axial hemorrhages.
  - Small contusions can be missed because of their proximity to overlying bone.
  - ICH may not be evident on CT scanning until hours or days after the injury, whereas contusions are usually visible immediately after the injury.
- Magnetic resonance imaging can be more sensitive for very small, or older, areas of bleeding (Fig. 12.1).

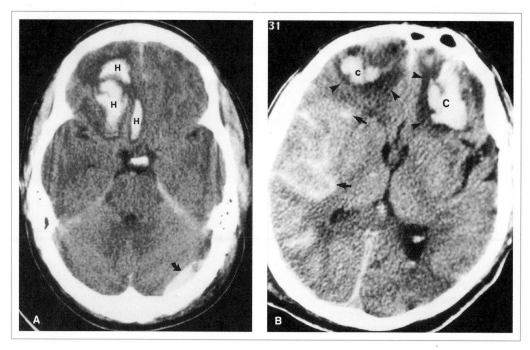

FIGURE 12.1: Cerebral contusions. **A:** Axial noncontrast computed tomographic study shows multiple acute hemorrhagic contusions (H) with hypodense surrounding edema in the right frontobasal region. There is a small acute epidural hematoma (curved arrow) in the left occipital region. **B:** In a different patient, computed tomography shows acute bilateral frontal hemorrhagic contusions (C) with surrounding edema (arrowheads) and acute subarachnoid hemorrhage (arrows) in the right sylvian fissure. (Reproduced with permission from Harris JH, Harris WH. *The Radiology of Emergency Medicine*, 4th ed. Philadelphia: Lippincott Williams & Wilkins, 2000.)

Evaluation

- Early diagnosis is crucial to improved mortality, thus head CT should be expedited.
- Particular attention should be paid to the patency of the patient's airway.
- A thorough neurological examination should be performed in all patients with head injury.
- Signs of Cushing's triad (bradycardia, hypertension, abnormal respiratory pattern), focal neurologic deficits, or uncal herniation (fixed, dilated pupil) mandate prompt imaging.

Management

- Increased ICP can lead to a decreased level of consciousness, and intubation should be strongly considered in patients who are actively vomiting, rapidly decompensating, or having a Glasgow Coma Scale score of ≤8. Hypoxemia should be avoided because it will lead to further brain damage.
- Blood pressure should be aggressively managed:
  - Hypotension (from other injuries) can lead to decreased cerebral perfusion.
  - Hypertension can lead to increased bleeding, edema, and mass effect.
- Neurosurgical consultation should be obtained immediately after diagnosis is made. If the patient presents with signs/symptoms of increased intracranial

pressure (Cushing's triad, anisocoria), neurosurgical consultation prior to imaging is appropriate.
- Seizure prophylaxis in the form of phenytoin or fosphenytoin (15–20 mg/kg) should be considered.
- Identify and correct coagulopahty.
- If there is evidence of increased ICP, the following short-term therapies should be considered:
  - Mannitol or hypertonic saline (if blood pressure permits).
  - Hyperventilation (goal pCO_2 in a range of 30–35).
  - Sedation with benzodiazepines or propofol.
- Drain placement by a neurosurgeon may be necessary to decrease ICP and to invasively measure cerebral perfusion pressure.

Special Considerations
- Repeat head computed tomography can be considered within the first few hours.
  - Risk factors for progression of bleeding include large initial size and associated (subarachnoid or subdural) bleeding.
  - Small contusions may not require any repeat imaging.

Best Evidence/Clinical Decision Rules

Are there any medications that can help decrease bleeding?

Recombinant factor VIIa is a prothrombotic agent that has been shown to limit the progression of ICH; however, it has not been definitively shown to decrease mortality or improve outcome. Since it is prothrombotic, rFVIIa has been associated with increased risk of deep vein thrombosis (DVT).

Obviously, coagulopathies should be corrected immediately with blood products (e.g., fresh frozen plasma) and/or vitamin K.

Suggested Readings
Chang EF, Meeker M, Holland MC. Acute traumatic intraparenchymal hemorrhage: risk factors for progression in the early post-injury period. *Neurosurgery.* 2006;58(4):647–655.

Maas AI, Stochetti N, Bullock R. Moderate and severe traumatic brain injury in adults. *Lancet Neurol.* 2008;7(8):728–741.

Narayan RK, Maas AI, Marshall LF, Servadei F, Skolnick BE, Tillinger MN. Recombinant factor VIIA in traumatic intracerebral hemorrhage: results of a dose-escalation clinical trial. *Neurosurgery.* 2008;62(4):776–786.

13 Diffuse Axonal Injury

Azita Hamedani

Definition

- Diffuse axonal injury (DAI) is one of the most common and devastating consequences of traumatic brain injury. It is a frequent cause of persistent vegetative state (PVS) in trauma patients.
- DAI often results from rotational-deceleration injuries. While such mechanism of injury is seen most commonly in motor vehicle accidents, DAI can also be seen in falls, assaults, and sporting injuries (e.g., soccer and hockey).
- Although DAI is labeled as "diffuse" brain injury, it is most appropriately characterized as multifocal.

Pathophysiology

- DAI results from axonal shear injury induced by rotational forces that affect the brain during sudden acceleration-deceleration.
- Injury typically occurs in areas where the density difference is greatest between neuronal structures. As such, the vast majority of DAI lesions occur in the lobar white matter, at the gray-white junction. (Fig. 13.1).

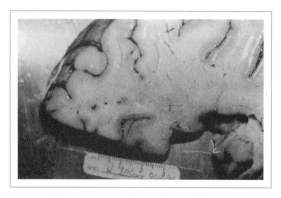

FIGURE 13.1: In this autopsy specimen, small hemorrhages are seen throughout the brain and corpus callosum consistent with diffuse axonal injury. (Reprinted with permission from Greenberg MI, Hendrickson RG, Silverberg M, et al. *Greenberg's Text-Atlas of Emergency Medicine*. Philadelphia: Lippincott Williams & Wilkins, 2005.)

- Axons lose their elasticity when rapidly stretched. Some axons are completely disrupted at the time of trauma (mechanical, primary injury). Other axons may not be completely torn, but alterations in axonal membrane that impair axoplasmic transport can lead to swelling and subsequent axonal splitting over the course of a couple weeks (biochemical cascade, secondary injury).
- A retraction ball can be seen after the axon splits into two—a histopathologic hallmark finding of DAI.
- Injured axons subsequently undergo Wallerian degeneration.

Diagnosis

- Multifocal white-matter lesions, measuring 1–15 mm, are found in a characteristic distribution. Lesions are typically ovoid, with the long-axis parallel to involved axonal tracts. Greatest injury occurs more centrally; peripheral lesions are usually smaller.
- Three stages have been defined on the basis of anatomic location of DAI lesions:
  - Grade 1 (mild): Involvement of frontal and temporal lobes; less likely, parietal and occipital lobes, internal and external capsules, and cerebellum.
  - Grade 2 (moderate): In addition to Stage 1 lesions, corpus callosum involvement.
  - Grade 3 (severe): In addition to Stage 1 and 2 lesions, brain stem involvement.
- Although computed tomographic (CT) imaging is most appropriate and accessible as part of initial trauma evaluation, more than half of patients with DAI have a normal head computed tomography on presentation.
- CT scan criteria include small intraparenchymal hemorrhages (petechial hemorrhages) in the cerebral hemispheres, corpus callosum, adjacent to the third ventricle, and potentially in the brain stem. However, fewer than 20% of patients with DAI demonstrate these characteristics of CT findings.
- The most sensitive imaging modality presently is magnetic resonance imaging (MRI). Recommended sequences include T1-weighted, T2-weighted, and diffusion-weighted images. Gradient-echo imaging is particularly useful, as it can demonstrate lesions not seen on T1- and T2-weighted sequences.

Evaluation

- As with other head injuries, facilitate rapid CT imaging to identify injuries that require acute intervention.
- DAI may or may not be associated with other evidence of head injury (skull fractures, subarachnoid hemorrhage, subdural or epidural hemorrhage).
- **DAI should be strongly suspected when the patient's clinical symptoms are disproportionate to his/her CT imaging and level of intoxication (Fig. 13.2).**

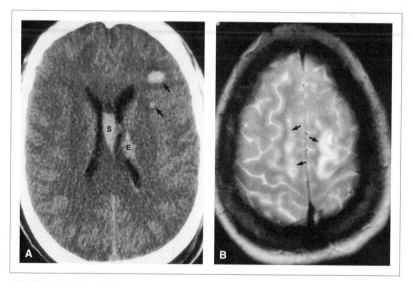

FIGURE 13.2: Shearing injuries. **A:** The axial computed tomography shows two left frontal hemorrhagic shearing injuries (arrows). There is a hemorrhagic shearing injury of the septum pellucidum (S) and a left subependymal hemorrhage (E) secondary to shearing of the subependymal veins. **B:** Magnetic Resonance T-2-weighted image (different patient) shows non-hemorrhagic shearing injuries (arrows) in both frontal lobes. (From Harris JH, Harris WH. *The Radiology of Emergency Medicine*, 4th ed. Philadelphia: Lippincott Williams & Wilkins, 2000.)

Management

- Attention should be directed to head injury diagnoses that require acute intervention.
- **There is currently no specific treatment for DAI beyond what is done for any type of head injury, including early intubation to protect the airway, preventing hypotension and hypoxia, and trying to mitigate increased intracranial pressure.**
- DAI rarely causes death since brain stem function is usually not affected. As such, the vast majority of patients remain in a PVS. For this reason, DAI can be an especially stressful diagnosis for patient's families.
- Supportive services for the family are an important component of long-term management plan.

Special Considerations

- Prognosis is somewhat associated with number of observed lesions. However, the extent of axonal injury is uniformly worse than what can be visualized by computed tomography or MRI.
- Recovery for the 10% of patients who escape PVS occurs over the course of the first year. Axonal disconnection represents a final event; the neuron has permanently lost its ability to communicate with its target. Functional recovery in DAI patients, therefore, is due to repair of damaged axons that did not completely disconnect.

Best Evidence/Clinical Decision Rules

- False-negative head computed tomographies are common, so MRI should be preformed in appropriate clinical context.
- False-negative MRI may occur when only routine sequences are performed, so gradient-echo sequences should be requested.
- It is likely that DAI is currently underdiagnosed given limitations of current imaging modalities. It is believed that DAI may be responsible for the global cognitive deficits evidenced after traumatic brain injury, even though these patients are currently not known to carry a DAI diagnosis.

Suggested Readings

Meythaler JM, Peduzzi JD, Eleftheriou E, Novack TA. Current concepts: diffuse axonal injury-associated traumatic brain injury. *Arch Phys Med Rehabil.* 2001;82: 1461–1471.

Smith DH, Meaney DF, Shull WH. Diffuse axonal injury in head trauma. *J Head Trauma Rehab.* 2003;18(4):307–316.

Toyama Y, Kobayashi T, Nishiyama Y, et al. CT for acute stage of closed head injury. *Radiat Med.* 2005;23(5):309–316.

Wasserman JR, Koenigsberg RA. Diffuse axonal Injury. www.emedicine.com.

Section Editor: Jay Lemery

14

Facial Trauma: The First 15 Minutes, Algorithm, and Decision Making

Hina Zafar Ghory

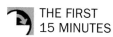 THE FIRST
15 MINUTES

ABCs and Vitals

- Do not be distracted by an obvious facial deformity. Be systematic about surveying the ABCs.
- Beware of maxillary fractures or a "flail mandible" which makes bag-valve mask ventilation difficult.
- If the chin lift or jaw thrust is unsuccessful, the tongue may need to be pulled forward with gauze, a towel clip, or a suture through the anterior tongue.
- Follow cervical spine injury precautions and consider concomitant injuries to carotid vessels. The facial injury itself may be a distracting injury. If the c-spine has been cleared, allow the patient to sit up and lean forward to clear blood and secretions, if possible.
- You should anticipate a difficult airway, including consideration of awake or fiberoptic intubations without paralytics.
- Avoid nasotracheal intubation and placement of nasogastric tubes because of the possibility of intracranial penetration made possible by some facial fractures.

History

- May be secondary to blunt or penetrating trauma.
- Listen to emergency medical services—they may have already discovered critical details of the airway prior to arrival.

Physical Examination

- Inspect the face for asymmetry.
- Palpate the entire face for step-offs, crepitus, tenderness, hypesthesia/anesthesia, or cranial nerve palsies.
- Assess for any abnormality of the orbital station, ocular movements, and visual acuity.
- Evaluate for cerebrospinal fluid (CSF) rhinorrhea or otorrhea.
- Check for midface facial stability by grasping and gently moving teeth and hard palate.
- Trismus or difficulty opening the mouth may be secondary to a zygomatic fracture with impingement of the temporalis muscle.

Emergency Interventions

- Assess the airway early. Edema and bleeding may make intubation more challenging as time progresses.
- Assess for intracranial penetration.
- Assess for vision loss. Perform a lateral canthotomy early if there is any suspicion of a retrobulbar hematoma.
- Identify associated injuries. While nasal and zygomatic fractures may be caused by low-impact trauma, other facial fractures require high impact and thus, multisystem involvement is common.
- For most facial injuries, computed tomography will be the imaging modality of choice; however, management of head, chest, and abdominal trauma takes precedence over facial imaging.

Memorable Pearls

- Domestic, elder, and child abuse are important causes of facial injuries.
- Blindness occurs in 0.5–3% of patients with facial fractures. Examine the eyes and extraocular motions carefully.
- Massive hemorrhage from facial fractures is rare. Control maxillofacial bleeding with direct pressure, packing, or manual reduction of displaced fractures.
- Intraoral palpation helps differential bony from soft tissue tenderness.
- CSF rhinorrhea is suggested by finding a double-ring or "halo" when nasal discharge is placed on filter paper, due to the separation of CSF from blood.

Essential Considerations

Know the anatomy of the face and the common facial fracture patterns.

- Nasal fractures: most common facial fractures; present with swelling and tenderness over the nasal bridge.
- Mandibular fractures: Second most common facial fractures; present with malocclusion and pain with jaw movement.
- Frontal sinus/frontal bone fractures: Require high forces and are frequently associated with orbital involvement and intracranial injury from disruption of posterior table of the sinus.
- Nasoethmoidal-orbital fractures: Result from trauma involving the bridge of the nose or medial orbital wall and are often associated with CSF leaks from dural tears.
- Orbital fractures: "Orbital blowout fractures" are the most common orbital fractures and result from direct trauma to the orbital rim or globe, leading to the herniation of orbital contents through the orbital floor. Extraocular muscle entrapment leading to inability to look up or double vision when looking in certain directions is not uncommon.
- Zygomatic fractures: The classic "tripod fracture" involves the infraorbital rim, zygomaticofrontal suture, and zygomaticotemporal junction leading to flattening of the cheek and eye tilt from tension on the lateral canthus.
- Maxillary fractures: Midface fractures, categorized as Le Fort I, II, and III, are high-energy injuries which can lead to airway compromise.

Consultations

- Facial fractures may involve several subspecialty services depending on the injury. These include trauma surgery, oral and maxillofacial surgery, ENT, plastic surgery, ophthalmology, and neurosurgery.

DECISION
MAKING

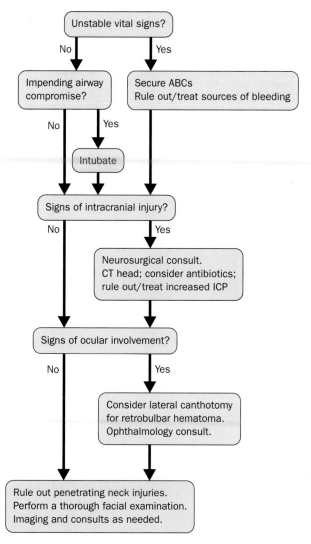

Facial fractures: Decision making algorithm. CT, computed tomography; ICP, intracranial pressure.

15 Midface Fractures

Elisabeth Gomes

Definition

- The face is divided into thirds (Fig. 15.1):
  - Upper third—forehead and frontal sinus.
  - Middle third—nose, maxillae, orbits, and zygomas.
  - Lower third—mandible and dentition.

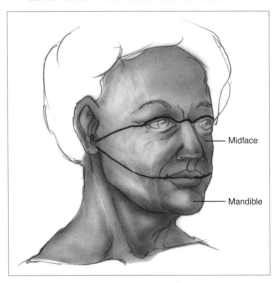

FIGURE 15.1: Midface and mandible zones for penetrating injuries to the face. (Reprinted from Chen AY, Stewart MG, Raup G, et al. Penetrating injuries of the face. *Otolaryngol Head Neck Surg* 1996;115:464–470, with permission.)

Pathophysiology

- The maxillary framework and horizontal and vertical bony bolstering provide strength and support. Maxillary fractures occur in about 6–25% of all facial fractures.
- Midfacial injuries result from high-energy trauma like motor vehicle accidents, assault, and falls.
- Fractures of the midface are commonly classified using the system developed by Rene Le Fort (Fig. 15.2):
  - Le Fort I: Horizontal maxillary fracture.
  - Le Fort II: Pyramidal-shaped fracture involving nose, maxillae, orbits, and zygomas.
  - Le Fort III: Complete craniofacial separation at the base of the skull.
- Most fracture lines are not so precise or confined, but the Le Fort classification is still used because it aids in communicating management plans.

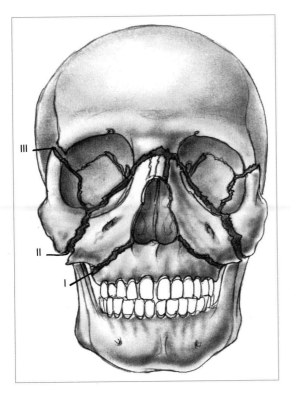

FIGURE 15.2: Le Fort fracture levels. Although these levels usually do not describe the extent or exact nature of midfacial fractures, they are still appropriately used for a general description of the injuries. (Reprinted with permission from Bailey BJ, Johnson JT, Newlands SD, et al. *Head & Neck Surgery— Otolaryngology*, 4th ed. Philadelphia: Lippincott Williams & Wilkins, 2006.)

Diagnosis

- History
  - Useful to know magnitude, location, and direction of impact.
  - Assess for clues in the history that suggest concomitant injuries: altered mental status (intracranial injury), focal neurologic deficit (c-spine injury), vision deficit, or double vision (orbital or cranial nerve involvement).
- Physical examination
  - Open and close jaw; inspect oropharynx and airway.
  - Assess vision, globe position, extraocular movement, and intercanthal distance.
  - Inspect for deformity, swelling, ecchymosis, gross blood, and cerebrospinal fluid from nose and ear.
  - Palpate for movement of any bony impairment and neurological deficit.
- Waters' view is a good screening tool for low pretest probability of skeletal injury (Fig. 15.3).
- In penetrating trauma, anteroposterior (AP) and lateral view may help assess depth of impaled object. Consider angiography to assess vascular compromise.
- Noncontrast computed tomographic (CT) thin cuts of both axial and coronal planes are the modality of choice.
  - Three-dimensional reconstruction may or may not be helpful, pending the area of injury.

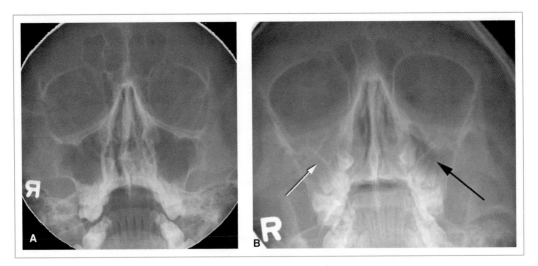

FIGURE 15.3: A: Normal Waters view of the sinus. The maxillary sinuses are clear. The sinuses are positioned just above the temporal bones to avoid the confusion of overlapping images. **B:** Opacified right maxillary sinus. A Waters view shows the lack of air in the right maxillary sinus (*white arrow*). Compare with the normal left side (*black arrow*). (Reprinted with permission from Bailey BJ, Johnson JT, Newlands SD, et al. *Head & Neck Surgery—Otolaryngology*, 4th ed. Philadelphia: Lippincott Williams & Wilkins, 2006.)

Evaluation
- Evaluate the patient for all injuries, including cervical spine and intracranial injury, prior to focus on the midface alone.
- Midfacial injuries result from high-energy impact.
  - For occluded oropharynx, attempt disimpaction of bone fragments to facilitate airflow and perform orotracheal intubation if possible.
  - Quickly move to cricothyrotomy if airway is unstable and oropharynx is obstructed.
- Control bleeding with pressure, packing, suturing, or cautery as necessary.
- **Rapid imaging once patient is *stable*.**

Management
- Attend all life-threatening injuries first.
- Nondisplaced or minimally displaced facial injuries without airway compromise can be treated as outpatient with delayed care for up to 7 days for adults and 3 days for children.
- In penetrating trauma, do not remove or disrupt any impaled objects. It may be acting as a tamponade for vascular structures.
- Penetrating trauma with vascular compromise requires exploration in the operating room.
- Tetanus vaccine, if needed.
- Antibiotics for open fractures or fractures involving the sinuses.
- Consider early consultation of ENT, ophthalmology, or OMFS (oral and maxillofacial surgery) as injuries are recognized.
- Assess for cerebrospinal fluid leak.
- Consider the cosmetic effects of these injuries. Facial deformities can have devastating psychological ramifications.

Special Considerations

- Imperative to recognize retrobulbar hematoma and perform emergent lateral canthotomy when appropriate.
- Identify and drain hematomas of the nasal septum and ear.
- Nerve injury can occur from the primary assault or secondary to surgical reconstruction and fixation devices; therefore, it is important to document deficits prior to surgery.
- Depending on the level of injury, recovery is a long process, up to 8 weeks. Attention to infection through this process is important in minimizing osteomyelitis.
- Shock is unlikely in patients with midfacial trauma alone, especially when gross bleeding had been controlled. Look for a secondary cause of shock.

Best Evidence/Clinical Decision Rules

Should all patients with suspected facial fractures be computed tomography scanned?

Several studies have shown that a single 30-degree occipitomental view (Waters' view) is sufficient for screening for midfacial injuries. CT scans are helpful in delineating the extent of injury once positive on Waters' view.

Suggested Readings

Bailey B, Johnson J, Newlands S, et al. *Head & Neck Surgery—Otolaryngology*, 4th ed. Philadelphia: Lippincott Williams & Wilkins, 2006.

Demetriades D, et al. Initial evaluation and management of gunshot wounds to the face. *J Trauma.* 1998;45(1):39–41.

Goh SH, Low BY. Radiologic screening for midfacial fractures: a single 30-degree occipitomental view is enough. *J Trauma.* 2002;52(4):688–692.

Mckay MP. Facial trauma. In: Marx JA, ed. *Rosen's Emergency Medicine: Concepts and Clinical Practice*, 6th ed. Philadelphia, PA: Mosby, 2006:382–398.

Merritt RM, Williams MF. Cervical spine injury complicating facial trauma: incidence and management. *Am J Otolaryngol.* 1997;18(4):235–238.

Moe KS, Kim DW. Facial trauma, maxillary and Le Fort fractures. emedicine.com.

Pogrel A, Podlesh SW, Goldman KE. Efficacy of a single occipitomental radiograph to screen for midfacial fractures. *J Oral Maxillofac Surg.* 2000;58(1):24–26.

16

Orbital Fractures

Peter Chen

Definitions

- Orbital fracture: fracture of any portion of the bones of the orbit encasing the eye.
- Blowout fracture: fracture of the orbital floor or medial wall. Can involve entrapment of orbital contents including the inferior or medial rectus muscles (Table 16.1).

Pathophysiology

- Blowout fractures of the orbital floor are caused by two mechanisms:
  - Blunt trauma to the orbit transmits force to the thinner and weaker orbital floor.
  - Direct trauma to the infraorbital rim causes buckling of the orbital floor.
- Fracture can lead to entrapment of the inferior rectus and inferior oblique muscles.
- Fracture can also lead to hypoesthesia of the ipsilateral cheek and lip due to injury of the infraorbital nerve.

Diagnosis

- Patients with significant orbital or facial trauma should receive computed tomographic (CT) imaging with thin cuts. **Remember that facial trauma often results in multiple injuries.**
- CT imaging can diagnose orbital fractures and evaluate the need for surgical intervention. Computed tomography also allows for the diagnosis of retrobulbar hematomas, intraocular foreign bodies, other facial fractures, and intracranial injuries (Fig. 16.1).
- Plain films have poor sensitivity and are of limited value.

TABLE 16.1: Characteristics of blowout fractures

Type of fracture	Clinical manifestation	Imaging choice	Management
Blowout fractures (floor)	Pain with upward gaze Limitation of upward gaze with severe diplopia suggests muscle entrapment	X-ray (Waters' view) Computed tomography	Ophthalmology consult Antibiotics and decongestants for patients with sinus fractures
Blowout fractures (medial wall)—more rare	Subcutaneous orbital emphysema suggests ethmoid sinus disruption	Same as above	Same as above

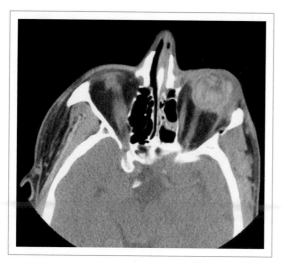

FIGURE 16.1: Computed tomography showing a left-sided orbital fracture in association with a ruptured globe and lens dislocation. (Courtesy of New York Presbyterian Hospital, New York, NY.)

Evaluation

- Careful examination of the orbit and surrounding soft tissue should begin with consideration of possible globe rupture, which precludes applying direct pressure to the orbit.
- A distorted anterior chamber, teardrop pupil, and extrusion of intraocular contents (including the pigmented iris or aqueous humor) are clues to a globe rupture.
- History and mechanism of injury are important to establish early to help focus the physical examination. Penetrating trauma to the orbit should raise suspicion of open globe lacerations with intraocular foreign bodies.
- The eyelids should be examined for high-risk lacerations involving the medial aspect (lacrimal ducts), lid margins, and upper lid. Exposed fat indicates perforation of the orbital septum.
- The facial bones surrounding the orbit should be inspected for signs of fracture. Extensive facial fractures such as tripod or LeFort fractures may accompany orbital blowout fractures. Crepitus may indicate fracture of the maxillary or ethmoid sinuses.
- Proptosis, painful vision loss, and limitation of extraocular movements (EOM) are clues to a retrobulbar hematoma. Intraocular pressure will be increased.
- Visual acuity should be assessed in all patients including testing for an afferent papillary defect, which indicates injury to the optic nerve (as in a retrobulbar hematoma).
- The eye should be inspected for specific injuries such as subconjunctival hemorrhage, corneal abrasion, hyphema, iridodialysis, and lens dislocation. Posterior injuries such as retinal detachment may be diagnosed with a careful fundoscopic examination or ultrasound.
- Slit-lamp and fluorescein examinations should be conducted on stable patients without extensive injuries. A positive Seidel test is streaming of aqueous from a corneal perforation. However, avoid any eye solutions in the case of a suspected open globe.

Management

- Management of associated injuries, such as hyphema, retrobulbar hematoma, and globe rupture, is discussed in separate chapters.

- Emergent ophthalmology consultation is necessary for severe and moderate injuries such as open globe, hyphema, lens dislocation, blowout fracture with entrapment, and high-risk lid lacerations.
- Prophylactic antibiotics are recommended for blowout fractures involving a sinus.

Special Considerations

- 30% of orbital fractures are associated with other facial fractures.
- 30% of orbital fractures are associated with serious intraocular injuries.

Best Evidence/Clinical Decision Rules

How good is computed tomography for diagnosis of serious orbital trauma?

CT scanning without contrast and with fine cuts through the orbit is the diagnosis of choice for the patient who has sustained significant facial trauma. The sensitivity and specificity for an open globe are about 70% and 95%, respectively. It is the modality of choice for orbital fractures as it provides far more sensitivity and clinical information than plain films, which have a sensitivity of only 50%. CT images will also find retrobulbar hemorrhages, lens dislocations, intraocular foreign bodies, and other facial fractures.

Suggested Readings

Brady SM, McMann MA, Mazzoli RA, et al. The diagnosis and management of orbital blowout fractures: update 2001. *Am J Emerg Med*. 2001;19:147.

Hasan N, Colucciello SA. Maxillofacial trauma. In: Tintinalli JE, Gabor KD, Stapczynski SJ, eds. *Emergency Medicine: A Comprehensive Study Guide*. 6th ed. New York: McGraw-Hill Co Inc, 2004:1583–1590.

Kreidl KO, Kim DY, Mansour SE. Prevalence of significant intraocular sequelae in blunt orbital trauma. *Am J Emerg Med*. 2003;21:525.

McKay MP. Facial trauma. In: Marx JA, Hockberger RS, Walls RM, eds. *Rosen's Emergency Medicine, Concepts and Clinical Practice*. Vol 1. 7th ed. Philadelphia: Mosby, 2010:323–337.

17

Mandibular Trauma: Fractures and Dislocations

Sam Gerson

Definition
- **Mandibular fracture** is a disruption of any part of the mandibular bone, including the alveolar portion supporting the dentition.
- **Mandibular dislocation** is a displacement of the mandibular condyle from the fossa of the temporomandibular joint.

Pathophysiology

Fractures
- Second most common type of facial fracture (after nasal).
- Ring-shaped structure, so multiple fractures occur in more than 50% of cases.
- Most commonly result from vehicular accidents, assaults, and falls.
- Classified by anatomic location: body (36%), angle (31%), condylar (18%), symphysis (8%), ramus (6%), and coronoid (1%) (Fig. 17.1).
- Fractures may be described as closed or open, displaced or nondisplaced, and favorable (stable) or unfavorable (unstable).

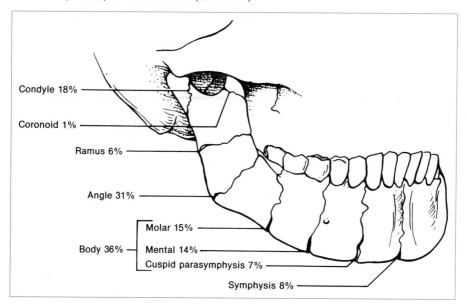

FIGURE 17.1: Mandible fracture sites and incidence. (Reprinted with permission from Wolfson AB, Hendey GW, Ling LJ, et al. *Harwood-Nuss' Clinical Practice of Emergency Medicine*, 5th ed. Philadelphia: Lippincott Williams & Wilkins, 2009.)

Dislocations
- Anterior—most common, may occur without significant trauma following extreme mouth opening (laughing, yawning).

- Posterior—blow to the chin, associated with damage to external auditory canal.
- Lateral—side blow to the jaw, associated with a condylar fracture.
- Superior—blow to partially open mouth, associated with cerebral contusion, facial nerve injury, and deafness.

Diagnosis

- Mandibular fractures/dislocations should be suspected in any trauma patient presenting with jaw deformity or deviation, jaw pain, trismus, or malocclusion.
- All trauma patients with findings suspicious for fracture/dislocation should have imaging to identify fracture locations and degree of displacement (Fig. 17.2).

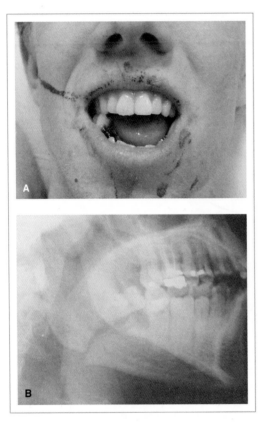

FIGURE 17.2: Open mandibular fracture as seen clinically **(A)** and radiographically **(B)**. (A, Courtesy of Madelyn Garcia, MD; **B,** Courtesy of Robert Hendrickson, MD.) (Reprinted with permission from Greenberg MI, Hendrickson RG, Silverberg M, et al. *Greenberg's Text-Atlas of Emergency Medicine.* Philadelphia: Lippincott Williams & Wilkins, 2005.)

- Panorex (panoramic) radiographs will identify the majority of fractures.
- If Panorex is not available, the following plain film views of the mandible should be ordered: lateral oblique, PA, Waters', and Towne.
- Consider noncontrast computed tomographic scan in patients with multiple facial injuries or in those with a suspicion for condylar fracture (poorly visualized on plain film) (Fig. 17.3).

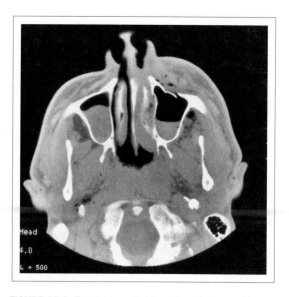

FIGURE 17.3: Facial computed tomographic image. There are multiple eggshell-like fractures involving the wall of both maxillary antra. Both maxillary antra are opacified with blood. The nasal passages are filled with soft-tissue density, suggesting blood and contused tissues. (From Harwood-Nuss A, Wolfson AB, et al. *The Clinical Practice of Emergency Medicine*, 3rd ed. Philadelphia: Lippincott Williams & Wilkins, 2001.)

Evaluation

- Perform a careful head, neck, and dental examination to identify any luxated or avulsed teeth, intraoral lacerations, or sensory deficits.
- Palpate along the mandible for tenderness, bony crepitance, step-off, and/or sensory loss of lips or gingiva.
- Place a finger in the external auditory canal during jaw motion to palpate the mandibular condyle.
- **Ecchymosis on the floor of the mouth is pathognomonic for a mandibular fracture.**
- Common signs of fracture/dislocation include malocclusion (most sensitive), pain, limited jaw opening, and jaw deviation.
- In dislocations with significant trauma, obtain radiographs to rule out fracture and confirm type of dislocation before attempting reduction.
- In suspected superior dislocation, consider noncontrast head computed tomography to rule out intracranial injury.
- Specific types of injuries and their indicative findings are outlined in Table 17.1.

TABLE 17.1: Findings and Specific Injuries in Mandibular Trauma

Finding	Specific injury
Displacement of the lower incisors	Symphysis fracture
Angulated or avulsed teeth	Alveolar fracture
Lateral crossbite	Unilateral condylar fracture
Anesthesia of lower lip	Injury of inferior alveolar or mental nerve

Management

- All mandibular fractures require prompt consultation with ENT or oral surgery for reduction and fixation.
  - Patients with closed, nondisplaced fractures may be discharged home (if there is no airway compromise) with recommendations for a soft diet, analgesia, and referral to an oral surgeon in 1–2 days.
  - Displaced fractures, open fractures, and associated dental trauma require emergent consultation in the emergency department.
  - Gingival lacerations indicate an open fracture requiring antibiotics (penicillin or clindamycin) and tetanus.
- Dislocations that are open, superior, unreducible, or those with associated fractures or nerve injury require surgical consultation.
- Admission is required for patients with airway compromise, excessive bleeding, severely displaced fractures, infected or open fractures, or significant comorbidities.
- Closed anterior dislocations without evidence for fracture may be reduced in the emergency department without imaging.
  - Manual reduction is achieved with downward and backward pressure on the posterior teeth.
  - Benzodiazepines, intra-articular lidocaine injections, and/or procedural sedation may be necessary.
  - Recommend 2 weeks with a soft diet, support of the chin during wide mouth opening, and follow-up with an oral surgeon.
  - Barton bandage (an ACE bandage wrapped around the jaw and head) is not required but may provide additional support and comfort.

Special Considerations

- Flail mandible is a potentially life-threatening complication of multiple jaw fractures that result in a loss of bony support to the tongue leading to airway obstruction. Initial management is to open the mouth, pull the tongue forward, and secure it with a towel clip or large suture. If the cervical spine is cleared, have the patient sit up and lean forward to assist in maintaining a patent airway. Consider early intubation if these techniques fail.
- **Warning**: facial fractures may prevent a successful seal with a bag mask, so be prepared with equipment for a rescue (LMA) or surgical airway (cricothyroidotomy).

Best Evidence/Clinical Decision Rules

Is there a clinical test that is helpful for detecting mandibular fractures in a patient with jaw pain but no instability or deformity?

Tongue-blade Test

Ask the patient to bite down on a tongue blade while twisting the blade in an attempt to break it. A patient with an intact mandible will be able to break the blade; a patient with a broken mandible will reflexively open the mouth (95% sensitive, 65% specific).

Suggested Readings

Alonso LL, Purcell TB. Accuracy of the tongue blade test in patients with suspected mandibular fracture. *J Emerg Med.* 1995;13:297.

Munter DW, McMuirk TD. Head and facial trauma. In: Knoop KJ, Stack LB, Storrow AB, eds. *Atlas of Emergency Medicine*, 2nd ed. New York: McGraw-Hill, 2002:3–27.

Nael H, Colucciello SA. Maxillofacial trauma. In: Tintinalli JE, Kelen GD, Stapczynski S, et al., eds. *Emergency Medicine: A Comprehensive Study Guide*, 6th ed. New York: McGraw-Hill, 2004:1583–1590.

18

Nasal Fractures and Epistaxis

Dana Sacco

Definition

- A nose fracture is a break in the bone or cartilage over the bridge, in the sidewall, or septum of the nose.
- Epistaxis is bleeding from the nose, usually with drainage out of the nostrils but occasionally with posterior drainage of blood into the oropharynx.
  - Sixty percent of people will experience epistaxis over the course of their lifetime although only 6% require medical attention.
- Epistaxis is classified as anterior or posterior depending on the source of bleeding:
  - **Anterior**—more common, largely self-limited; 80% bleed from Kiesselbach's plexus in the septum.
  - **Posterior**—can result in significant hemorrhage; bleeding is from posterior branches of sphenopalatine artery (Fig. 18.1).

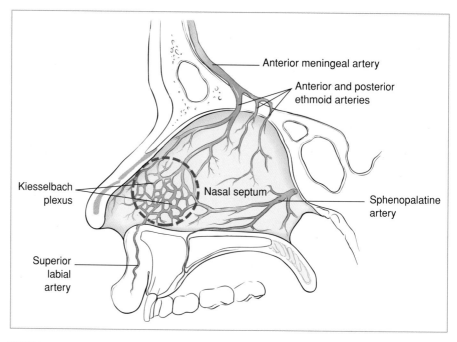

FIGURE 18.1: Anatomy of nasal septum. (From Kost SI, Post JC. Management of epistaxis. In: Henretig FM, King C, eds. Textbook of pediatric emergency procedures. Philadelphia: Williams & Wilkins; 1997:663, with permission.)

Pathophysiology

- The nose is susceptible to trauma because there is no soft tissue to dissipate the force, especially in older patients due to more brittle bones.

TABLE 18.1: Signs of nasal fracture

Direct signs	Indirect signs
Swelling	Periorbital ecchymosis
Tenderness	Epistaxis
Crepitance	Rhinorrhea
Ecchymosis	
Nasal deformity	

- Because of the mechanism, associated C-spine and closed head injuries are common.
- Mucosal blood vessels in the nose are superficial and relatively unprotected.

Diagnosis
- **Nasal fracture**
  - The diagnosis is clinical. Signs of nasal fracture are outlined in Table 18.1.
  - X-ray is not required for diagnosis or management.
  - Obtain a computed tomographic scan if other fractures are suspected.
- **Epistaxis**
  - Diagnosis is made with direct visualization, first attempted with a nasal speculum.
  - Determine whether the source of bleeding is anterior or posterior (see below).

Evaluation
- Suspected associated C-spine and head injuries should be evaluated immediately in the acute setting.
- **Nasal fractures**
  - Palpate the nose looking for evidence of crepitance, step-offs, or instability, which may indicate associated orbital/midface fractures.
  - Thoroughly examine structures surrounding the nose, including orbits, mandible, and C-spine.
- **Epistaxis**
  - To evaluate the source of bleeding, the patient should lean forward and apply pressure to both nares below the level of the nasal bones for 20 minutes. If bleeding persists, have the patient blow nose to remove clots.
  - Apply a topical anesthetic and vasoconstrictor, for example, gauze soaked in lidocaine with epinephrine, or oxymetazoline (Afrin) nasal spray.
  - Insert nasal speculum and spread vertically; use suction to remove clots as necessary. This will allow visualization of most **anterior** sources.
  - Source of bleeding is likely **posterior** if no anterior source is identified **and**:
    - Bleeding is from both nares.
    - Blood is draining into the posterior pharynx.
    - Anterior packing of both nares fails to control bleeding.
  - Laboratory testing: routine coagulation studies are not recommended unless a coagulation disorder is suspected or the patient is on anticoagulation.

Management

- Follow usual trauma guidelines, ensure adequate airway in the setting of trauma to the face, and follow spinal precautions when indicated.
- **Nasal fractures**
  - Nothing needs to be done for simple nasal fractures. Just provide nasal decongestants and analgesia and either plastic surgery or ENT follow-up.
  - Complications should be anticipated and evaluated:
    - ▶ Septal hematoma—rare, easily visualized with otoscope as bluish fluid-filled sac overlying the nasal septum. Classic teaching recommends that these hematomas must be incised and drained to prevent abscess formation or avascular necrosis from developing within several days (despite any significant evidence).
    - ▶ Cribriform plate fracture—associated with cerebrospinal fluid rhinorrhea, which may occur up to a week after. If suspected, place the patient in upright position and obtain neurosurgical consultation.
- **Epistaxis**
  - Bleeding may be hemodynamically significant, especially in the elderly, so first address the need for volume resuscitation.
  - Bleeding from **anterior** source that is visualized:
    - ▶ **Cauterize** with direct visualization using silver nitrate sticks. (Only one side of the septum should be cauterized because of a small chance of septal perforation.)
    - ▶ **Electric cautery** is usually performed in ENT clinic with local anesthesia.
    - ▶ **Anterior nasal packing**-commercially available products or layered petrolatum gauze can be used if bleeding is not controlled with cautery or if an anterior source is suspected but not visualized.
- Patients will need ENT follow-up for packing removal and should be discharged on antibiotics (typically first-generation cephalosporin).
  - Bleeding from **posterior** source:
    - ▶ **Balloon tamponade** can be accomplished by placing a Foley catheter through the nostril with the tip in the oropharynx, inflating the balloon with 3–4 mL water or air, then pulling forward until the balloon tamponades the posterior choana. The nasal cavity should then be packed anteriorly. Alternatively, balloon tamponade can be achieved with a commercially available epistaxis balloon.
    - ▶ **Posterior nasal packing** applies direct pressure to the choana by threading a gauze pad sutured to a catheter into the nostril, through the nasopharynx into the oral cavity.
- These patients should always be admitted, usually to a monitored setting, and placed on prophylactic antibiotic coverage with opiate analgesia.

Special Considerations

- Fractures frequently associated with nasal fractures include fractures of the orbital wall, zygoma, and sinuses.
- For extreme nasal displacement, consult ENT for realignment.
- In cases of epistaxis where it is necessary to pack both nostrils anteriorly, the patient should be admitted for observation.
- Warfarin does not need to be stopped if the levels are therapeutic.
- Aspirin is associated with epistaxis and hospitalization.
- Risks of infection, septal damage, and ulceration exist with packing.
- Risks of balloon migration, airway obstruction, and tissue necrosis exist with posterior packing.

Best Evidence

Is there an association between hypertension and epistaxis?

Frequently, patients present to the emergency department with epistaxis and hypertension. The link between the two has been debated for quite some time. In an evaluation of more than 1,000 patients with epistaxis in a 2003 paper, Fuchs and colleagues showed that any history of epistaxis was not associated with hypertension. However, it was associated with a history of allergic rhinitis.

Suggested Readings

Fuchs FD, Moreira LB, Pires CP, et al. Absence of association between hypertension and epistaxis: a population-based study. *Blood Press*. 2003;12:145–148.

Hsiao J. Epistaxis. In: Shah K, Mason C, eds. *Essential Emergency Procedures*. Philadelphia: Lippincott Williams & Wilkins, 2008:303–309.

Pope L, Hobbs C. Epistaxis: an update on current management. *Postgrad Med J*. 2005; 81:309–314.

Waters TA, Peacock WF. Nasal Emergencies and Sinusitis. In: Tintinalli J, Gabor KD, Stapcyynski SJ, eds. *Emergency Medicine: A comprehensive Study Guide*, 6th ed. New York: McGraw Hill, 2004:1476–1480.

19 Ear Trauma

Jesse Borke

Definition

- Injuries to the ear (Fig. 19.1) may be associated with serious injuries of the head, face, or neck.
- Ear injuries can result in hearing loss, poor cosmetic outcome, vertigo, and loss of balance.

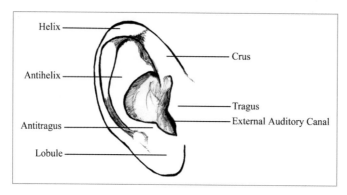

FIGURE 19.1: Anatomy of the ear.

Pathophysiology

- **Auricle trauma**
  - Human bites are the most common injury, then falls, MVAs, and dog bites.
  - Blunt trauma → hematoma → infection or avascular necrosis → deformity.
- **Barotrauma**
  - Barotrauma results from the expansion or contraction of gases in an enclosed space, such as from diving, flying, blast injuries, lightning, or acoustic trauma.
  - Middle ear barotrauma is the most common; inadequate clearance via the eustachian tube → overpressure of the middle ear causes serous fluid and blood to leak into the middle ear → tympanic membrane (TM) rupture.
- **Tympanic membrane perforation**
  - TM perforation commonly results from barotrauma, penetrating injuries, or blunt trauma to the head. It is the most common sequela of lightning strikes.
  - Associated displacement of the ossicles may cause a conductive hearing loss that requires surgical correction.
- **Thermal injuries**
  - Frostbite: Temperatures of −19°F or lower usually cause injury. Superficial frostbite results in erythema and edema of the skin without (first degree) or with bullae (second degree). Third- and fourth-degree frostbite results in necrosis of the skin and leads to gangrene and tissue loss.
  - Burns: Burns of the face and neck comprise almost 30% of reported burn injuries. Many patients sustaining significant facial burns suffer burns to the ears.

- **Temporal bone fractures:** Ear injuries are often associated with head trauma, especially with fractures of the temporal bone.
  - Cerebrospinal fluid (CSF) otorrhea can result from seemingly minor head injuries. Disruptions of the ceiling of the middle ear allow CSF to enter the cavity and flow out across a ruptured TM. If the TM is not ruptured, the fluid may pass through the eustachian tube and produce CSF rhinorrhea.
  - The facial nerve passes through the middle ear and is susceptible to injury and resultant paralysis from temporal bone fractures or foreign bodies.
  - Head injuries with or without temporal bone fractures may result in disarticulation of the ossicular chain and conductive hearing loss.
  - Temporal bone fractures may go across the cochlea and cause sensorineural hearing loss. Such injuries often result in total permanent loss of hearing and severe vertigo for the first few days following injury.

Diagnosis
- Barotrauma is diagnosed on the basis of history, gross and otoscopic inspection, and hearing tests and should be suspected in diving, blast, lightning, or acoustic injuries.
  - Patients with barotitis media may have a feeling of fullness or fluid inside the ear, congestion, muffled hearing, or hearing loss. On otoscopy, fluid may appear behind the TM, causing it to bulge and appear red.
  - Barotraumatic injuries to the ear may result in TM perforation. There may or may not be pain, bleeding, hearing loss, tinnitus, discharge, or vertigo.
- TM perforation is seen on otoscopic examination. Severe pain, complete hearing loss, or non–water-related vertigo suggests additional injury.
- Thermal Injuries
  - In frostbite, the ear will initially appear pale, progressing to erythema, edema, and eventually necrosis. In superficial frostbite injuries, the underlying tissue remains soft and pliable. In deep injuries, the underlying tissue is very hard.
  - Burns are classified by depth. Management depends on accurate grading.
- Head trauma/temporal bone fractures
  - Have a high suspicion for major injury in head trauma patients presenting with ear injuries. It is important to evaluate for CSF otorrhea or rhinorrhea, facial nerve paralysis, conductive or sensorineural hearing loss, and vertigo, as these may be suggestive of temporal bone fracture or other serious injury.

Evaluation
- Initial evaluation should focus on ABCs, trauma examination, resuscitation if necessary, and identifying associated injuries of the head and face. Emergent imaging as needed.
- Examination of the ear should include:
  - Inspection for auricular trauma, frostbite or burns, bleeding or discharge, CSF otorrhea or rhinorrhea, and signs of internal trauma. Mastoid ecchymosis indicates the presence of a basilar skull fracture (Battle's sign).
    - CSF otorrhea is best demonstrated with the patient's head down. If the TM is not ruptured, the fluid may pass through the eustachian tube and produce CSF rhinorrhea.
  - Otoscopic examination of the canals for lacerations and otorrhea and direct visualization of the TMs. Evaluate the TM for perforation, bulging, dullness,

barotitis media, CSF, or hemotympanum. **Hemotympanum appears as a purple (not red), often bulging TM.**

▶ A step-off at 12 o'clock at the medial end of the ear canal is evidence of a temporal bone fracture and suggestive of ossicular dislocation. Bone conduction will be greater than air conduction in such injuries.

- Evaluate gross hearing and test for any conductive or sensorineural hearing loss (Rinne and Weber tests): Partial hearing loss in trauma suggests TM rupture. Complete hearing loss suggests additional injuries to ossicles or inner ear. Sudden severe vertigo, tinnitus, or sensorineural hearing loss suggests inner ear damage.
- Evaluate the facial nerve by examining the face for paralysis, decreased lacrimation, numbness, or paresthesias to the affected side.
- History of barotrauma necessitates examination of the TM and auditory canal, neurologic examination to assess for inner ear damage, and a pulmonary examination looking for subcutaneous emphysema or pneumothorax.

Management

■ Auricle trauma: Untreated open auricular injuries result in deformity and infection.
- Antibiotics should be prescribed for high-risk injuries, including pseudomonas coverage for contaminated wounds.
- For regional anesthesia, infiltrate local anesthetic circumferentially around the base of the auricle in the subcutaneous plane.
- Abrasions: Clean and thoroughly irrigate; reevaluate wound in 24 hours.
- Lacerations (no missing skin or cartilage).
  ▶ Simple lacerations not involving the perichondrium or cartilage can be approximated with nylon.
  ▶ For lacerations involving the cartilage, the perichondrium should be sutured using 5-0 or 6-0 absorbable sutures. For complex lacerations or if debridement is necessary, a specialist should be consulted.
  ▶ After skin closure, an antimicrobial ointment and a firm, contoured, nonpressure dressing should be applied. A bolster dressing may be required to avoid hematoma formation.
- Avulsion/amputation (missing skin or cartilage).
  ▶ Isolated traumatic ear amputation is uncommon and frequently occurs in conjunction with serious head and neck trauma.
  ▶ Complete or partial avulsions are repaired by a specialist.
- Hematoma: Acute treatment involves drainage of the effusion via needle aspiration or incision followed by application of a pressure dressing.

■ Otic barotrauma/TM perforation
- Remove debris from the ear canal and fully visualize the entire TM. Do not irrigate; irrigation may force debris into the middle ear.
- Document patient's hearing status.
- If clinically indicated, obtain computed tomographic scan to rule out temporal bone fracture and ossicular disarticulation.
- Prescribe antibiotics if there is evidence of infection (broad-spectrum if the patient has been scuba diving). Prophylactic antibiotics are not indicated. Ototopical medicines are controversial, with suspensions preferred over solutions.
- Indications for urgent ENT consultation include vertigo, sensorineural hearing loss, severe tinnitus, active and significant bleeding, and facial paralysis.
- Treatment of middle ear barotraumas without perforation consists of decongestants, analgesics, and antihistamines. Antibiotics should be used if purulent otorrhea is observed.

- Disposition.
  - ▶ Most perforations heal spontaneously but refer to a specialist for surgical evaluation and formal audiogram.
  - ▶ Admit patients with associated injuries or severe vertigo.
- Thermal injuries
  - The therapy for frostbite is rewarming. The ear should be aseptically and quickly rewarmed with saline-soaked gauze that has been warmed to 38°–40°C (100.4°–104°F). With rewarming, the ear will become painful. If blisters form, they should be allowed to reabsorb spontaneously.
  - If the burn is an isolated injury and superficial partial-thickness, treatment in the emergency department should consist of cleansing and irrigation, nonsulfa antimicrobial ointment, and a nonpressure dressing. Referral should be within 24 hours.
  - Burns more severe than first-degree should be seen in consultation with a burn specialist or ENT. Deep partial-thickness burns with blistering or any full-thickness burns should be managed at a burn center.
  - *Pseudomonas aeruginosa* is present in 95% of burn infections.
- Head trauma/temporal bone fractures
  - CSF otorrhea
    - ▶ Emergent computed tomographic scan to diagnose the injury and detect intracranial blood or injury.
    - ▶ Admission and urgent neurosurgical consultation are indicated for all patients with CSF leakage.
    - ▶ Meningitis is a potential complication but prophylactic antibiotics do not have proven benefit.
  - Facial nerve paralysis
    - ▶ Consult a maxillofacial surgeon in the emergency department.
  - Conductive hearing loss
    - ▶ Patients without serious concomitant injuries (e.g., temporal fracture) can be discharged with ENT follow-up within a few days for surgical reconstruction of the ossicular chain.
  - Sensorineural hearing loss
    - ▶ Control vertigo with diazepam. Consult ENT in the emergency department.

Special Considerations

- Traumatic ear injuries may be found in association with injuries of the face or head, which may need to be evaluated first. Immobilize cervical spine and investigate for intracranial injury or fracture when indicated, including temporal bone fractures.
- Consider nonaccidental trauma in pediatric patients.

Best Evidence/Clinical Decision Rules

What method of treatment is best to treat auricular hematoma?

A 2004 Cochrane review reports that there is no good evidence to suggest which method of treatment is best in the treatment of acute auricular hematoma. The classic teaching, however, generally recommends that treatment is better than leaving a hematoma untreated and potentially developing into "cauliflower ear."

Should I prescribe antibiotics for auricle trauma?

A 2001 Cochrane review reports that there is evidence that there is a decrease in infection rates after human bites (the most common cause of auricle trauma). There is no evidence that the use of prophylactic antibiotics is effective for cat or dog bites to the ear.

Suggested Readings

Jones SEM, Mahendran S. Interventions for acute auricular haematoma. *Cochrane Database Syst Rev.* 2004;(2):CD004166.

Medeiros IM, Saconato H. Antibiotic prophylaxis for mammalian bites. *Cochrane Database Syst Rev.* 2001;(1):CD001738.

Snyder B, Neuman T. Dysbarism and complications of diving. In: Tintinalli JE, Kelen GD, Stapczynski JS, eds. *Emergency Medicine: A Comprehensive Study Guide*, 6th ed. New York: McGraw-Hill, 2004:1213–1217.

Templer J, Renner GJ. Injuries of the external ear. *Otolaryngol Clin North Am.* 1990;23(5):1003–1018.

Tintinalli A, Lucchesi M. Common disorders of the external, middle, and inner ear. In: Tintinalli JE, Kelen GD, Stapczynski JS, eds. *Emergency Medicine: A Comprehensive Study Guide*, 6th ed. New York: McGraw-Hill, 2004:1464–1471.

Section Editor: Emily Senecal

20

Eye Trauma: The First 15 Minutes, Algorithm, and Decision Making

Emily Senecal

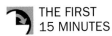 THE FIRST
15 MINUTES

ABCs and Initial Steps

- Evaluate for other life-threatening injuries using ATLS guidelines.
- For eye trauma patients requiring intubation, consider premedication to minimize the rise in intraocular pressure and alternatives to succinylcholine for paralysis.
- Protect the injured eye from further injury during initial trauma assessment.
- Elevate the head of the bed as soon as it is safe to do so.
- Provide antiemetics and analgesics in symptomatic patients to mitigate a rise in intraocular pressure.

Physical Examination

- Inspect for periorbital edema, ecchymoses, gross deformity, proptosis, laceration, facial fracture, or other overt abnormality.
- Avoid applying pressure to the globe when attempting lid retraction and avoid tonometry measurements until globe rupture has been ruled out.
- Assess direct and consensual pupillary reactivity with special attention to the possibility of an afferent pupillary defect.
- Assess extraocular movements. Determine whether the patient has pain with extraocular movements.
- Assess visual acuity. In bed-bound patients, evaluate each eye individually for light perception, hand motion, counting fingers, and reading printed material, or utilize a pocket vision card. In ambulatory patients, utilize a standard vision chart.
- Check for visual field defects.
- Perform a fundoscopic examination.
- Once the patient has been stabilized (which may be after the first 15 minutes), perform a slit lamp examination, first with the eye in the native state and then after fluorescein staining. Perform tonometry once globe rupture has been ruled out. Noteworthy slit lamp findings are listed in Table 20.1.

Emergency Interventions

- Provide rapid evaluation and treatment for other potentially life-threatening injuries.
- Perform immediate, copious irrigation for all ocular chemical exposures.

TABLE 20.1: Noteworthy slit lamp findings

Corneal clouding, corneal abrasion, or corneal ulceration
Seidel sign: rivulets of aqueous humor flowing from a site of globe perforation
Subconjunctival hemorrhage and ciliary flush
Anterior chamber for cells and flare, hyphema, and hypopyon
Ocular foreign body, including the use of lid eversion

- Consult ophthalmology immediately for suspected cases of globe rupture, retrobulbar hematoma, muscle entrapment, retinal detachment, and orbital compartment syndrome.
- **Perform emergent lateral canthotomy in patients with proptosis, worsening visual acuity, and rising intraocular pressures (signs and symptoms of retrobulbar hematoma).**

Memorable Pearls

- Do not perform magnetic resonance imaging on any patient with suspected or confirmed metallic intraocular foreign body.
- Avoid maneuvers that may increase intraocular pressure in suspected cases of globe rupture.
- Maintain a high level of suspicion for retinal detachment in all patients with vision loss.

Essential Considerations

- Ocular trauma is rarely life-threatening in and of itself; however, acute vision loss is a cause of major morbidity. Prompt, thorough action on the part of emergency physicians will provide eye trauma patients the best possible chance of maintaining long-term vision.

Consultations

- Emergent ophthalmology consultation is mandatory for all patients with globe rupture, retrobulbar hematoma, muscle entrapment orbital compartment syndrome, and retinal detachment.
- Urgent ophthalmology follow-up is indicated in many ocular traumatic injuries (e.g., corneal abrasion or ulceration, ocular foreign body with residual rust ring, hyphema, traumatic iritis).

DECISION
MAKING

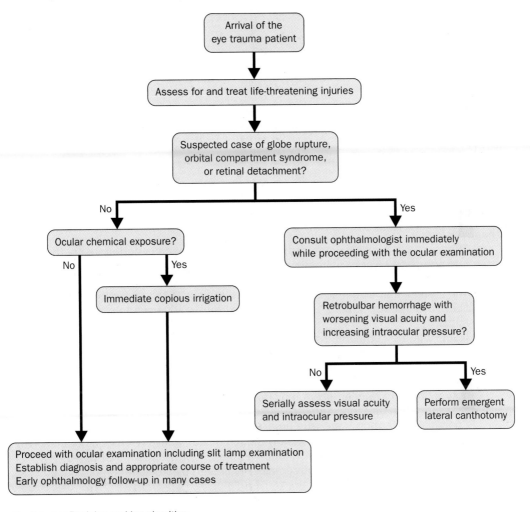

Eye trauma: Decision making algorithm.

21 Corneal Trauma

Benjamin White

Definition

- Corneal injury is damage to the corneal epithelium or matrix, most commonly in the form of abrasions, lacerations, burns, and irritations.
- Corneal injuries result from myriad causes, most frequently from foreign bodies or substances that come into contact with the eye.
- The management of corneal injury is based in large part on the cause of injury, with a stepwise approach to diagnosis and treatment being most prudent.

Pathophysiology

- The cornea is a highly organized, avascular matrix of cells and proteins, divided into a surface layer of epithelium and four deeper, stromal layers of connective tissue.
- The corneal epithelium contains some of the highest concentrations of nerve fibers of any body structure, and thus is extremely sensitive to nocioceptive stimuli.
- Given that the cornea is avascular, nourishment and immune protection are provided only by the tear fluid and aqueous humor, predisposing it to rapid progression of certain infections.
- While the corneal epithelium has the capacity to heal very rapidly (within 24 hours), injury to deeper layers may take significantly longer to heal and result in scar formation and long-term sequelae.
- Chemical ocular burns are true emergencies. *Alkaline chemicals* (e.g., drain cleaners, industrial solvents) rapidly induce a liquefactive necrosis that dissolves ocular tissue. *Acidic chemicals* induce a coagulation necrosis that is less devastating because the depth of injury is limited by precipitation of tissue proteins.

Diagnosis

- Corneal injury may be suspected in any patient complaining of a painful and/or red eye.
- Patients frequently describe blurry vision, foreign-body sensation, photophobia, tearing, and a sharp or "scratchy" pain that can be made worse with blinking or eye movements.
- History taking should include detailed recall of events surrounding the injury, exposure to chemicals or other substances, sensation of foreign body, symptoms of visual change, and habits of contact lens use.
- The diagnosis may not be obvious in cases of minor trauma (e.g., digital), small, high-velocity foreign bodies (e.g., machining, lawn-mower debris), and certain foreign substances (e.g., cosmetics). Thus, maintaining an appropriate level of clinical suspicion is in the best interest of the patient.

Evaluation

- In cases of ocular chemical exposure, copious irrigation must be initiated immediately, prior to a complete ocular evaluation.
- Meticulous examination of the cornea and periorbital structures, with the aid of a slit lamp, will often identify the extent of injury and may identify the causative agent. Slit lamp examination is performed first with the eye in the native state, then with the aid of fluorescein staining, in which a cobalt blue light reveals increased staining wherever the corneal epithelial cells are damaged or denuded (Fig. 21.1).

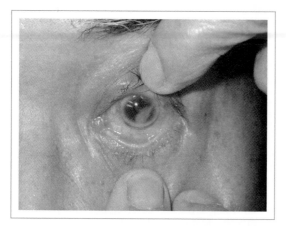

FIGURE 21.1: Fluorescein-stained large central corneal abrasion. (Courtesy of Anthony Morocco, MD.) (Reprinted with permission from Greenberg MI, Hendrickson RG, Silverberg M, et al. *Greenberg's Text-Atlas of Emergency Medicine*. Philadelphia: Lippincott Williams & Wilkins, 2005.)

- **Excluding full-thickness injury and globe rupture is of highest priority. Evidence of these diagnoses are listed in Table 21.1.**
- Adequate analgesia is both humane and frequently required to achieve a complete examination. Topical ester anesthetics (0.5% tetracaine) are rapidly absorbed through the corneal epithelium and are both diagnostically and therapeutically useful.
- Corneal ulcers need to be excluded, especially in patients who report contact lens use, as they can rapidly (over hours) erode through the corneal matrix, threatening vision (Fig. 21.2).
- If an intraocular foreign body is suspected on the basis of symptoms, history, or physical findings, plain film or computed tomographic (preferred) imaging should be performed.

TABLE 21.1: Indicators of full-thickness injury or globe rupture

Flat-appearing cornea
Air bubbles in anterior chamber
Stream of aqueous humor flowing from injury site (Seidel sign: fluorescein-stained stream)

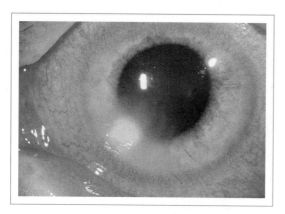

FIGURE 21.2: Infected corneal ulcers are characterized by corneal infiltrates associated with overlying epithelial defects and an anterior chamber reaction. (Reprinted with permission from Tasman W, Jaeger EA, eds. *The Wills Eye Hospital Atlas of Clinical Ophthalmology,* 2nd ed. Philadelphia: Lippincott Williams & Wilkins, 2001.)

Management

- Management of corneal injuries begins with copious irrigation (especially in the case of foreign substances) and may be facilitated by a Morgan lens.
- If foreign-body sensation persists, or vertical abrasions are noted on examination, lid eversion should be performed using a moist cotton-tipped swap, which may then be used to extract the foreign body if visualized.
- Superficial abrasions most often heal spontaneously, and there is little evidence to confirm or refute topical antibiotic administration. **Contact lens wearers should discontinue use and may benefit from topical agents that treat *Pseudomonas.*** In addition, although patients may experience relief from topical analgesics, these should not be prescribed for home use as they can delay healing. Eye patching should be avoided.
- If suspicion of corneal ulcer exists, patients require antibiotic treatment and observation at minimum, with some patients (depending on presentation and provider level of comfort) requiring emergent ophthalmologic consultation.
- Globe rupture, intraocular foreign bodies, and deep or extensive corneal lacerations mandate specialist consultation.
- Disposition: Most patients with corneal injury are candidates for discharge with close follow-up, after a thorough evaluation has been performed. Given the varying propensity for delayed complications (e.g., corneal ulcer), explicit discharge instructions are paramount.

Special Considerations

- Metallic foreign bodies need be removed urgently with an eye spud or 25- or 27-gauge needle. If a rust ring has formed, the patient should be referred for ophthalmologic consultation and removal (Fig. 21.3).
- Contact lens use, especially long-term use or in those with poor hygiene, predisposes patients to corneal irritation, injury (digital), and infection (corneal ulcer).

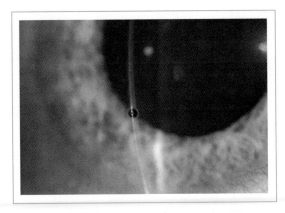

FIGURE 21.3: Corneal rust ring. (Reprinted with permission from Tasman W, Jaeger EA, eds. *The Wills Eye Hospital Atlas of Clinical Ophthalmology,* 2nd ed. Philadelphia: Lippincott Williams & Wilkins, 2001.)

Best Evidence/Clinical Decision Rules

Should I give my patient with a corneal injury an eye patch?

A recent 2006 Cochrane review of 11 randomized, controlled trials found that the use of occluding patches placed over the injured eye both slows healing on the first day and makes no difference in pain levels. In addition, patching results in loss of binocular vision. In summary, the practice of patching simple corneal abrasions may be abandoned, as it is not evidence-based.

Suggested Readings

Aronson AA, Yang NM. Corneal laceration. www.emedicine.com.

Bhatia K, Sharma R. Eye emergencies. In: Adams JG, Barton ED, Collings J, et al, eds. *Emergency Medicine*. Philadelphia: Saunders Elsevier, 2008:213–233.

Turner A, Rabiu M. Patching for corneal abrasions. *Cochrane Database Syst Rev.* 2006;(2):CD004764. Review.

22

Globe Trauma

Sara Nelson

Definition

- Globe injury is a traumatic injury to the sclera and cornea, which are the external fibrous layers of the eye.
- Open globe rupture results from a sudden increase in intraocular pressure in the setting of blunt trauma.
- Open globe laceration is a penetrating injury to the eye by a sharp object or projectile. Globe lacerations can be either penetrating, in which there is an entry wound but no exit wound, or perforating, in which there is both an entry and an exit wound.

Pathophysiology

- The eye sits in a rigid and protective structure made of the orbital bones. High-impact blunt force on the eye causes an acute rise in intraorbital pressure. This rise in pressure can lead to both scleral rupture and fracturing of the walls of the orbit.
  - Scleral ruptures are most common where the sclera is thinnest and weakest, including at the insertions of the intraocular muscles, at the limbus (the junction of the cornea and sclera), at the optic nerve, and at the sites of prior surgeries.
  - Orbital wall fractures commonly occur at the orbital floor and the medial wall, where the bones are thinnest. Fractures of the orbital rim are also common and occur through direct force.
- The majority of globe lacerations involve the cornea. Scleral and limbic lacerations occur in about one-third of cases.

Diagnosis

- High-impact blunt trauma, high-velocity projectile (including hammering metal on metal), or injury with a sharp object, should raise the suspicion for an open globe injury (Fig. 22.1).

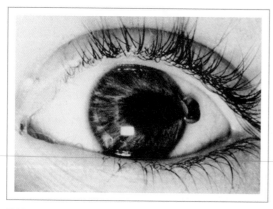

FIGURE 22.1: Penetrating corneal foreign body with entrapment of the iris, forming a teardrop pupil. This was a metallic chip projectile that resulted from hammering metal on metal. (Reprinted with permission from Wolfson AB, Hendey GW, Ling LJ, et al. *Harwood-Nuss' Clinical Practice of Emergency Medicine*, 5th ed. Philadelphia: Lippincott Williams & Wilkins, 2009.)

- Gross deformity of the eye with evidence of volume loss is highly suggestive of globe rupture.
- Obvious corneal lacerations may be seen by direct illumination with a penlight. Smaller lacerations may require indirect ophthalmoscopy. Bloody chemosis, severe subconjunctival hemorrhage, or hyphema may suggest an occult laceration or rupture.
- **Other physical findings suggestive of an open globe injury (Fig. 22.2) include:**
  - Extrusion of vitreous humor
  - External prolapse of the uvea (iris, ciliary body, choroid) or other internal structures
  - Peaked or irregular pupil
  - Tenting of the cornea or the sclera at puncture site
  - Marked decrease in visual acuity
  - Relative afferent pupillary defect
  - Low intraocular pressure—checked by an ophthalmologist only!
    - ▶ **Intraocular pressure should not be checked by the emergency physician if there is suspicion of an open globe.**
  - Seidel sign—fluorescein streams in a teardrop pattern away from the puncture site. This may be seen when fluorescein is used by the emergency physician/ophthalmologist to assess for a presumed corneal abrasion or to specifically look for globe injury.

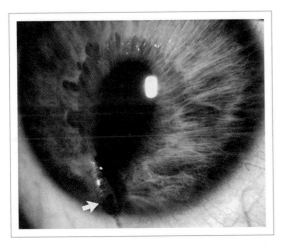

FIGURE 22.2: Corneal laceration (ruptured globe). Note the iris protruding through wound (arrow) and teardrop-shaped pupil pointing in direction of laceration. (Reprinted with permission from Fleisher GR, Ludwig S, Henretig FM, et al. *Textbook of Pediatric Emergency Medicine*, 5th ed. Philadelphia: Lippincott Williams & Wilkins, 2005.)

Evaluation

- Examination in high-risk patients should avoid maneuvers that apply pressure to the globe, such as lid retraction and intraocular pressure measurement with tonometry.
  - Children and uncooperative patients might need sedation to facilitate the examination.
- Evaluate visual acuity and assess for a relative afferent papillary defect.
- Assess for restricted extraocular movement suggesting extraocular muscle entrapment and for proptosis that suggests possible orbital compartment syndrome.

- Computed tomography of the orbit using fine cuts is the preferred radiographic modality for assessing open globe injuries, intraocular foreign bodies, and orbital wall fractures.
- Magnetic resonance imaging should not be used in any patient suspected of having a metallic foreign body.
- Once the diagnosis of open globe injury is made, further examination should be deferred until the time of the surgical repair in the operating room.

Management

- Increases in intraocular pressure may lead to further extrusion of ocular contents after an open globe injury. Measures must be taken to avoid external pressure on the eye and to avoid intraocular hypertension.
  - Avoid manipulation of the eye and use an eye shield to protect the eye.
  - Maintain patient bed rest with elevation of the head to at least 30 degrees.
  - Provide antiemetic therapy and pain control.
  - Use sedation as needed.
- Avoid placing any medication or eye drops into the eye (including fluorescein).
- Protruding foreign bodies should be left in place until evaluation by an ophthalmologist.
- Patients with open globe injuries should be given tetanus toxoid as needed and antibiotic prophylaxis.
  - Antibiotics should be targeted at organisms that cause posttraumatic endophthalmitis, including *Staphylococcus* and *Streptococcal* species, gram-negative organisms, and *Bacillus* species.
  - Appropriate regimens include vancomycin and ceftazidime, vancomycin and a fluoroquinolone, or ampicillin/sulbactam. For children, administer cefazolin and gentamicin.
- Patients should be kept NPO (nothing per mouth) in anticipation of surgery.
- Patients with open globe injuries require emergent evaluation by an ophthalmologist. Ideally, surgical repair of an open globe injury should occur within 24 hours of the injury.

Special Considerations

- Intraocular foreign bodies occur in 20–40% of open globe injuries. Most of these are small projectiles from the use of machine tools, hammering on stone or metal, explosions, and motor vehicle accidents.
- Infection occurs in 2–10% of all open globe injuries and is more common in injuries complicated by an intraocular foreign body. Organic intraocular foreign bodies are particularly prone to infection.

Best Evidence/Clinical Decision Rules

If my patient requires an emergent airway, is it appropriate to use succinylcholine?

In patients requiring intubation, the classic teaching is to avoid succinylcholine as this may lead to an increase in intraocular pressure and extrusion of intraocular contents. The literature contains many conflicting studies on the reality of this risk and on the efficacy of pretreatment. One case series by Libonati of 73 patients undergoing open eye surgery who were intubated with succinylcholine after pretreatment with nondepolarizing agents reported no adverse events. Although the risks and benefits must always be weighed, the prudent use of succinylcholine after pretreatment with nondepolarizing agents such as vecuronium or rocuronium is appropriate for rapid airway management in patients with ocular trauma.

Suggested Readings

Andreoli CM. Open globe injuries: emergent evaluation and initial management. www.UpToDate.com. Accessed December 10, 2008.

Casson RJ, Walker JC, Newland HS. Four-year review of open eye injuries at the Royal Adelaide Hospital. *Clin Experiment Ophthalmol.* 2002;30:15.

De Juan E Jr, Sternber P Jr, Michel RG. Penetrating ocular injuries. Types of injuries and visual results. *Ophthalmology.* 1983;90:1318.

Duch-Samper AM, Chaqués-Alepuz V, Menezo JL, Hurtado-Sarrió M. Endophthalmitis following open-globe injuries. *Curr Opin Ophthalmol.* 1998;9(3):59–65.

Kunimoto DY, Kanitkar KD, Makar MS, Friedberg MA, Rapuano CJ, eds. *The Wills Eye Manual: Office and Emergency Room Diagnosis and Treatment of Eye Disease*, 4th ed. Philadelphia: Lippincott, 2004.

Libonati MM, Leahy JJ, Ellison N. The use of succinylcholine in open eye surgery. *Anesthesiology.* 1985;62:637.

Parver LM, Dannenberg AL, Blacklow B, et al. Characteristics and causes of penetrating eye injuries reported to the National Eye Trauma System Registry, 1985–1991. *Public Health Rep.* 1993;108:625.

Rostomian K, Thach AB, Isfahani A, et al. Open globe injuries in children. *J AAPOS.* 1998;2:234.

Thompson WS, Rubsamen PE, Flynn HW Jr, et al. Endophthalmitis after penetrating trauma. Risk factors and visual acuity outcomes. *Ophthalmology.* 1995;102:1696.

Vachon CA, Warner DO, Bacon DR. Succinylcholine and the open globe. Tracing the teaching. *Anesthesiology.* 2003;99(1):220–223.

23

Hyphema

Mariah McNamara

Definition

- Traumatic hyphema is the accumulation of blood in the anterior chamber between the cornea and the iris after injury (Fig. 23.1).

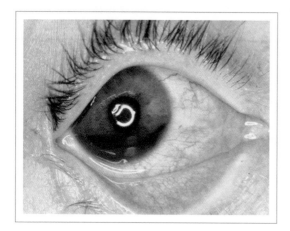

FIGURE 23.1: Grade 1 traumatic hyphema with blood layering in the anterior chamber. (Reprinted with permission from Harwood-Nuss A, Wolfson AB, et al. *The Clinical Practice of Emergency Medicine*, 3rd ed. Philadelphia: Lippincott Williams & Wilkins, 2001.)

- The hyphema grading system is based on the amount of layered blood in the chamber (Table 23.1).

Pathophysiology

- Sudden posterior displacement or shifting and stretching of the tissues results in a tear at the iris or ciliary body. Majority of cases are due to a tear at the anterior aspect of the ciliary body. The usual duration of an uncomplicated hyphema is 5–6 days.
- The blood accumulates in the anterior chamber and then exits via the trabecular meshwork and the canal of Schlemm or the juxtacanalicular tissue.
- Elevated intraocular pressures (IOPs) occur in approximately one-third of all hospitalized patients with hyphemas because of trabecular plugging by erythrocytes. The mean duration of elevated IOP is 6 days.

TABLE 23.1: Hyphema grading system

Microhyphema	Grade 1	Grade 2	Grade 3	Grade 4
No formation of layered clot	<1/3 of anterior chamber	1/3–1/2 of anterior chamber	1/2—less than total anterior chamber	Anterior chamber filled, also called "8-ball" hyphema

- Secondary hemorrhage occurs in approximately 25% of cases.
  - Results in a worse prognosis and is thought to be due to lysis and retraction of the clot that initially occludes the traumatized vessel.
  - Higher incidence in grade 3 or 4 hyphemas, younger patients, African American patients, and in those with sickle-cell anemia or trait.
  - Usually occurs between the 2nd and 7th day after trauma with most occurring on the 3rd or 4th day.
- The most serious complications are synechiae formation, corneal blood staining, and optic atrophy.

Diagnosis

- Traumatic hyphema should be suspected in all cases of orbital trauma. Midfacial fractures are associated with a 17% incidence of serious concomitant ocular injury.
- Diagnosis is most often made by gross inspection. Sitting the patient upright at 30 degrees allows the hyphema to settle and create a fluid level.
- A history of blurred vision when the patient is supine and progressive clearing of vision as the patient sits upright may indicate a previously undiagnosed hyphema.

Evaluation

- Initial evaluation should focus on identifying associated injuries including facial fractures, retrobulbar hematomas, and head and C-spine injuries.
- Careful inspection for gross ocular injury should be accompanied by documentation of visual acuity, visual fields, pupillary function, ocular motility, and the position of the globes.
- More than 75% of patients with a traumatic hyphema have more than one structural injury from the initial traumatic incident.
- Documentation of the size and shape of the hyphema is important for identifying and quantifying secondary hemorrhage.
- Daily tonometry is recommended for uncomplicated hyphemas.

Management

- Treatment is directed at reducing the risk of secondary hemorrhage, corneal blood staining, and optic atrophy from secondary glaucoma. Treatment decisions should be made in consultation with an ophthalmologist.
- Protection of the injured eye should include patching and shielding, and activity should be limited to quiet ambulation.
- Elevation of the head of the bed 30–45 degrees will facilitate the settling of the hyphema, improve visual acuity, and allow earlier visualization of posterior structures.
- Avoid aspirin and other nonsteroidal anti-inflammatory drugs because of their antiplatelet effects, which may increase the incidence of rebleeding.
- Topical atropine 1% is indicated to reduce ciliary spasm, prevent posterior synechiae formation, and facilitate posterior segment evaluation.
  - Avoid in patients with narrow chamber angles.
- Additional therapies (in conjunction with ophthalmology consultation).
  - Topical or systemic aminocaproic acid prevents recurrent hemorrhages by delaying clot lysis to allow the injured vessel to heal more completely.
    - Avoid in pregnancy, renal or hepatic dysfunction, or thrombotic disease.

TABLE 23.2: Indications for surgical management of hyphema

Uncontrolled elevated intraocular pressure

Early corneal bloodstaining

Hyphemas >50% for more than 10 days' duration

Patients with sickle-cell trait or anemia

- Topical corticosteroids such as 0.1% dexamethasone can be used to reduce intraocular inflammation and prevent the incidence of secondary hemorrhage.
- Elevated IOP can be controlled with topical beta-blockers, carbonic anhydrase inhibitors, or methazolamide in the case of sickle-cell trait or anemia.
- Surgical management is necessary in 5–7% of hyphemas. Indications are listed in Table 23.2.

Special Considerations

- Patients with sickle-cell disease or trait have higher incidence of increased IOP, optic nerve atrophy, and secondary hemorrhage related to traumatic hyphemas. **Ophthalmology should be involved and strongly consider admission for these patients.**
  - Avoid systemic carbonic anhydrase inhibitors to treat increased IOP. If this is not possible, methazolamide is preferred over acetazolamide.
- Reversal of any coagulopathy should be considered.
- Factors impacting disposition decision (especially for children and elderly).
  - Home safety
  - Activity restrictions
  - Medication delivery
  - Adequacy of follow-up
- Development of amblyopia as a result of corneal bloodstaining is a complication unique to the pediatric population.

Best Evidence/Clinical Decision Rules

- Consider outpatient management if:

  - No other injury mandating admission.
  - Hyphema <½ of anterior chamber.
  - Normal IOP.
  - Safe home environment.
  - Patient is able to comply with activity restrictions and medication administration.
  - Reliable follow-up.

- Consider surgery to evacuate hyphema if:

  - Sickle-cell disease or trait: if IOP is >24 mm Hg over 24 hours or if recurrent spikes of IOP over 30 mm Hg.
  - IOP >60 mm Hg for 2 days.
  - IOP >25 mm Hg with total hyphema for 5 days.
  - Corneal bloodstaining.
  - Failure to resolve to <50% of the anterior chamber volume by 8 days.

Suggested Readings

Brandt MT, Haug RH. Traumatic hyphema: a comprehensive review. *J Oral Maxillofac Surg.* 2001;59:1462–1470.

Recchia FM, Saluja RK, Hammel K, Jeffers JB. Outpatient management of traumatic microhyphema. *Ophthalmology.* 2002;109(8):1465–1470.

Sheppard JD, Crouch ER, Williams PB, Crouch ER Jr. Hyphema. eMedicine, Volume: 1, Update November 2006, http://www.emedicine.com/oph/topic765.htm#section%7Ebibliography.

Shiuey Y, Lucarelli MJ. Traumatic hyphema: outcomes of outpatient management. *Ophthalmology.* 1998;105(5):851–855.

Walton W, Von Hagen S, Grigorian R, Zarbin M. Management of traumatic hyphema. *Surv Ophthalmol.* 2002;47(4):297–334.

24

Traumatic Iritis

Monique Sellas

Definition

- Traumatic iritis, also referred to as iridocyclitis, is inflammation of the iris and/or ciliary body as a result of direct blunt traumatic injury to the globe. It can also be seen as a result of the following traumatic means:
  - Ocular burns
  - Foreign bodies
  - Corneal abrasions

Pathophysiology

- The iris is a heavily pigmented muscular structure located posterior to the cornea and anterior chamber and anterior to the lens. It controls the amount of light entering the eye via changes in pupillary size. The iris is an extension of the ciliary body.
- The ciliary body produces the aqueous humor that bathes the anterior chamber. Its muscle fibers contract to change the shape of the lens to allow different focal lengths.
- Blunt trauma to the globe may contuse and inflame the iris and ciliary body. Inflammation of these structures produces a classic clinical presentation in the affected eye:
  - Conjunctival injection in a perilimbal distribution (ciliary flush).
  - Deep aching pain that may radiate to the periorbital or temporal area and that is worse with extraocular movement.
  - Pupillary constriction that may be irregular, with sluggish papillary reflexes due to ciliary spasm.
  - **Consensual photophobia.**
    - ▶ Pain in affected eye when shining light in unaffected eye.
    - ▶ Helpful distinguishing feature as it is not seen in other superficial causes of photophobia.
  - Blurred vision.
  - Tearing without purulent discharge or crusting.
  - Variable intraocular pressure (IOP).

Diagnosis

- Diagnosis is confirmed by slit lamp examination of the anterior chamber using high-magnification (25–40×) and a small intense beam directed obliquely through the aqueous humor. Pathognomonic findings include:
  - Cells: white blood cells (WBCs) floating in the aqueous humor.
    - ▶ With significant inflammation, hypopyon can be seen which represents the layering of WBCs in the anterior chamber.
  - Flare: increased protein in the aqueous causes it to appear cloudy.
  - Keratitic precipitates, deposits of WBCs on the endothelium, are a hallmark of iritis (Fig. 24.1).

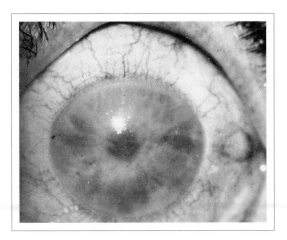

FIGURE 24.1: Acute iritis. This eye demonstrates the perilimbal injection and corneal edema that is common to both acute iritis and acute angle-closure glaucoma. The constricted miotic pupil seen here is characteristic of acute iritis. (Reprinted with permission from Harwood-Nuss A, Wolfson AB, et al. *The Clinical Practice of Emergency Medicine*, 3rd ed. Philadelphia: Lippincott Williams & Wilkins, 2001.)

Evaluation
- Perform a thorough physical examination of the eye with an emphasis on:
  - *Visual acuity*—may be reduced because of corneal clouding and high amounts of anterior chamber cells and flare.
  - *Cornea*—presence of a corneal abrasion or ulceration will change management of iridocyclitis.
  - *Pupils*—assess for asymmetry and consensual photophobia.
  - *Slit lamp examination*—assess for cells and flare.
  - *IOP measurement*—significantly elevated intraocular measurements should always prompt an ophthalmology consultation.

Management
- Treatment consists of paralyzing the iris and ciliary body with a long-acting cycloplegic agent.
  - Homatropine 5% qid, cyclopentolate 2% qid, or scopolamine 0.25% tid.
- Steroid drops are not first-line agents in the treatment of traumatic iridocyclitis.
  - May be considered to help inflammation if there is no improvement after 5–7 days.
  - Should be completely avoided in patients with a corneal epithelial defect.
  - This decision should be made in conjunction with the ophthalmologist.
- Ibuprofen reduces inflammation and pain and can be useful.
- Resolution usually occurs in 1 week.
- Ophthalmologic referral for follow-up is recommended.

Special Considerations
- If IOP is elevated, topical beta-blocker therapy (timolol [Timolol maleate], 0.5%) should be prescribed if there are no contraindications, and ophthalmology consultation and follow-up should be arranged.

Best Evidence/Clinical Decision Rules

Does a normal-shaped pupil exclude the diagnosis of iritis?

A Best Evidence Topic Report by Hunsley in 2006 found that patients who present with acute iritis often have no change in pupil size or shape, that is, their pupil appears normal compared with their other eye. Thus, the full constellation of symptoms and signs must be taken into consideration when making the diagnosis.

Suggested Readings

American Optometric Association Consensus Panel. *Optometric Clinical Practice Guideline: Care of the Patient With Anterior Uveitis*. St. Louis: American Optometric Association, 1994.

Bord SP, Linden J. Trauma to the globe and orbit. *Emerg Med Clin N Am.* 2008;26:97–123.

Hunsley T, Lee C. Does a normal-shaped pupil exclude the diagnosis of iritis. *Emerg Med J.* 2006;23:872–873.

Mahmood AR, Narang AT. Diagnosis and management of the acute red eye. *Emerg Med Clin N Am.* 2008;26:35–55.

Robinett DA, Kahn JH. The physical examination of the eye. *Emerg Med Clin N Am.* 2008;26:1–16.

Weisman RA, Savino PJ. Management of patients with facial trauma and associated ocular/orbital injuries. *Otolaryngol Clin N Am.* 1991;24:37.

Ehlers JP, Shah C, eds. *The Wills Eye Manual: Office and Emergency Room Diagnosis and Treatment of Eye Disease*. Philadelphia: Lippincott Williams & Wilkins, 2004.

25

Traumatic Retinal Detachment

Ronak Patel

Definition

- Retinal detachment (RD) is defined as a separation of the inner sensory layer of retina from the underlying tissue called the retinal pigment epithelium (RPE).
- Traumatic retinal detachment (tRD), rather than being a distinct entity, simply refers to the etiology of the detachment but is most often associated with a specific pathophysiology (see below).

Pathophysiology

- RD usually occurs via one of three mechanisms, with tRD occurring mostly through the first.
  - Rhegmatogenous: This most common method of tRD occurs when a tear or hole in the retina allows vitreous fluid to leak into the potential space between the sensory layer of the retina and the RPE.
  - Tractional: Occurs when vitreous humor adhesions to the retinal surface pull the retina off the wall of the eye as the vitreous contacts. While most adhesions result from chronic disease (e.g., diabetic retinopathy), penetrating trauma can also result in such adhesions.
  - Exudative: Occurs when fluid, usually from an inflammatory or neoplastic process, accumulates under the sensory layer of the retina in the absence of a full-thickness retinal break.
- The physical lifting of the sensory retinal layer off its supporting RPE and accompanying circulation causes direct ischemia to the photoreceptors, rapidly leading to permanent loss of vision.

Diagnosis

- Because tRD can progress more rapidly than nontraumatic RD, immediate diagnosis and treatment is crucial to preserve vision.
- tRD should be suspected in anyone complaining of painless unilateral vision loss, though bilateral and gradual vision loss does not rule out tRD.
- Patients do not always complain of vision loss early in the process but often describe floaters or flashers in the eye, loss of acuity or distortions of vision in discrete areas of the visual field, or irregular shapes such as the classic "curtain," or shadow, coming down.
- Diagnosis requires a dilated pupil examination of the retina by an ophthalmologist.
- Ultrasound is the best imaging modality to use as it can identify RD and can determine the type of detachment if tears or exudative buildup is visualized (Fig. 25.1).

Evaluation

- Facilitate rapid consultation and evaluation by an ophthalmologist, as tRD is one of the few ocular emergencies requiring therapeutic intervention within hours to preserve vision.

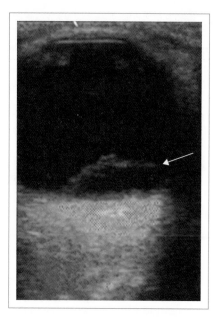

FIGURE 25.1: Ultrasound demonstrating detachment of the retina in the inferior portion of the image (white arrow). (Courtesy of St. Luke's Roosevelt Emergency Medicine Ultrasound Division, New York, NY.)

- Visual field defects can help localize the area of detachment.
- Ocular pressure may be reduced by about 5 mm Hg in the pathologic eye.
- Slit lamp examination may demonstrate the pathognomonic dust-like pattern of Shafer's sign for retinal tears in the vitreous.
- Fundoscopic examination sometimes reveals a grayish hue of the detached retina.
- Laboratory workup and advanced imaging should focus on completing a trauma evaluation and preparing the patient for potential emergent surgery.

Management
- Immediate ophthalmologic consultation is recommended in suspected tRD.
- Management should focus of completing a focused trauma evaluation and preparing for emergent surgery.

Special Considerations
- Although some cases may not need emergent surgical repair, all need immediate ophthalmologic evaluation.
- Symptoms of RD may present months after the traumatic event and anyone with ocular trauma should be given precautions for tRD.

Best Evidence/Clinical Decision Rules

Can emergency physicians (EPs) diagnose RD with bedside ultrasonography?

A 2002 study published in *Academic Emergency Medicine* compared diagnoses made by bedside ocular ultrasonography performed by EPs for ocular pathology with final diagnosis by ophthalmologist, computed tomographic scan, or both. In 60 of 61 cases, the EP ultrasound diagnosis agreed with the ophthalmologist or computed tomographic diagnosis or both. Nine of these cases were of RD, and all were detected by bedside EP ultrasonography. While in no way definitive, this study points to a potential future role of bedside ultrasonography by EPs in the diagnosis of tRD.

Suggested Readings

Blaivas M, Theodoro D, Sierzenski P. A study of bedside ocular ultrasonography in the emergency department. *Acad Emerg Med*. 2002;9:791–799.

Kang HK, Luff AJ. Management of retinal detachment: a guide for non-ophthalmologists. *BMJ*. 2008;336(7655):1235–1240.

Larkin GL. Retinal detachment. http://emedicine.medscape.com/article/798501-overview.

26

Retrobulbar Hematoma

Sayon Dutta

Definition

- Retrobulbar hematoma (RH) is a collection of blood in the potential space posterior to the globe in the orbit.
- RH occurs most commonly after facial trauma but also may occur after eyelid surgery and retrobulbar anesthesia.
- Spontaneous RH has been reported in patients with hemophilia, von Willebrand disease, and infraorbital aneurysm of the ophthalmic artery.

Pathophysiology

- The globe is enclosed within a continuous cone-shaped fascial envelope surrounded on all sides except anteriorly by the rigid bones that comprise the orbit.
- Anteriorly, the globe is constrained by the orbital septum and the eyelids.
- Traumatic RH occurs from bleeding of the infraorbital artery or one of its branches.
- As bleeding continues posterior to the globe, there is little room for the hematoma to accumulate, and the pressure within the orbital compartment begins to rise.
- The increased pressure within the orbital compartment directly compresses the optic nerve, central retinal artery, and other vessels that enter the eye.
- **Irreversible optic and retinal ischemia leading to blindness can occur within 90–120 minutes.**

Diagnosis

- RH should be suspected in trauma patients with decreased visual acuity, proptosis, eye pain, ophthalmoplegia, and a tense hard eye (Fig. 26.1).

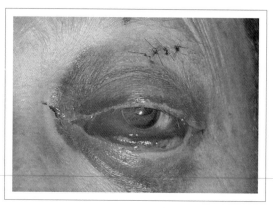

FIGURE 26.1: A 59-year-old man was hit in the left eye with a wrench and suffered a retrobulbar hemorrhage. His decreased vision, increased intraocular pressure, lid edema, ecchymosis, proptosis, and a subconjunctival hemorrhage improved with conservative treatment. (Reproduced with permission from Tasman W, Jaeger E. *The Wills Eye Hospital Atlas of Clinical Ophthalmology*, 2nd ed. Philadelphia: Lippincott Williams & Wilkins, 2001.)

- On fundoscopic examination, patients with RH may have a pale optic disc and, rarely, a cherry red macula.
- Pupillary examination may reveal an afferent pupillary defect.
- RHs can be seen on computed tomographic imaging (Fig. 26.2).

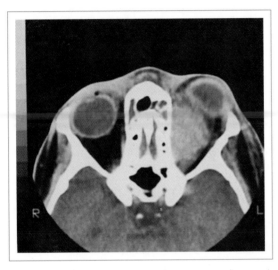

FIGURE 26.2: Computed tomography demonstrates a large retrobulbar hemorrhage along the medial orbital wall, compressing the optic nerve and distorting the globe. (Reproduced with permission from Tasman W, Jaeger E. *The Wills Eye Hospital Atlas of Clinical Ophthalmology*, 2nd ed. Philadelphia: Lippincott Williams & Wilkins, 2001.)

Evaluation

- Patients with traumatic injury to the eye should have serial visual acuity testing, intraocular pressure (IOP) measurements, and fundoscopic examinations.
- **IOP of >40 mm Hg in patients with facial trauma indicates acute orbital compartment syndrome, likely secondary to RH.**
- The diagnosis can be made clinically; however, a maxillofacial computed tomographic scan can confirm the diagnosis.
- Prompt diagnosis of RH is critical, as successful emergent decompression is time-sensitive.
- Patients with suspected RH and rapidly increasing IOP and decreasing visual acuity should have emergent therapy initiated without delaying for confirmatory imaging studies.
- All patients with RH warrant emergent ophthalmology consultation.

Management

- RH has both medical and surgical treatments.
- Once RH has been identified, medical therapy should be initiated immediately to decrease IOP and reduce ischemic injury.
- Medical therapeutic options to decrease IOP in adults include:
  - Acetazolamide 500 mg IV bolus followed by 125–250 mg IV q4–6 hours.
  - Mannitol 1–2 g/kg of 20% solution IV over 30–60 minutes.
  - Timolol 1–2 gtt of 0.25–0.5% solution to affected eye bid.

- Steroids have been shown to reduce inflammation and stabilize cell membranes against ischemic injury, with dosing options including:
  - Methylprednisolone 1 g IV one-time dose.
  - Hydrocortisone 100 mg IV one-time dose.
- The patient's head should be elevated to decreased IOP, and ice packs can be used to decrease swelling.
- Patients with severe symptoms such as decreased visual acuity or IOP of >40 mm Hg require emergent surgical decompression of the orbit by performing lateral orbital canthotomy and inferior cantholysis.
  - See lateral orbital canthotomy and inferior cantholysis chapter 98 for detailed description of procedure.
- Consult ophthalmology for definitive management.

Special Considerations

- If ophthalmology consultation is not available at your facility, medical therapies and lateral canthotomy and cantholysis should be performed prior to transfer of patients with RH.

Best Evidence/Clinical Decision Rules

Does the performance of lateral canthotomy actually improve a patient's IOP?

Although data lack on true traumatic models, a 2008 experimental cadaveric model of retrobulbar hemorrhage performed by Zoumalan and colleagues showed that the performance of lateral canthotomy and cantholysis decreased IOP by 59%.

Suggested Readings

Bailey W, Kuo P, Evans LS. Diagnosis and treatment of retrobulbar hemorrhage. *J Oral Maxillofac Surg*. 1993;51:780–782.

Goodall K, Brahma A, Bates A, et al. Lateral canthotomy and inferior cantholysis: an effective method of urgent orbital decompression for sight threatening acute retrobulbar haemorrhage. *Injury*. 1999;30:485–490.

Hislop W, Dutton G. Retrobulbar haemorrhage: can blindness be prevented? *Injury*. 1994;25:663–665.

Winterton JV, Patel K, Mizen KD. Review of management options for a retrobulbar hemorrhage. *J Oral Maxillofac Surg*. 2007;65:296–299.

Zoumalan CI, Bullock JD, Warwar RE, et al. Evaluation of intraocular and orbital pressure in the management of orbital hemorrhage. *Arch Ophthalmol*. 2008;126:1257–1260.

Section Editor: Bret Nelson

27
Spine Trauma: The First 15 Minutes, Algorithm, and Decision Making

Bret Nelson

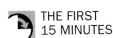

THE FIRST
15 MINUTES

ABCs

- Follow ATLS guidelines.
- Suspect spine injuries in the setting of head trauma, multiple organ system trauma, or altered mental status.
- Maintain spinal immobilization throughout the primary and secondary survey.
- Airway suction, jaw thrust, chin lift, and use of an oral airway may help alleviate upper airway obstruction.
- Early intubation, using rapid sequence intubation, should be considered when clinically indicated.
- Ensure adequate ventilation.
  - Cervical spinal cord injuries may be associated with diaphragmatic or intercostal muscle paralysis.
  - Spinal injuries are often associated with other injuries such as pneumothorax, cardiac or lung contusions, or other injuries which impair breathing or circulation.
- Evaluate for shock. Spinal injury may impair vascular tone but always rule out hemorrhage and hypovolemia in polytrauma first.

Spinal Immobilization

- Patients should be transported on a long rigid board with an appropriately sized rigid cervical collar in place. Padded blocks or "neck rolls" may be placed on both sides of the patient's head and neck for additional stability.
- The patient may be rolled into a lateral position (while maintaining spinal immobilization) in the setting of:
  - Vomiting (to reduce the risk of aspiration).
  - Third trimester of pregnancy (to reduce compression of the inferior vena cava by the gravid uterus, which causes hypotension).
- Patients should be removed from the rigid long board as soon as possible after transfer, and any hard surfaces should be padded. Skin breakdown occurs very rapidly in areas of pressure.
- With the cervical collar in place, patients may be "logrolled" to move them in the emergency department:
  - One operator stabilizes the head and cervical spine with his or her hands and forearms. This operator controls the timing of the roll by verbalizing instructions to the other operators.

- At least two additional operators stabilize the thoracic and lumbar spine, keeping the entire spinal column fixed against axial rotation during the roll.

Physical Examination

- Palpate the entire spine to identify any obvious fractures, depressions, or step-offs (Fig. 27.1).

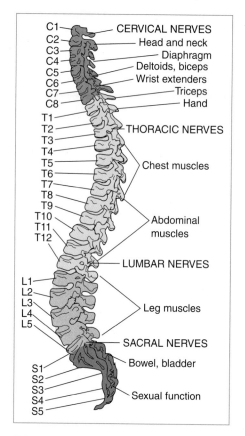

FIGURE 27.1: Structures affected by spinal nerves. (From Timby B, Smith N. Instructor's resource CD-ROM to accompany essentials of nursing: care of adults and children. Philadelphia: Lippincott Williams & Wilkins, 2005.)

- Thorough neurologic examination:
  - Assess motor function in trunk and all extremities (Table 27.1). Assess sensory function in trunk and all extremities (Fig. 27.2).
  - Reflexes.
    - Biceps (musculocutaneous nerve, C5–6)
    - Triceps (radial nerve, C6–8)
    - Patella (femoral nerve, L2–4)
    - Achilles (tibial nerve, S1–2)
  - Rectal examination, noting sphincter tone and perineal sensation (pudendal nerve, S2–4).

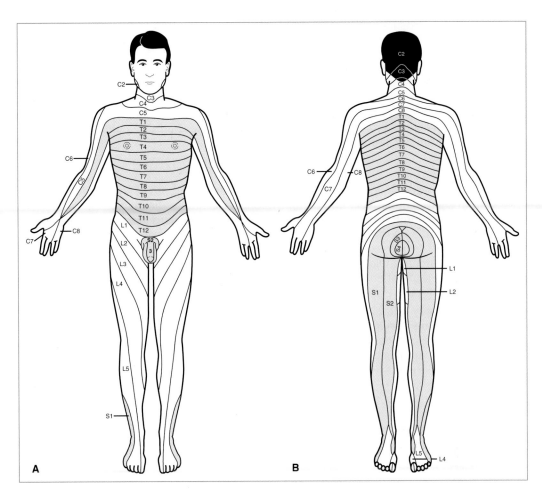

FIGURE 27.2: Anterior (**A**) and posterior (**B**) cervical, thoracic, lumbar, and sacral dermatomes. (From McDonald JV, Welch WC. Patient history and neurologic examination. In: Welch WC, Jacobs GB, Jackson RP, eds. *Operative Spinal Surgery*. Stamford: Appleton & Lange, 1999:3:15.)

Emergency Interventions
- Address abnormal vital signs, shock, and active bleeding.
- Provide rapid evaluation and assessment for other potentially life-threatening injuries.
- Arrange for rapid neuroimaging when indicated.

TABLE 27.1: American Spinal Injury Association Motor Strength Scale

0—No contraction or movement
1—Minimal movement
2—Active movement, not against gravity
3—Active movement against gravity
4—Active movement against light resistance
5—Active movement against full resistance

- Involve neurosurgical consultants early.
- Although very controversial, consider high-dose intravenous steroids in the setting of isolated blunt spinal cord injury within 8 hours.
  - Treatment as described in the National Acute Spinal Cord Injury Studies (NASCIS).
    - Methylprednisolone bolus of 30 mg/kg within 3 hours of injury, followed by 5.4 mg/kg/hr for 23 hours.
  - There is no role for steroids in the treatment of penetrating spinal injury.
  - **High-dose steroids may have a deleterious effect on the multitrauma patient and are not recommended in this scenario.**

Memorable Pearls
- Neurogenic shock may manifest as hypotension, bradycardia, and hypothermia with significant sensory and motor dysfunction distal to the injury.
- Deep vein thrombosis is a significant risk after spinal cord injury and should be addressed as part of the ongoing management of these patients.
- Priapism, decreased rectal tone, bladder dysfunction, and decreased perineal sensation may indicate serious spinal cord lesions.
- Up to 25% of patients with spinal injuries will have concomitant head injury.

National Emergency X-Radiography Utilization Study (NEXUS)
Criteria for Avoiding Cervical Spine Imaging (Clinical Clearance of C-spine)
- No midline cervical tenderness
- No focal neurologic deficit
- Normal alertness
- No intoxication
- No painful, distracting injury

Canadian Cervical Spine Rules
Are there any high-risk factors that mandate radiography?

- Age >65 years
- Dangerous mechanism of injury
  - Fall from height >1 meter
  - Axial loading injury
  - High-speed motor vehicle crash (more than 100 km/hr)
  - Rollover
  - Ejection
  - Motorized recreational vehicle or bicycle collision
- Presence of paresthesias

Are there any low-risk factors that allow safe assessment of range of motion?

- Simple rear-end crashes
- Ability to sit up in the emergency department
- Ability to ambulate
- Delayed onset of neck pain
- Absence of midline neck tenderness

Is the patient able to actively rotate the neck 45 degrees to the left and right?

Essential Considerations
- Adequate spinal immobilization is critical.
- Consideration of neuroimaging in the setting of minor injury can be guided by the NEXUS criteria and the Canadian Cervical Spine Rules. Patients who fulfill the criteria described in these rules are generally considered low-risk and do not require emergent cervical spine imaging.

Consultations

- Neurosurgical consultation is indicated for most spinal injuries involving the vertebrae or spinal cord. Some centers may alternatively involve spine specialists from the orthopedic service.

DECISION
MAKING

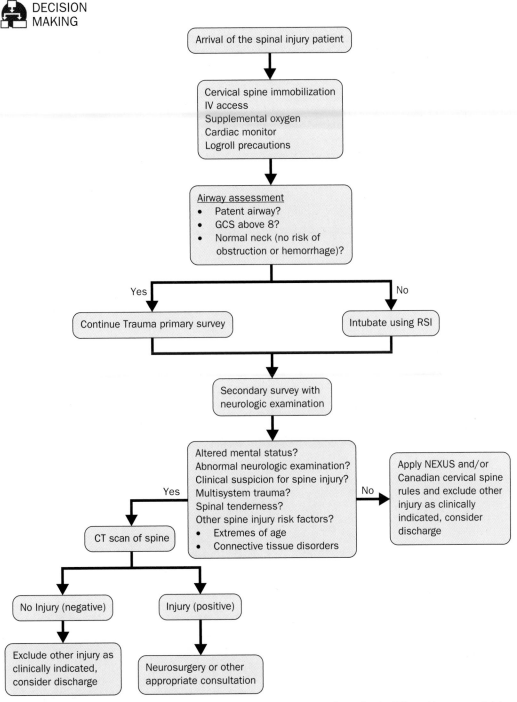

Spinal trauma: Decision making algorithm. IV, intravenous; GCS, Glasgow Coma Scale; RSI, rapid sequence intubation; CT, computed tomographic; NEXUS, National Emergency X-Radiography Utilization Study.

Suggested Readings

Bracken MB, Shepard MJ, Holford TR, et al. Administration of methylprednisolone for 24 or 48 hours or tirilazad mesylate for 48 hours in the treatment of acute spinal cord injury. Results of the third National Acute Spinal Cord injury randomized controlled trial. *JAMA*. 1997;277:1597–1604.

Hockberger RS, Kaji AH, Newton EJ. Spinal injuries. In: *Rosen's Emergency Medicine: Concepts and Practice*, 7th ed. Philadelphia: Mosby, 2010:337–377.

Malhotra NR, Thomas PG, Grady MS. Injury to the spine. In: Flint L, Meredity JW, Schwab CW, et al, eds. *Trauma: Contemporary Principles and Therapy*. Philadelphia: Lippincott Williams & Wilkins, 2008:297–304.

28 Dens and Odontoid Trauma

Lisa Jacobson

Definition

- The dens, or odontoid process, is the coronally projecting bone originating from the body of the second cervical vertebra.
- Dens fractures are divided into three groups (Figs. 28.1 and 28.2).
  - Type I—occurring above the attachment of the transverse ligaments.
  - Type II—occurring through the base of the odontoid process.
  - Type III—extending into the body of the second cervical vertebra.

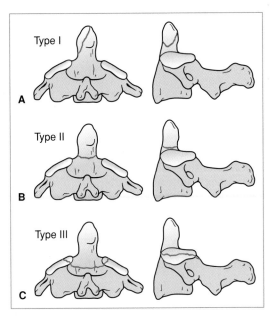

FIGURE 28.1: The odontoid fracture classification of Anderson and D'Alonzo. **A:** Type I fractures of the odontoid tip represent alar ligament avulsions. **B:** Type II fractures occur at the odontoid waist, above the C2 lateral masses. **C:** Type III fractures extend below the odontoid waist to involve the body and lateral masses of C2. Hadley has added the type IIA fracture with segmental comminution at the base of the odontoid (not shown). (Reprinted with permission from Bucholz RW, Heckman JD, Court-Brown C, et al., eds. *Rockwood and Green's Fractures in Adults*, 6th ed. Philadelphia: Lippincott Williams & Wilkins, 2006.)

Pathophysiology

- Spinal injury patterns depend upon the direction of force applied to the spine.
- Typically shearing anterior/posterior forces cause odontoid fractures.

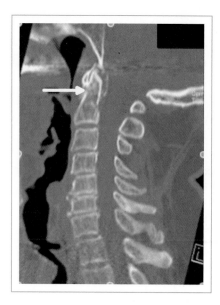

FIGURE 28.2: Computed tomographic scan demonstrating fracture line through the dens. (Courtesy of Mount Sinai Medical Center, New York, NY.)

Diagnosis
- While dens injuries can be suspected on the basis of mechanism of injury, confirmation requires radiographic imaging.
- Often these injuries can be seen on plain films:
  - Lateral—look for fracture and alignment of lordotic curves.
  - Anterior/posterior (AP)—look for fracture and spinous process alignment.
  - Odontoid—look for fracture and alignment of C1 with C2.
  - Predental space—the distance between the posterior aspect of anterior arch of C1 and the anterior aspect of odontoid process as seen on the lateral view. The space should be <3 mm in adults and <5 mm in children (Fig. 28.3).
- Computed tomography has increased sensitivity and is the imaging modality of choice.

Evaluation
- Maintain a high level of suspicion in motor vehicle accidents at high speed and when patients have obvious facial trauma.
- After completing your ABCs of trauma management, palpate the cervical spine while maintaining alignment to evaluate for step-offs and tenderness.
- With any suspicion of C-spine injury, assess neurological function distally.
- Facilitate rapid plain films or computed tomographic (CT) scan to identify injury.

Management
- The first and most important component of management is C-spine stabilization.
- Always manage the ABCs and identify life-threatening injuries first. Then do a complete neurological examination paying specific attention to:
  - Asymmetrical movements or weakness.
  - Changes in breathing patterns.

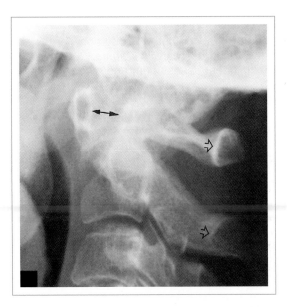

FIGURE 28.3: Atlantoaxial subluxation in a patient with rheumatoid arthritis. Lateral radiograph in flexion shows anterior subluxation of C1 on C2. Notice the widening of the predental space (double arrows) and malalignment of the spinolaminar lines of C1 and C2 (open arrows). (Reprinted with permission from Daffner RH. *Clinical Radiology: The Essentials*, 3rd ed. Philadelphia: Lippincott Williams & Wilkins, 2007.)

- Paresthesias, weakness, or paralysis—especially shoulder shrug and torticollis.
- Rectal tone.
- Proceed with appropriate imaging.
- The goal of management in the emergency department is to prevent cord injury while stabilizing the patient for evaluation of fracture stability and need for neurosurgical intervention.

Special Considerations

- Os odontoideum is the incomplete fusion of the odontoid onto the body of C2. This is a congenital defect often found incidentally with C-spine imaging in the setting of trauma.
- Patients with rheumatoid arthritis are more likely to injure the transverse ligaments of C2 even with minor trauma.

Best Evidence/Clinical Decision Rules

What is the preferred imaging modality for the initial evaluation of suspected spine injury?

A study in the *Journal of Trauma* (2005) found the sensitivities and specificities of CT scan for thoracolumbar fracture of 100% and 97%, respectively, with a negative predictive value of 100%. Plain radiographs were 73% sensitive, 100% specific, with a negative predictive value of 92%. Another study in 2006 compared x-ray and CT scan findings in acute spinal trauma, as well as the utility of using plain films versus CT scan as the initial imaging modality in trauma. The authors found a sensitivity of 70% for plain films of the spine, compared with 100% for CT scan. Patients evaluated by CT scan alone spent less time in radiology than those screened by plain films first (1.0 vs. 1.9 hours). Thus, CT scan should be used in any patient where spinal injury is suspected, and it may be feasible for Computed tomography to be the primary modality (over the use of plain films).

Suggested Readings

Antevil JL, Sise MJ, Sack DI, et al. Spiral computed tomography for the initial evaluation of spine trauma: a new standard of care? *J Trauma*. 2006;61(2):382–387.

Beattie LK, Choi J. Acute spinal injuries: assessment and management. *Emerg Med Pract*. 2006;8(5):1–28.

Berry GE, Adams S, Harris MB, et al. Are plain radiographs of the spine necessary during evaluation after blunt trauma? Accuracy of screening torso computed tomography in thoracic/lumbar spine fracture diagnosis. *J Trauma*. 2005;59(6): 1410–1413; discussion 1413.

Hockberger RS, Kaji AH, Newton EJ. Spinal injuries. In: Marx JA, Hockberger RS, Walls RM, eds. *Rosen's Emergency Medicine: Concepts and Clinical Practice*. 7th ed. Philadelphia: Mosby, 2010:337–377.

Hoffman JR, Mower WR, Wolfson AB, et al. Validity of a set of clinical criteria to rule out injury to the cervical spine in patients with blunt trauma. National Emergency X-Radiography Utilization Study Group. *NEJM*. 2000;343(2):94–99.

Stiell IG, Clement CM, McKnight RD, et al. The Canadian C-spine rule versus the NEXUS low-risk criteria in patients with trauma. *NEJM*. 2003;349(26):2510–2518.

29 Traumatic Spondylolisthesis (Hangman's Fracture)

Suzanne K. Bentley

Definition

- Hangman's fracture is defined as a bilateral C2 pars interarticularis fracture (the bone segment between the superior and inferior facet joints of the vertebrae).
- This fracture type is most commonly caused by hyperextension injury, such as during motor vehicle or diving accidents, but is named for its historic occurrence after judicial hangings caused by noose placement under the angle of the jaw (Fig. 29.1).

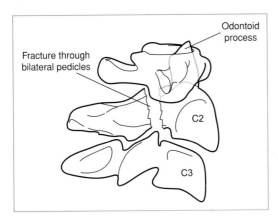

FIGURE 29.1: Lateral view of a hangman's fracture. (Reprinted with permission from Mick N, Peters JR, Egan D, et al. *Blueprints Emergency Medicine*, 2nd ed. Philadelphia: Lippincott Williams & Wilkins, 2005.)

Pathophysiology

- Hangman's fracture results in traumatic spondylolisthesis of C2 anteriorly on C3 resulting in the loss of bony connection between C1 and C3 (Fig. 29.2).
- The anatomy of C2 results in passage of the superior facets anteriorly and the inferior facets posteriorly causing stress through the pars interarticularis.
- Because of the relatively large size of the spinal canal versus the size of the spinal cord at the cervical level, neurologic damage is rarely associated.

Diagnosis

- Imaging is indicated to investigate all significant cervical spine injuries and in patients whose clinical presentation includes neck stiffness or pain, midline tenderness to palpation, or neurologic symptoms such as focal deficits, paresthesias, and abnormal deep tendon reflexes.
- Imaging may include cervical spine x-rays including anterior-posterior, lateral, open-mouth, and oblique views. However, computed tomographic imaging better visualizes these structures (Fig. 29.3).

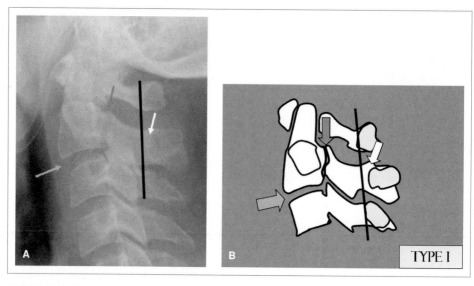

FIGURE 29.2: Type I hangman's fracture. **A:** Lateral radiograph and **(B)** type I hangman's fracture illustration demonstrate a nondisplaced subtle fracture line through the pars interarticularis of the axis (dark grey arrow) and posterior offset of the C2 spinolaminar line (black line/bright white arrow). The second intervertebral disc is intact (off-white arrow). (Reprinted with permission from Schwartz ED, Flanders AE. *Spinal Trauma: Imaging, Diagnosis, and Management.* Philadelphia: Lippincott Williams & Wilkins, 2007.)

- Magnetic resonance imaging may additionally be indicated to better evaluate ligaments, soft tissues, and spinal cord compression.

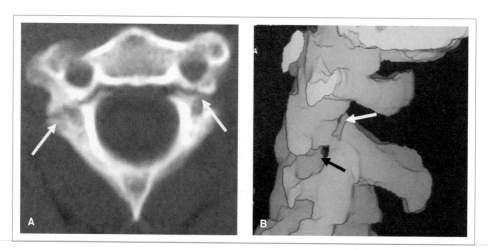

FIGURE 29.3: Type I hangman's fracture. **A:** Axial computed tomography demonstrates the bilateral pars fracture of C2 (white arrows) without significant fragment displacement. **B:** Computed tomography reformatted 3D surface-rendered lateral view shows the nondisplaced subtle fracture line through the pars interarticularis of the axis (white arrows) and normal C2–3 disc space (black arrow). (Reprinted with permission from Schwartz ED, Flanders AE. *Spinal Trauma: Imaging, Diagnosis, and Management.* Philadelphia: Lippincott Williams & Wilkins, 2007.)

Evaluation

- Immediate C-spine immobilization on patient arrival is obligatory if not previously done with special care during patient transfers, positioning, and intubation.
- Facilitate rapid imaging of the spine.
- Obtain early neurosurgical consultation when fractures are identified.
- Careful neurologic examination should focus on sensory and motor function, perineal sensation, rectal tone, and other signs of cord compromise.

Management

- Hangman's fractures generally heal well with external immobilization. Surgery is indicated if there is spinal cord compression or after failure of external immobilization.
- Neurosurgical consultation is mandated when hangman's fractures (like all cervical spine fractures) are identified.
- Hangman's fractures are classified into several types. Types and treatment are listed in Table 29.1.

Special Considerations

- A number of studies have shown relatively low rates of associated neurologic damage from hangman's fractures (due to the relatively large size of the spinal canal versus the spinal cord at the cervical level). However, postmortem studies by Bucholz showed that traumatic spondylolisthesis was second only to occipitoatlantal dislocations in cervical injuries leading to fatalities. Whenever a C-spine injury is identified, remember to always consider and address associated injuries.

TABLE 29.1: Classification and treatment of hangman's fractures

Classification	Description	Treatment
Type I	Hyperextension with or without additional axial load. No angulation of the deformity and the fracture fragments are separated by <3 mm	Immobilization in a cervical collar or halo vest until union occurs
Type II	Hyperextension and axial load with secondary flexion causing displacement of the fracture	Reduction of anterior angulation of fracture, typically via traction therapy followed by use of a halo vest until union occurs
Type IIA	Same as Type II with an additional component of distraction during injury that causes disruption of the C2–C3 disk space making the fracture unstable	Immediate halo vest placement and traction should be avoided
Type III	Fracture through the neural arch, facet dislocation, and disruption of the C2–C3 disk space making this fracture type unstable	Early closed reduction of the facet dislocation followed by halo vest to maintain reduction. If closed reduction cannot be obtained or maintained, open reduction is indicated

Best Evidence/Clinical Decision Rules

Should I obtain angiography of the neck on a patient with suspected or confirmed hangman's fracture?

- Kral et al. (2002) reported that vertebral artery injury is rarely symptomatic and therefore easily overlooked. Thromboembolic complications, however, may result in permanent morbidity or mortality due to brainstem ischemia and infarction.
- Willis et al. (1994) reported that vertebral artery injury after cervical spine fracture or dislocation is more prevalent than previously believed. The possibility of vertebral artery injury should be considered during the establishment of clinical management of the cervical spine.
- In a 2002 case report, Takahashi reported that preoperative or intraoperative angiography was useful in preventing brain-related ischemic complications during reduction of dislocated hangman's fractures.
- **Bottom line: Consider angiography of neck vessels in the setting of hangman's fracture.**

Suggested Readings

Bucholz RW, Burkhead WZ, Graham W, Petty C. Occult cervical spine injuries in fatal traffic accidents. *J Trauma.* 1979;19(10):768–771.

Kral T, Schaller C, Urbach H, Schramm J. Vertebral artery injury after cervical spine trauma: a prospective study. *Zentralbl Neurochir.* 2002;63:153–158.

Laron JL. Injuries to the Spine. In: Tintinalli JE, Kelen GD, Stapczynski JS, eds. *Emergency Medicine: A Comprehensive Study Guide,* 6th ed. New York: McGraw-Hill, 2004:1702–1712.

Skinner HB. Disorders, diseases, and injuries of the spine. *Current Diagnosis & Treatment in Orthopedics,* 4th ed. New York, NY: The McGraw-Hill Companies, Inc., 2006:221–298.

Takahashi T, Tominaga T, Ezura M, et al. Intraoperative angiography to prevent vertebral artery injury during reduction of a dislocated hangman fracture. Case report. *J Neurosurg.* 2002;97:355–358.

Willis BK, Greiner F, Orrison WW, Benzel EC. The incidence of vertebral artery injury after midcervical spine fracture or subluxation. *Neurosurgery.* 1994;34:435–441.

30 C1 Fracture (Jefferson Burst Fracture)

Elizabeth Cho

Definition
- A Jefferson fracture is defined as a burst fracture of the ring of C1 (the atlas) that occurs from an axial load to the head.
- Classically described as having two fractures in the anterior arch and posterior arch of C1, though fracture variants include two and three part fractures.

Pathophysiology
- C1 is a closed ring with no vertebral body. Thus, a fracture of this ring would result in a disruption (fracture) in at least two segments of the ring.
- The injury is often seen in diving injuries, where the axial load occurs from the diver striking his/her head on the ground or other object in shallow water.
- The axial loading force on the occiput of the head is transmitted to the superior articular surfaces of the lateral masses of the atlas. The lateral masses are then driven outward, causing fractures of the anterior and posterior arches of C1.
- Approximately 50% of C1 fractures are associated with other cervical spine injuries. These associated injuries commonly involve the dens, the C2 posterior arch, or C2 vertebral body.
- **Rupture of the transverse ligament should be suspected if the combined displacement of the lateral masses is >7 mm.** This finding is significant for C1–C2 instability since the ligament stabilizes C1 with respect to C2. A Jefferson fracture is considered to be unstable if this ligament is ruptured (Fig. 30.1).

Diagnosis
- If obtaining cervical spine radiographs, the anterior-posterior, open mouth view (odontoid), and lateral view should be obtained
  - If the open mouth view shows a >7 mm combined lateral displacement of the lateral masses of C1 with respect to C2, suspect a transverse ligament tear.
  - On lateral view, a widening of the predental space (>3 mm in adults, >5 mm in children) between the anterior arch of C1 and the odontoid is suggestive of prevertebral hemorrhage and retropharyngeal swelling. This is also a sign of transverse ligament disruption (Fig. 30.2).
- Computed tomographic (CT) scan is the preferred modality to diagnose cervical fractures.
  - CT imaging can detect a transverse ligament tear and/or avulsion fractures not seen on the plain film.
  - Any associated spinal cord injuries would only be seen on computed tomography/magnetic resonance imaging (Fig. 30.3).

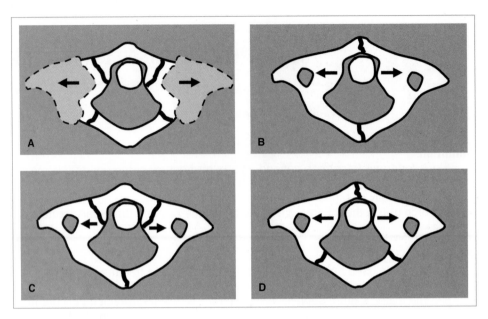

FIGURE 30.1: Jefferson fracture. The classic Jefferson fracture (JF) is a four-point injury with fractures occurring at the junctions of the anterior and posterior arches with the lateral masses, the weakest structural portions of the atlas (C1), with resultant bilateral offset or spreading of the lateral articular masses of C1 **(A)** (arrows indicate offset of lateral masses). However, computed tomography has shown that JF requires only one anterior and one posterior arch fractures **(B)**, although any combination of anterior and posterior arch fractures may occur **(C,D)**. Most commonly, there are two fractures in the posterior arch (one on each side) and a single fracture in the anterior arch off the midline **(D)**. (Reprinted with permission from Harris JH Jr, Mirvis SE. Vertical compression injuries. *The Radiology of Acute Cervical Spine Trauma*, 3rd ed. Baltimore: Williams & Wilkins; 1996:340–345; Landells CD, Van Pethegem PK. Fractures of the atlas: classification, treatment and morbidity. *Spine.* 1988;13:450–452.)

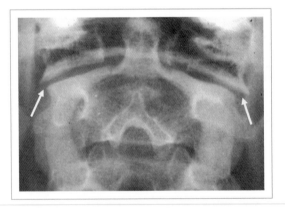

FIGURE 30.2: Jefferson fracture. Anteroposterior (AP) open-mouth view demonstrates lateral displacement of the lateral masses of C1 bilaterally (arrows) in relation to the superior facets of C2. (Reproduced with permission from Schwartz ED, Flanders AE. *Spinal Trauma: Imaging, Diagnosis, and Management*. Philadelphia: Lippincott Williams & Wilkins, 2007.)

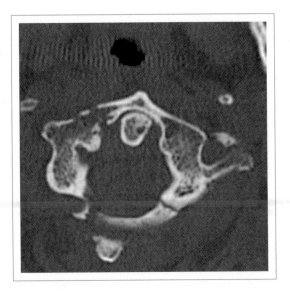

FIGURE 30.3: Computed tomographic scan demonstrating characteristic fracture pattern. (Courtesy of Mount Sinai Medical Center, New York, NY.)

Evaluation

- Patients with any C-spine fracture or suspected cervical injury should be immediately stabilized at the scene. These patients are often victims of major trauma and can have multiple injuries.
- In the emergency department, assess airway, breathing, circulation, and disability; apply hard c-collar if not already done by prehospital personnel.
- If possible, the patient should be asked whether he/she has any pain and to move both upper and lower extremities to rule out any gross neurologic deficit.
- A more thorough neurologic examination should be performed during the secondary survey once the patient is stabilized to assess for any possible motor or sensory deficits.
- Consider neurogenic shock in anyone with possible spinal injury if vital signs show hypotension and bradycardia, assuming other etiologies of shock (i.e., hemorrhage) have been ruled out.
- Facilitate rapid CT scan and/or plain film for evaluation of C-spine injury.
- Careful and frequent reassessment of the patient is needed to assess for any change in mental or neurologic status.

Management

- Neurosurgical consultation is mandated when a C1 burst fracture is identified.
- Administer intravenous fluids and pain medication as needed.
- If intubation is needed, it is essential to minimize movement of the head to protect the C-spine. Use jaw thrust maneuver instead of a head-tilt method and perform orotracheal intubation with in-line stabilization.
- Nondisplaced or minimally displaced fractures of the lateral mass and Jefferson fractures can be treated nonoperatively. C-collar immobilization is the treatment of choice to allow for healing and to prevent displacement.
- Fractures where the combined lateral mass displacement is >7 mm will likely require halo traction stabilization by neurosurgical colleagues.

- Internal fixation/fusion of C1–C2 after the fracture is reduced in traction is an alternative treatment.

Special Considerations
- Spinal cord injuries rarely occur with Jefferson fractures because the spinal canal is widest with respect to the spinal cord at this level. However, it should always be considered, especially when other cervical spine fractures are associated with it.
- Vertebral artery injuries have been seen in C1 fractures leading to associated stroke symptoms. Suspect in any patient with symptoms suggesting vascular compromise.

Best Evidence/Clinical Decision Rules

Is it appropriate to clear the cervical spine in an obtunded or unconscious patient with a normal computed tomography?

There is some controversy over whether a normal computed tomography and plain radiographs are sufficient to rule out cervical injury in patients with persistently altered mental status. A 2008 study by Meanker in the *Journal of Trauma* found that a normal CT scan of the cervical spine in blunt trauma victims with persistently altered mental status was not sufficient to rule out cervical spine injury. Magnetic resonance imaging was found to be the most reliable and accurate test to rule out any cervical spine injury including ligamentous injury in obtunded patients despite a normal CT c-spine.

Suggested Readings

Hecht AC, Silcox III DH, Whitesides TE. Injuries of the cervicocranium. In: Browner B, Jupiter J, Levine A, Trafton P, eds. *Skeletal Trauma: Basic Science, Management, and Reconstruction*, 3rd ed. Philadelphia: Elsevier Science, 2003:820.

Hockberger RS, Kaji AH, Newton EJ. Spinal injuries. In: Marx J, Hockberger R, Walls R, eds. *Rosen's Emergency Medicine: Concepts and Clinical Practice*, 7th ed. Philadelphia: Mosby Elsevier, 2006:349–374.

Larson JL. Injuries to the spine. In: Tintinalli JE, Kelen GD, Staczynski JS, Ma OJ, Cline DM, eds. *Emergency Medicine: A Comprehensive Study Guide*, 6th ed. New York: The McGraw-Hill Companies, Inc, 2004:1702–1711.

Meanker J, Philp A, Boswell S, Scalea TM. Computed tomography alone for cervical spine clearance in the unreliable patient—are we there yet? *J Trauma*. 2008;64(4):898–903.

Schwartz DT. Cervical spine injuries. In: Schwartz D, ed. *Emergency Radiology: Case Studies*. New York: The McGraw-Hill Companies, Inc, 2008:397–404.

Wood GW. Fractures, dislocations, and fracture-dislocations of the spine. In: Canale S, Heaty J, eds. *Campbell's Operative Orthopaedics*, 11th ed. Philadelphia: Mosby Elsevier, 2008:1784–1785.

31

Facet Dislocation and Vertebral Subluxation

Marisa L. Oishi

Definition

- Facet dislocations occur when there is complete anterior displacement of the inferior articular facet of one vertebral body with respect to the superior articular facet of the vertebral body below.
- Dislocations can be unilateral or bilateral and are often accompanied by anterior vertebral subluxation.

Pathophysiology

- Unilateral facet dislocations (Fig. 31.1).
  - Usually results from **flexion-rotation injuries**, most commonly at the C5/C6 and C6/C7 levels.
  - Unilateral facet dislocations are **typically stable** and *infrequently associated with neurologic impairment*.
  - The facet joint on the side of the direction of rotation acts as a pivot, while the superior facet of the contralateral joint rides up and forward relative to the inferior facet, and then rests in the intervertebral foramen.
  - Dislocation causes damage to the interspinous ligament, ligamentum flavum, and ipsilateral joint capsules. The adjacent posterior longitudinal ligament or disc annulus may also be damaged.
  - May be associated with mild anterior subluxation of the vertebral body up to 25% of the disc space.
- Bilateral facet dislocations (Fig. 31.2).
  - Classically considered a **pure hyperflexion injury**, although it can occur from several mechanisms.
  - This **highly unstable** injury is *commonly associated with neurologic deficit*.
  - Bilateral dislocation results in significant injury to all posterior ligamentous structures, the posterior longitudinal ligament, and disc annulus.
  - Anterior subluxation of the vertebral body of 50% or greater may result in cord impingement and neurologic injury.
  - Severe dislocations can result in injury to the vertebral artery and death.

Diagnosis

- Suspicion for facet dislocation should be raised in any patient with hyperflexion or extension injuries. Occipital lacerations often suggest flexion injuries, whereas frontal or superior injuries reflect extension and axial compression injuries, respectively.
- Clinical presentation usually includes pain and neurological symptoms (i.e., radiculopathies).

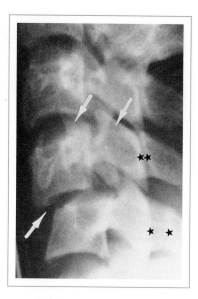

FIGURE 31.1: Unilateral facet dislocation. C4 is offset anteriorly on C5 less than 50% of the width of the vertebral body and apophyseal joints. The disc space between C4 and C5 is narrowed. Note that the distance between the posterior cortex of the apophyseal joint facet and the anterior cortex of the spinous process tip is wider below the level of dislocation than above the level (stars). Anterior vertebral offset of more than 50% would denote a bilateral facet dislocation. (Reprinted with permission from Swischuk L. *Emergency Radiology of the Acutely Ill or Injured Child*, 2nd ed. Baltimore: Williams & Wilkins, 1986:697.)

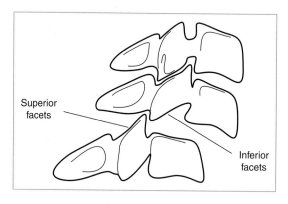

FIGURE 31.2: Lateral view of a bilateral facet dislocation. (Reprinted with permission from Mick N, Peters JR, Egan D, et al. *Blueprints Emergency Medicine*, 2nd ed. Philadelphia: Lippincott Williams & Wilkins, 2005.)

- Standard anterior/posterior (AP) and lateral radiographs commonly miss small unilateral facet dislocations because of the rotational nature of the injury. Trauma oblique radiographs may help visualize dislocations.
  - The "bowtie" sign on the lateral view is pathognomonic for unilateral facet dislocation: the two cranial facets are seen while the caudal facets overlap and are seen as a single facet (Fig. 31.3).

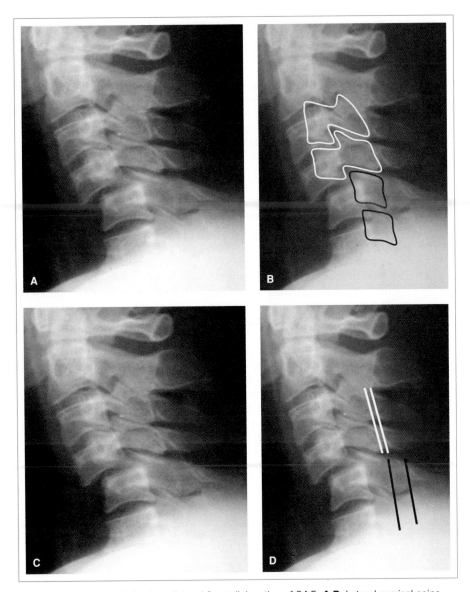

FIGURE 31.3: "Bowtie" sign in unilateral facet dislocation of C4-5. **A,B:** Lateral cervical spine radiographs show anterolisthesis of C4-5 with about 25% displacement. The articular pillars are offset from C4 above (white lines in **B**) and are seen in oblique profile giving the "bowtie" appearance; the "bowtie" sign indicates rotation. The articular pillars are superimposed at C5 and below and are seen in lateral profile (black lines in **B**). (Reprinted with permission from Schwartz ED, Flanders AE. *Spinal Trauma: Imaging, Diagnosis, and Management*. Philadelphia: Lippincott Williams & Wilkins, 2007.)

- Computed tomographic scans have the additional capability of reformatting images in sagittal and oblique planes to better display the facet alignments.
- Magnetic resonance imaging (MRI) can be useful to evaluate foraminal encroachment and to evaluate for disc herniation, which can occur in 15% of bilateral dislocations.

Evaluation

- Facilitate rapid C-spine imaging to identify injury.
- Initial evaluation should focus on identifying associated injuries and preventing further injury.
- Special consideration should be given to early intubation, especially when impaired ventilation is suspected because of C-spine or other injuries.
- Identify signs of neurogenic shock.
  - Hypotension and bradycardia due to loss of sympathetic innervation and unopposed vagal stimulation.

Management

- **Neurosurgical consultation is essential** when facet dislocation is identified and should be considered earlier with high clinical suspicion.
- Reduction and stabilization should be performed as soon as possible to minimize continued neurologic injury.
- The goal of management of patients with facet dislocation and vertebral subluxation is to minimize further spinal cord injury from secondary insults.
  - Immediate spinal immobilization to protect the spinal cord.
  - Early reduction and stabilization.
- Reduction and stabilization.
  - Unilateral facet dislocation.
    - <3.5-mm subluxation: Philadelphia collar for 6 weeks with close follow-up to ensure that progression of subluxation does not occur.
    - >3.5-mm subluxation: Closed reduction and halo stabilization (surgery usually reserved for cases in which closed reduction fails, or signs of middle column disruption).
  - Bilateral facet dislocation.
    - High rate of redislocation after closed reduction.
    - Operative stabilization and fixation is often required.

Special Considerations

- Delays in diagnosis of unilateral facet dislocations may occur in up to 40% of patients.
- Disc herniations may occur in 10–40% of patients with facet dislocations. These patients can deteriorate after closed reduction, resulting in neurologic deficit. MRI may be beneficial to help determine who may benefit from anterior discectomy and fusion.

Best Evidence/Clinical Decision Rules

Should an MRI be obtained prior to closed reduction of the cervical spine to evaluate for disc herniation and prevent postreduction neurologic deterioration?

In large studies of awake, cooperative patients, closed reduction without pretraction MRI has not shown to result in worsened neurologic function. If an MRI can be obtained quickly and safely, pretraction MRI is reasonable; however, this is difficult to obtain in many centers. MRI is required in uncooperative patients or operative candidates. If disc herniation is evident on MRI, anterior discectomy and fusion is performed.

Suggested Readings

Browner BD, et al. *Skeletal Trauma: Basic Science, Management, and Reconstruction*, 3rd ed. Philadelphia: Elsevier Science, 2003.

Laron JL. Injuries to the Spine. In: Tintinalli JE, Kelen GD, Stapczynski JS, eds. *Emergency Medicine: A Comprehensive Study Guide*, 6th ed. McGraw-Hill: New York, 2004:1702–1712.

Wheeless CR, Nunley JA, Urbaniak JR. *Wheeless' Textbook of Orthopaedics. Data Trace Internet Publishing*, 2007. http://www.wheelessonline.com.

32

Teardrop Fracture

Mary P. Eldridge

Definition

- Teardrop fractures are characterized by the distinct triangular fragment of the anteroinferior aspect of the vertebral body involved that is said to resemble a teardrop (Fig. 32.1).
- They are classified as either extension or flexion teardrop fractures (Table 32.1).

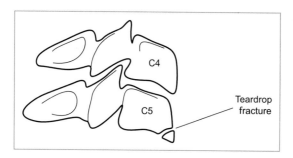

FIGURE 32.1: Lateral view of a teardrop fracture. (Reprinted with permission from Mick N, Peters JR, Egan D, et al. *Blueprints Emergency Medicine*, 2nd ed. Philadelphia: Lippincott Williams & Wilkins, 2005.)

Pathophysiology

- Extension teardrop fractures
  - The hyperextension mechanism causes the anterior longitudinal ligament to avulse the inferior portion of the anterior vertebral body at its insertion.
  - More common in:
    - Older patients with osteoporosis due to fusion deformities in the lower cervical spine.
    - Trauma caused by the forehead or face striking the dashboard or steering wheel in a motor vehicle collision.
    - Unbelted patients after the deployment of an air bag.
  - If unstable, it may be associated with a central cord syndrome caused by buckling of the ligamentum flavum into the spinal cord.

TABLE 32.1: Teardrop fracture classifications and characteristics

Extension teardrop fractures	Flexion teardrop fractures
Caused by hyperextension	High-energy hyperflexion injury
True avulsion fractures of anteroinferior vertebral body	Nonavulsion fracture of anteroinferior corner of vertebral body
Associated with discoligamentous disruption, most commonly C2/C3.	Leads to both bony and ligamentous disruption Often associated with spinal cord injury

- Flexion teardrop fractures
  - Occur when the neck is flexed, creating a straight spinal column, which is then forcibly loaded in compression.
  - They are common in:
    - Tackling injuries in football players.
    - Motor vehicle collisions.
    - Diving accidents in shallow water.
  - Associated anterior cord syndrome following a flexion teardrop fracture is due to impingement of the spinal cord by the fracture hyperkyphosis.

Diagnosis
- Extension teardrop fracture
  - Computed tomographic (CT) imaging is not necessary for the diagnosis but should still be obtained to delineate the extent of injury, differentiate between other similar appearing pathology, and evaluate for associated injuries.
  - Characteristically, the vertical height of the extension teardrop fragment equals or exceeds its horizontal width.
  - In younger patients with a lower cervical hyperextension teardrop fracture and significant soft-tissue swelling on plain films, computed tomography is required to better characterize the fracture and to evaluate for additional injuries.
  - A frequent source of confusion is osteophyte formation.
- Flexion teardrop fractures
  - CT imaging is particularly useful.
  - The anterior height of the vertebral body is reduced.
  - Diffuse prevertebral soft-tissue swelling is common.
  - Posterior displacement of the fractured vertebra and diastasis of the interfacetal joints indicate disruption of the longitudinal ligaments, intervertebral disc, and posterior ligament complex.
- Radiographically, flexion- and extension-type teardrop fractures are distinguishable.
  - In an extension teardrop fracture, the fragment is rotated 35 degrees anteriorly.
  - Conversely, a flexion teardrop fracture remains aligned with the anterior margin of the spine (Fig. 32.2).

Evaluation
- Follow typical ATLS guidelines and protect the airway of patients when indicated.
- Obtain a CT scan to identify injury as soon as the patient is stable.
- Extension teardrop fractures.
  - **Usually stable in flexion and unstable in extension.**
  - When unstable, they may cause a central cord syndrome.
- Flexion teardrop fractures.
  - **Unstable** and are associated with neurological injury 75% of the time if they involve the axis.
  - The classic neurological syndrome is anterior cord syndrome.

Management
- **Neurosurgical consultation is mandated** when a cervical spine fracture is identified.
- All patients should have strict cervical spine precautions in the emergency department.

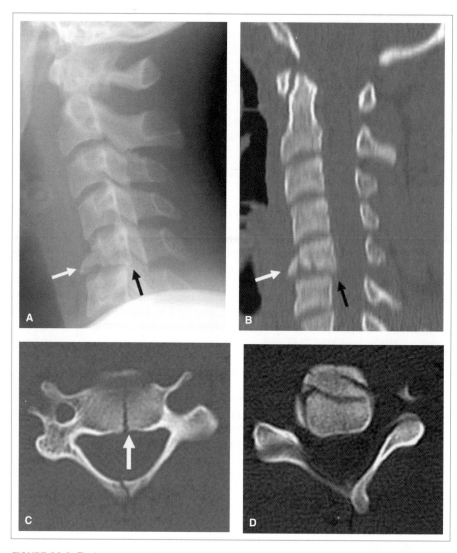

FIGURE 32.2: Flexion teardrop fracture of C5. Lateral radiograph of cervical spine **(A)** and sagittal multiplanar computed tomographic (CT) reformation **(B)** show compression of the body of C5 associated with a mild posterior subluxation of C5 upon C6 (black arrows in **A,B**). The fragment from the anterior inferior surface of C5 (white arrow) is the "teardrop." **C:** Axial CT image through the top of C5 demonstrates a sagittal fracture of the vertebral body (white arrow) and sagittal fracture of the spinous process. **D:** Axial CT image through the lower half of C5 shows a comminuted fracture of the anteroinferior end plate. (Reprinted with permission from Schwartz ED, Flanders AE. *Spinal Trauma: Imaging, Diagnosis, and Management.* Philadelphia: Lippincott Williams & Wilkins, 2007.)

- Extension teardrop injuries are managed with a hard collar.
  - Treatment involves cervical brace immobilization for 3 months, with lateral flexion-extension radiographs obtained to document stability.
- Flexion teardrop injuries treatment and prognosis are dependent on the degree of disruption of the posterior osteoligamentous structures.
  - The initial treatment of patients with this injury is skeletal tongs traction.
  - Unless the degree of instability is mild, surgery is usually indicated.

Special Considerations

- Stretching of the vessels during hyperextension or rotation may cause intimal disruption, with resultant dissection or thrombotic occlusion.
- Accompanying craniofacial and intracranial injury are frequently present, as are injuries to the trachea, esophagus, and other soft-tissue structures of the neck.
- Patients should be managed in a neurologic or surgical intensive care unit.

Best Evidence/Clinical Decision Rules

Is computed tomography angiography recommended in the setting of a teardrop fracture?

A study of hyperextension injuries of the cervical spine by Rao (2005) found that soft-tissue and vascular injures are not infrequent in the setting of teardrop fracture, and computed tomography angiography should be considered.

Suggested Readings

Bracken MB. Steroids for acute spinal cord injury. *Cochrane Database Syst Rev.* 2002;(3):CD001046.

Hecht AC, Silcox DH III, Whitesides TE Jr. Injuries of the cervicocranium. In: Browner BD, Jupiter JB, Levine, AM, Trafton PG, eds. *Skeletal Trauma: Basic Science, Management, and Reconstruction*, 3rd ed. Philadelphia: Saunders, 2003:777–814.

Hockgerger RS, Kaji AH, Newton EJ. Spinal injuries. In: Marx JA, Hockberger RS, Walls RM, eds. *Rosen's Emergency Medicine: Concepts and Clinical Practice,* 7th ed. Philadelphia: Mosby, 2010:337–377.

Larson JL Jr. Injuries to the spine. In: Tintinalli JE, Kelen GD, Stapczynski JS, eds. *Emergency Medicine: A Comprehensive Study Guide,* 6th ed. New York: McGraw-Hill, 2004.

Lindsey RW, Pneumaticos SG, Gugala Z. Management techniques for spinal injuries. In: Browner BD, Jupiter JB, Levine AM, Trafton PG, eds. *Skeletal Trauma: Basic Science, Management, and Reconstruction*, 3rd ed. Philadelphia: Saunders, 2003:746–777.

Mirvis SE. Spinal imaging. In: Browner BD, Jupiter JB, Levine AM, Trafton PG, eds. *Skeletal Trauma: Basic Science, Management, and Reconstruction*, 3rd ed. Philadelphia: Saunders, 2003:708–746.

Mirza SK, Anderson PA. Injuries of the lower cervical spine. In: Browner BD, Jupiter JB, Levine AM, Trafton PG , eds. *Skeletal Trauma: Basic Science, Management, and Reconstruction*, 3rd ed. Philadelphia: Saunders, 2003:814–875.

Rao SK, Wasyliw C, Nunez DB. Spectrum of imaging findings in hyperextension injuries of the neck radiographics. *Radiographics.* 2005;25:1239–1254.

33

Anterior Cord Syndrome

Daniel J. Singer

Definition

- Anterior spinal cord syndrome (ASCS) is a spinal cord injury characterized by paralysis and loss of temperature and pain sensation.
- ASCS is caused by disruption of the spinothalamic and cortical spinal tracts in the anterior spinal cord, often secondary to hyperflexion trauma injuries.
- The posterior column is unaffected, with preservation of proprioception, vibratory, and crude touch.

Pathophysiology

- ASCS is often caused by hyperflexion traumatic injuries. The acute spine trauma may cause contusion, disc herniation, or bony fragment displacement and secondary compression of the anterior compartment of the spinal cord.
- Vascular disruption, such as laceration or thrombosis of the anterior spinal artery, affects the spinothalamic and corticospinal tracts and may result in ASCS (Fig. 33.1).

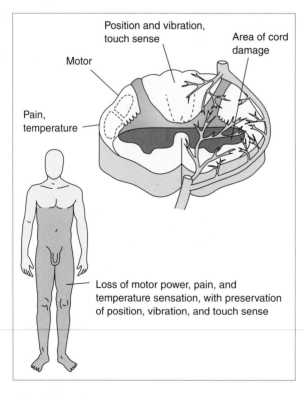

FIGURE 33.1: Anterior cord syndrome. Cord damage and associated motor and sensory loss are illustrated. (Reprinted with permission from Hickey JV. *The Clinical Practice of Neurological and Neurosurgical Nursing*, 3rd ed. Philadelphia: JB Lippincott, 1997.)

Diagnosis
- **Anterior spinal cord injury should be suspected on physical examination in any trauma patient who presents with paralysis and loss of pain and temperature sensation.**
- ASCS is a clinical diagnosis; however, computed tomography (CT) and/or magnetic resonance imaging (MRI) are necessary to evaluate underlying injuries.
  - CT will delineate bony injuries such as vertebral fractures and bone fragments.
  - MRI will delineate soft-tissue injuries such as contusions, herniated disks, and impingement of the spinal cord.

Evaluation
- Evaluation should focus on stabilizing the patient's airway, breathing, and circulation and identifying associated injuries.
- Complete neurological examination to identify the level and extent of injury.
- Immediate evaluation with CT or MRI when patient is stable to evaluate injuries amendable to surgery.

Management
- **Neurosurgical consultation is mandated** when ASCS is identified. Consider early involvement of neurosurgery or trauma surgery teams when index of suspicion is high.
- Perform immediate and aggressive resuscitation to stabilize and optimize patient hemodynamically.
- When stable, patients should be taken for spine imaging and subsequently to the operating room if a lesion amendable to surgery is discovered.
- Consider treating with methylprednisolone to minimize inflammation and secondary spinal cord injury (very controversial).

Special Considerations
- Patients with ASCS have a poor prognosis for recovery of neurological function. As reported by Kirschblum (1998), only 10–20% will have recovery of motor function, with a small percentage of those regaining purposeful, coordinated movement.

Suggested Readings
Bracken MB, Shepard MJ, Collins WF, et al. A randomized, controlled trial of methyl-prednisolone or naloxone in the treatment of acute spinal cord injury: results of the second national acute spinal cord study. *New Engl J Med*. 1990;322:1405.

Kirschblum SC, O'Connor KC. Predicting neurologic recovery in traumatic cervical spinal cord injury. *Arch Phys Med Rehabil*. 1998;79:1456.

34 Central Cord Syndrome

Christopher Tainter

Definition

- Acute central spinal cord injury preferentially affecting motor strength in the **upper extremities more than the lower.**
- Commonly associated with bladder dysfunction (usually retention).
- Various degrees of sensory loss below the affected level.

Pathophysiology

- Preferentially affects centrally located fibers of the corticospinal and spinothalamic tracts.
- Upper extremity tracts are most medial, lower extremity tracts are more lateral.
- Usually caused by hyperextension injuries, especially with underlying spondylosis.
- Atraumatic causes include syringomyelia or intramedullary tumor (Fig. 34.1).

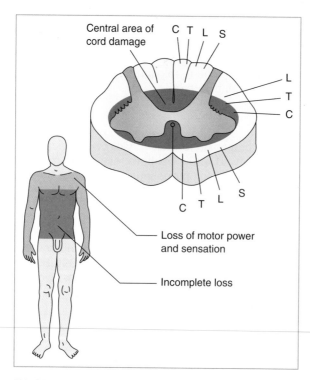

FIGURE 34.1: Central cord syndrome. A cross-section of the cord shows central damage and the associated motor and sensory loss (C, cervical; T, thoracic; L, lumbar; S, sacral). (Reprinted with permission from Hickey JV. *The Clinical Practice of Neurological and Neurosurgical Nursing,* 3rd ed. Philadelphia: JB Lippincott, 1997.)

Diagnosis

- Classically occurs with hyperextension injuries with underlying cervical spondylosis.
- Suspect in patients with disproportionate neurological findings affecting upper limbs more than lower.
- Sensory deficits may or may not be present.
- Bowel and bladder function may be preserved.
- Neck and/or back pain are common complaints.
- Suspected injury can be confirmed with magnetic resonance imaging (MRI) (Fig. 34.2).

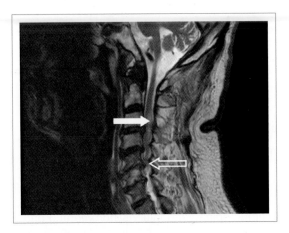

FIGURE 34.2: T2-weighted magnetic resonance imaging of cervical spine showing enhancement in the center of the cord (solid arrow) and preexisting spondylosis (outlined arrow). (Courtesy of Mount Sinai Medical Center, New York, NY.)

Evaluation

- Careful initial neurological examination for baseline comparison.
  - Neck or back pain/tenderness
  - Motor function (graded 0–5)
  - Sensory level must be determined
  - Vibratory/proprioception indicates posterior column function
  - Deep tendon reflexes
  - Bulbocavernosus reflex to evaluate for spinal shock
- Computed tomographic or radiographic imaging may show spinal canal compromise but may not be sensitive to transient stenosis capable of causing cord damage.
- Imaging often demonstrates spondylosis, which may be preexisting.
- MRI confirms central cord injury.

Management

- Spinal immobilization for anyone with suspected spinal cord injury.
- Intubate (with in-line stabilization) any patient with injury above C5, which may compromise diaphragmatic innervations.
  - If possible, perform neurologic examination prior to intubation.
- Support hemodynamics to maintain perfusion of spinal cord.

- Monitor for signs of neurogenic shock characterized by both hypotension and bradycardia.
- Evaluate for blood loss: hemoperitoneum, hemothorax, pelvic injury, thigh hematoma, and so forth.
- Triage/transfer to trauma center or designated spine center.
- Emergent MRI and spine surgery (orthopedic or neurosurgery) consult.
- Consider initiation of steroids within 8 hours for *nonpenetrating* spinal trauma (very controversial).

Special Considerations

- Central cord syndrome is the most common spinal cord injury syndrome, accounting for approximately 9% of traumatic spinal cord injuries.
- Generally favorable prognosis.
- Factors associated with worse prognosis: increasing age, presence of spasticity, and lower functional ability at the time of admission.
- Progressive neurological deterioration is usually an indication for immediate surgery.

Best Evidence/Clinical Decision Rules

What is the prognosis of patients with central cord syndrome?

A review published by McKinley et al. in the *Journal of Spinal Cord Medicine* in 2007 looked at outcomes from 839 consecutive admissions to the spinal cord injury unit at a major tertiary care center with an inpatient rehabilitation unit. They found that central cord syndrome was the most common spinal cord injury syndrome and had the worst functional status at admission, presumably due to the upper extremity (hand) weakness. At discharge, these patients showed marked improvement in motor and self-care assessment scores.

Suggested Readings

Baron B, Scalea T. Spinal cord injuries. In: Tintinalli J, Kelen G, Stapczynski J, eds. *Emergency Medicine: A comprehensive Study Guide*. New York: The McGraw-Hill Companies, Inc. The American College of Emergency Physicians, 2004:1569–1583.

Bracken MB, Shepard MJ, Collins WF, et al. A randomized, controlled trial of methylprednisolone or naloxone in the treatment of acute spinal cord injury: results of the second national acute spinal cord injury study. *New Engl J Med.* 1990;322:1405–1411.

McKinley W, Santos K, Meade M, Brooke K. Incidence and outcomes of spinal cord injury clinical syndromes. *J Spinal Cord Med.* 2007;30(3):215–224.

Merriam WF, Taylor TK, Ruff SJ, McPhail MJ. A reappraisal of acute traumatic central cord syndrome. *J Bone Joint Surg Br.* 1986;68(5):708–713.

Newey ML, Sen PK, Fraser RD. The long-term outcome after central cord syndrome: a study of the natural history. *J Bone Joint Surg Br.* 2000;82(6):851–855.

Schneider RC, Cherry G, Pantek H. The syndrome of acute central cervical spinal cord injury: with special reference to the mechanisms involved in hyperextension injuries of the cervical spine. *J Neurosurg.* 1954;11:546–577.

35 Brown-Séquard Syndrome

Jennifer Galjour

Definition

- Brown-Séquard Syndrome is hemisection of the spinal cord, resulting in a constellation of symptoms characterized by the following neurologic abnormalities distal to the level of injury: (Fig. 35.1).
  - Ipsilateral motor paralysis and loss of proprioception and vibratory sense.
  - Contralateral pain and temperature sensory loss.

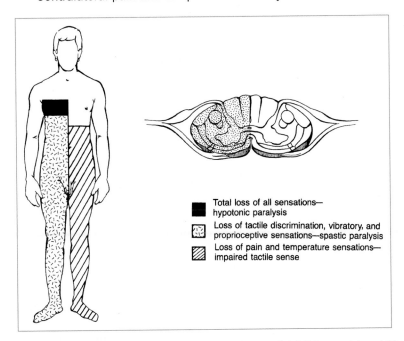

FIGURE 35.1: Involved tracts and the superimposed areas of deficit from an injury at T4, resulting in the Brown-Séquard syndrome. (Reprinted with permission from Wolfson AB, Hendey GW, Ling LJ, et al. *Harwood-Nuss' Clinical Practice of Emergency Medicine*, 5th ed. Philadelphia: Lippincott Williams & Wilkins, 2009.)

- Either sensory or motor symptoms may predominate, but nearly all patients retain continence.

Pathophysiology

- Understanding Brown-Séquard syndrome requires knowledge of spinal cord anatomy and the location and pathway of each spinal tract.
- The symptoms of Brown-Séquard syndrome may be the result of either functional (e.g., infarct, demyelination) or anatomic insults, with the latter being far more common. These can include penetrating trauma such as a stab wounds or gunshots, or vertebral fractures.

Diagnosis

- When suspecting Brown-Séquard syndrome, a good neurologic examination can help establish a diagnosis. Although some deficits are ipsilateral and others contralateral due to crossing of tracts within the spinal cord, all deficits are distal to the cord lesion.
- **Ipsilateral deficits.**
  - Use a tuning fork to evaluate vibratory sensation. Remember to place the tuning fork over a bony prominence so that vibration is adequately transmitted.
  - A simple test to evaluate proprioception, or perceived position sense, is to ask the patient which direction you are moving his or her fingers or toes (up or down) with his or her eyes closed.
  - To evaluate motor loss in patients, compare the patient's ability to move bilateral extremities, noting any unilateral weakness.
- **Contralateral deficits.**
  - There are a number of ways to evaluate pain sensation. Judging a patient's reaction to application of pressure to the nail bed is generally sufficient.
  - A metal tuning fork can be used to assess for temperature (cold) sensation.
- Bowel and bladder continence is usually unaffected in Brown-Séquard syndrome.
- When evaluating for neurologic deficits, remember to **always test both sides**. Comparison is key when determining relative unilateral deficits.

Evaluation

- Because Brown-Séquard syndrome can be caused by a number of different processes, the need to image and imaging modality will vary by suspected etiology.
  - Vertebral body fractures and penetrating trauma can be approached with a number of modalities. However, computed tomographic scan is generally most readily available to emergency departments, with magnetic resonance imaging as a later option to attain more detailed information.
- Arguably the most practical and effective tool in evaluating a patient with suspected Brown-Séquard syndrome is a thorough neurologic examination.

Management

- Although there are many causes of Brown-Séquard syndrome, management of traumatic spinal cord injury will be discussed here.
- Patients with spinal cord trauma often arrive at the emergency department immobilized. Any airway, breathing, and circulation resuscitation measures should be executed carefully, maintaining immobilization as much as possible until spinal injury can be carefully assessed.
- Neurogenic hypotension, a common sequela of spinal cord injury, is typically mild and responsive to fluid resuscitation, except in high cervical injuries. Neurogenic hypotension in the setting of a high cervical lesion may require more aggressive blood pressure management with pressors.
- Although high-dose steroids have classically been associated with improved outcomes, literature is variable and the issue remains controversial.

Special Considerations

- Very rarely do spinal injuries, infarcts, or other spinal cord insults result in a perfect, complete hemisection of the spinal cord. Therefore, patients with Brown-Séquard syndrome may have variations in their symptoms and deficits.

Best Evidence/Clinical Decision Rules

Besides fluid resuscitation, what other medications should be administered in the early management of penetrating spinal cord trauma due to stab wounds or gunshots?

Empiric broad-spectrum antibiotics should be added to the arsenal of early pharmacologic treatment to avoid complications such as meningitis or spinal cord abscess. An article in the journal *Orthopedic Clinics of North America* (1996) cites antibiotics and tetanus toxoid as mainstays of treatment in penetrating injuries to the thoracic and lumbar spine.

Suggested Readings

Hammerstad JP. Strength and reflexes. In: Goetz CG, ed. *Textbook of Clinical Neurology*, 3rd ed. Philadelphia: Saunders, 2007:243–289.

Heary RF, Vaccaro AR, Mesa JJ, et al. Thoracolumbar infections in penetrating injuries to the spine. *Orthop Clin North Am*. 1996;27(1):69–81.

Hockberger RS, Kaji AH, Newten EJ. Spinal injuries. In: Marx JA, Hockberger RS, Walls RM, eds. *Rosen's Emergency Medicine: Concepts and Clinical Practice*, 7th ed. Philadelphia: Mosby, 2010:337–377.

36

Thoracic Spine Fracture

Matthew Constantine

Definition

- Traumatic thoracic fractures may be defined as traumatic disruption of bony and/or ligamentous structures of the thoracic vertebral column including the T12-L1 junction.
- Generally classified by fracture or mechanism pattern (see below) with further discernment of level of stability.
- Classification is partially based on specific mechanism of injury (Table 36.1).

Pathophysiology

- Often occur as a result of high-energy mechanisms as the articulation with the rib cage provides additional stability. Examples include high-speed motor vehicle collisions, falls from height, pedestrians struck by automobiles, and direct blows (either blunt or penetrating).
- At extremes of age or with underlying pathology (such as spinal metastatic disease, osteoporosis), mechanism of injury can be more insidious.
- Thoracic column is divided into three subcolumns:
  - Anterior—anterior half of vertebral body.
  - Middle—posterior half of vertebral body including the posterior longitudinal ligament.
  - Posterior—supra- and interspinous ligaments, facets, and spinous processes.

TABLE 36.1: Classification of thoracic fractures

Wedge fracture	Flexion injury causes compression of anterior column. No middle or posterior involvement. May be stable or unstable. >50% reduction in vertebral height considered severe.
Burst fracture	Compression by flexion or axial load. Fracture of entire bony endplate. Both anterior and middle columns involved. Unstable.
Flexion-distraction fracture	Anterior flexion with distraction. Causes disruption of posterior elements. May involve compression of anterior column depending on axis point of flexion. Very unstable.
Translational injuries	Large shearing forces leading to fracture dislocation, translocation, and/or rotational injuries. Highly associated with neurologic injury.
Minor fracture	Includes fractures to spinous process, transverse process, facets, and pars interarticularis. Stable.

Diagnosis

- Clinical suspicion for these fractures will depend upon understanding the mechanism of injury and the forces involved. If the patient is awake and alert then a neurologic examination may reveal severe deficits indicating spinal cord injury secondary to fractures.
- Diagnosis is made by imaging with plain film, computed tomography (CT) or magnetic resonance imaging.
  - Plain film may be able to rule out fracture if suspicion is low and there are no other clinical indicators of pathology.
  - Fractures found on x-ray film (Fig 36.1) will likely require further delineation by CT.

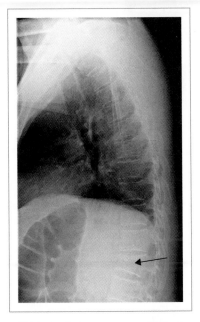

FIGURE 36.1: Plain film radiograph demonstrating a wedge fracture of the thoracic spine (arrow). (Courtesy of Mount Sinai Medical Center, New York, NY.)

- Patients for whom suspicion is higher secondary to mechanism will likely undergo computed tomographic scan to evaluate for other pathology. Coronal and sagittal reconstructions using bone window settings can very accurately diagnose spinal injury (see Fig. 36.2).
- Overall CT has been found to be more sensitive than x-ray for fractures.

Evaluation

- Careful examination of the entire spine should include direct visualization and palpation of spine. Findings may include step-offs from translocation or dislocation, paraspinal swelling, and point tenderness.
- Neurological evaluation is critical as well, including motor, sensory, and reflex examinations.
- The magnitude of force required to damage the thoracic spine will often cause other visceral injuries, which should not be overlooked.

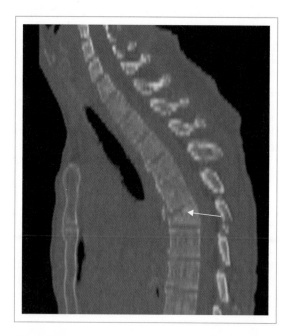

FIGURE 36.2: Computed tomographic scan demonstrating similar wedge fracture of the thoracic spine (arrow) and preservation of the spinal cord canal posteriorly. (Courtesy of Mount Sinai Medical Center, New York, NY.)

- Although neurologic/spinal shock may present with neurogenic hypotension and concomitant bradycardia, this diagnosis should not be made until hemorrhagic shock has been ruled out.

Management
- Consultation with spine specialist for any fracture. Determination of stability and disposition is better made with specialist involvement.
- Spinal immobilization throughout evaluation and management is standard practice; however, as discussed in a Cochrane review from 2001, it is based more in historical precedent and consensus than scientific evidence. Hard spine boards are not necessary for adequate spinal immobilization and may rapidly lead to pressure ulcers. Logrolling precautions and cervical collar are adequate.
- Agitated or obtunded patients may require further physical or chemical restraints for immobility.
- If the spinal cord is injured through a blunt trauma mechanism, corticosteroids are frequently used (although still very controversial).

Special Considerations
- Patients with thoracic spine injuries may require transfer to a trauma center if spine specialist consultation is not available.

Best Evidence/Clinical Decision Rules

Is there a widely used clinical decision rule to select patients who require imaging of the thoracic spine based on mechanism of injury and physical examination?

A study by Diaz (2007) sought to develop an evidence-based practice guideline to address the following questions:

1. Does a patient who is awake, nonintoxicated, and without distracting injuries require radiographic workup or a clinical examination only?
2. Does a patient with a distracting injury, altered mental status, or pain require radiographic examination?
3. Does the obtunded patient require radiographic examination?

After selecting 27 studies of traumatic spinal injury for analysis, the authors found insufficient evidence to establish clear guidelines for these clinical questions. No prospective, randomized controlled trials support a particular selection criteria or method of evaluation for thoracic injuries. Twenty-five percent of patients meeting criteria for CT evaluation after blunt trauma will have a thoracolumbar spine (TLS) injury, but the scans are often ordered to evaluate for other pathology. The study also found a sensitivity and specificity of 60% and 70% for plain x-rays, suggesting that computed tomographic scan is a better modality for the evaluation of TLS injury.

Suggested Readings

Diaz JJ, Cullinane DC, Altman DT, et al. Practice management guidelines for the screening of thoracolumbar spine fracture. *J Trauma*. 2007;63(3):709–718.

Hockgerger RS, Kaji AH, Newton EJ. Spinal injuries. In: Marx JA, Hockberger RS, Walls RM, eds. *Rosen's Emergency Medicine: Concepts and Clinical Practice*, 7th ed. Philadelphia: Mosby, 2010:337–377.

Inaba K, Munera F, McKenney M, et al. Visceral torso computed tomography for clearance of the thoracolumbar spine in trauma: a review of the literature. *J Trauma*. 2006;60(4):915–920.

Kwan I, Bunn F, Roberts I, on behalf of the WHO Pre-Hospital Trauma Care Steering Committee. Spinal immobilisation for trauma patients. *Cochrane Database Syst Rev*. 2001;(2):CD002803.

Larson JL Jr. Injuries to the spine. In: Tintinalli JE, Kelen GD, Stapczynski JS, Ma OJ, Cline DM, eds. *Emergency Medicine: A Comprehensive Study Guide*, 6th ed. New York: McGraw Hill, 2004:1702–1712.

37

Lumbar Spine Fracture

Nicholas Genes

Definition

- Lumbar fractures can arise from blunt or penetrating trauma when the forces applied to the lower spine exceed its strength and stability.
- Lumbar fractures are usually associated with high-energy mechanisms such as falls from height, motor vehicle crashes, and gunshot wounds. They can also be seen with relatively minor trauma and abnormal bony architecture (e.g., malignancy, osteoporosis, or Pott disease).
- There are five major lumbar fracture types, listed in order of progressive clinical concern (the latter two fractures are inherently unstable and are frequently associated with neurologic deficits):
  - Wedge (flexion) compression fracture.
  - Burst (axial compression) fracture.
  - Chance (distractive) fracture.
  - Flexion-distraction fracture.
  - Translation fracture

Pathophysiology

- The type of fracture depends on the applied forces of compression, distraction, and translation.
- Fractures of the lumbar spine can cause debilitating pain, limitations to movement, radiculopathies, and spinal cord deficits.
- The lumbar spinal cord has a richer blood supply than the thoracic cord (due largely to the artery of Adamkiewicz) and more generous spinal canal, so it is less susceptible to ischemia or direct trauma.
- The lumbar spine, however, is more mobile than the thoracic spine or pelvis and for this reason it is more susceptible to injury—despite its wider, larger vertebral bodies.

Diagnosis

- Lumbar spine fracture should be suspected in any trauma patient with sufficient mechanism complaining of back pain or focal neurologic deficit.
- A distracting injury or altered mental status can render clinical assessment of spine tenderness unreliable.
- **In the setting of trauma, a flaccid paralysis of the lower extremities, with loss of deep tendon reflexes and bulbocavernosus reflex, signifies the acute phase of a complete cord syndrome.** Incomplete lesions have some degree of motor or sensory function below the level of injury. Ileus may accompany and further suggests spinal cord injury.
- Lumbar fractures can also lead to caudal equinal syndromes (bladder and bowel control irregularities, lower limb nerve deficits) and anterior cord syndromes from direct compression or disruption of the spinal cord's blood supply.

■ Although history may predict fracture type, lumbar spine fractures are diagnosed radiographically via computed tomography or plain films (Fig. 37.1). Magnetic resonance imaging may be necessary to delineate associated ligamentous and soft-tissue injuries, as well as assess cord compression.

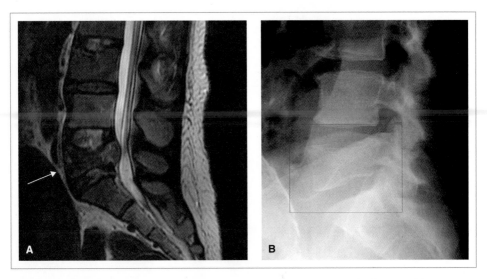

FIGURE 37.1: A: Magnetic resonance image demonstrating an L5 compression fracture with retropulsion. **B:** Plain film shows a different L5 compression fracture. (Courtesy of Mount Sinai Medical Center, New York, NY.)

Evaluation

■ Facilitate rapid imaging via computed tomography.
■ Lumbar fractures are evaluated through the perspective of "stability." The definition is somewhat controversial. A "stable" spinal fracture is one that, under physiologic stress, will not progress to cord damage or cause incapacitating pain.
■ Stability can be evaluated radiographically, using a traditional three-column model.
  ● The *anterior column* encompasses the anterior longitudinal ligament to the middle of the vertebral body.
  ● The *middle column* runs from the midvertebral body to the posterior longitudinal ligament.
  ● The *posterior column* consists of the neural arch, facet joint capsules, spinous process, and supraspinous and intraspinous ligaments.
■ **A fracture is generally considered unstable if there is involvement of the middle column plus one other column.**
■ The so-called **"Lap Belt" sign** is highly associated with intestinal and mesenteric injuries and also with Chance fractures. In patients using lap-only restraints, clinicians should be vigilant for these injuries (Fig. 37.2).

Management

■ Patients should have their pain controlled and spinal movements minimized.
■ All potentially unstable lumbar fractures and dislocations require consultation with a spine specialist. These patients may require braces, body casts, or surgical fixation.

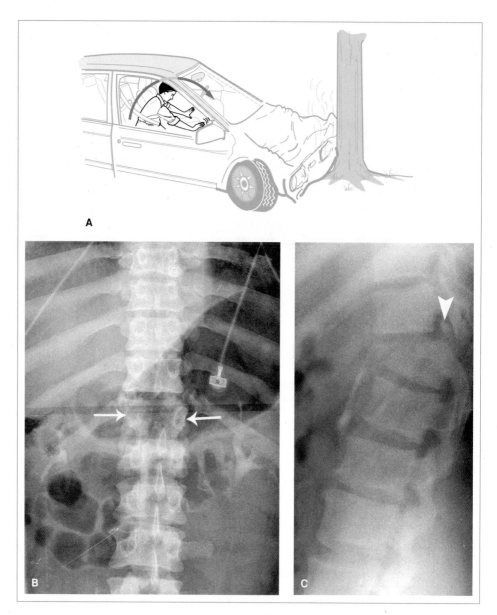

FIGURE 37.2: Flexion distraction mechanism of injury. **A:** This mechanism involves the classic "lap belt" injury. The flexion force is centered anterior to the spine, resulting in distraction extending through the posterior elements to the anterior column. The distractive nature of injury often leaves patients neurologically intact, although there may be significant abdominal organ injury. This leads to the classic Chance fracture (purely osseous) and Chance variants (soft tissue or combined osseous/soft tissue). AP **(B)** radiograph demonstrates widening of the interpediculate (arrows) and interspinous distance of T12, findings consistent with a flexion-distraction fracture. Acute hyperflexion deformity is appreciated on the lateral radiograph **(C)** with decrease in vertebral body height anteriorly, characteristic of the flexion vector. (Reprinted with permission from Schwartz ED, Flanders AE. *Spinal Trauma: Imaging, Diagnosis, and Management*. Philadelphia: Lippincott Williams & Wilkins, 2007.)

- Any lumbar fracture with neurologic deficit mandates admission or transfer to a referral center.
- One lumbar fracture that can be safely discharged is an isolated anterior wedge compression fracture with less than 50% loss of height and no neurologic deficits. These patients may require a brace or pain control and will need follow-up with a spine specialist.
- Isolated transverse pedicle fractures, without neurological deficit, instability, or associated injuries, can be managed symptomatically with outpatient follow-up.

Special Considerations
- Chance fracture (Fig. 37.3).

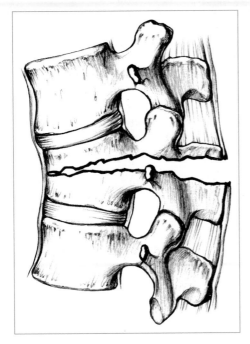

FIGURE 37.3: Chance fracture. (Reprinted with permission from Hansen ST, Swiontkowski MF. *Orthopaedic Trauma Protocols*. New York: Raven, 1993:221.)

- Fracture of the spine caused by extreme flexion (often the body around a lap belt during sudden deceleration) that disrupts the posterior elements.
- Rarely causes neurologic deficit unless vertebral bodies are displaced.
- Associated with hollow viscus injuries.
- Pediatric patients, because of their immature skeleton and elastic ligaments, are far more susceptible to spinal cord injury without radiographic abnormality (SCIWORA). Any report of neurologic deficit or suspicion for significant injury mandates consultation and computed tomography or magnetic resonance imaging. It is also important to be mindful of abuse and neglect in this population.

Best Evidence/Clinical Decision Rules

Do I need plain films of the TLS spine in my patients with significant blunt trauma who are going to get a chest-abdomen-and-pelvis CT?

A recent review (Berry, 2005) of 103 patients presenting with high-risk blunt abdominal trauma who underwent routine CT of chest, abdomen, and pelvis at a level 1 trauma center showed that CT was more sensitive than plain films of the thoracic and lumbar spine in identifying fractures (100% vs. 73%) and took less time to perform. The authors recommend omitting plain films to expedite patient evaluation.

Should I maintain complete spinal immobilization in patients with suspected thoracolumbar trauma?

A Cochrane review (Kwan, 2001) noted no randomized controlled trials on spinal immobilization strategies in trauma patients. It should be noted, however, that the emergency medical services (EMS) longboard is intended for extrication and transport, does not conform to the physiologic shape of the spine, and can cause pressure sores and distracting pain after limited use.

Suggested Readings

Berry GE, Adams S, Harris MB, et al. Are plain radiographs of the spine necessary during evaluation after blunt trauma? Accuracy of screening torso computed tomography in thoracic/lumbar spine fracture diagnosis. *J Trauma.* 2005;59: 1410–1413.

Kwan I, Bunn F, Roberts I. Spinal immobilisation for trauma patients (review). *Cochrane Database Syst Rev.* 2001;(2).

Patel RV, DeLong W, Vresilovic EJ. Evaluation and Treatment of Spinal Injuries in the Patient with Polytrauma. *Clinical Orthop Relat Res.* 2004;422:43–54.

Savitsky E, Votey S. Emergency department approach to acute thoracolumbar spine injury. *J Emerg Med.* 1997;15:49–60.

Section Editor: Jonathan Wassermann

38
Neck Trauma: The First 15 Minutes, Algorithm, and Decision Making

Jonathan Wassermann

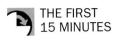 THE FIRST
15 MINUTES

ABCs
- Check vital signs and determine stability
- Follow ATLS guidelines and Neck Trauma Algorithm

History
- Most penetrating trauma to neck that presents to the emergency department is secondary to stab, slash, or gunshot wounds.
- Most blunt trauma to the neck is due to motor vehicle accidents or falls. Strangulation or compression injuries of the neck are different than blunt trauma due to motor vehicle accidents and should be treated as such.

Physical Examination
- Inspection
  - Critical signs of penetrating trauma are listed in Table 38.1. Zones of injury are listed in Table 38.2.
  - Zone II penetration of the platysma is an indication for operative exploration.

TABLE 38.1: Critical signs of penetrating trauma

Hard signs	Soft signs
Expanding hematoma	Hemoptysis/hematemesis
Severe active bleeding	Oropharyngeal blood
Shock not responding to fluids	Dyspnea
Decreased/absent radial pulse	Dysphonia/dysphagia
Vascular bruit/thrill	Subcutaneous/mediastinal air
Cerebral ischemia	Chest tube air leak
Airway obstruction	Nonexpanding hematoma Focal neurologic deficit

TABLE 38.2: Penetrating neck trauma: Zones of injury

Zone	Location	Considerations
I	Defined inferiorly by clavicles and superiorly by the cricoid cartilage	May affect both thoracic and neck structures
II	Extends from the cricoid cartilage inferiorly to the angle of mandible superiorly	Injuries in Zone II are more common and easily accessible surgically
III	Includes the area superior to the angle of the mandible to the base of the skull	Should be considered head injuries in addition to neck injuries

- Very important to frequently reassess the neck for all types of injuries, ideally 10–15 minutes after first inspection and/or immediately before patients leave the resuscitation room for ancillary testing.
- Bubbling or air emanating from wound is very concerning for a tracheal injury.
- Auscultation
  - Bruits or thrills may be heard with vascular injuries.
- Palpation
  - Tenderness: Its location may identify an injury and midline cervical tenderness may indicate a cervical spine injury.
  - Crepitus indicates that air has moved into the soft tissue space and presupposes that an injury has occurred to the trachea, esophagus, or pulmonary tree.
  - Mobility or tenderness of the laryngeal cartilage may indicate a laryngeal fracture, with possible airway compromise and difficulty with endotracheal intubation.

Emergency Interventions
- Loss of the airway is the most significant complication of neck trauma, and early intervention to secure the airway should be considered as determined by the clinical scenario.
- Bleeding should be managed by direct compression. While inspection is important to discern whether the wound penetrated the plastysma muscle, avoid the inclination to probe neck wounds blindly as this may dislodge clots.
- If central venous access is necessary, place cordis through the subclavian vein (avoid predominate side of injury) or femoral vein.
- Unstable patients should be transferred to the operating room for definitive care depending on the type and location of injury as well as associated injuries.

Memorable Pearls
- Early airway intervention and control should always be considered when warranted.
- Always consider the possibility of blunt cervical-spine injuries. Remove the C-collar to examine the neck and then replace while maintaining in-line stabilization. All these patients should be considered to have a cervical spine injury until cleared.
- With improvements in multidetector computed tomography (CT) angiography, "mandatory" neck exploration for platysma violation and "mandatory" arteriography for Zone I and III injuries are falling out of favor. Hemodynamic instability and hard signs should prompt immediate neck exploration but other patients may benefit from CT-angiography initially.

- Especially in blunt trauma, neck injuries are uncommonly isolated injuries—always identify any associated injuries.
- Other injuries are more likely to cause severe hemorrhage. After airway is secure if there is a suspicion of intra-abdominal or other major injury and the patient is unstable, patient may need laparotomy prior to further diagnostic workup of neck injuries.

Diagnostic Evaluations

- In the age of CT-angiography, stable patients rarely go directly to the OR for exploration.
- Plain films
  - Should be considered in the trauma room if suspected cervical spine injury or warranted on the basis of location of projectile.
  - In-line stabilization should always be maintained when there is concern for a cervical spine injury.
  - In Zone 1 neck injuries always obtain a chest x-ray to evaluate for pneumothorax or hemothorax.
- Computed tomographic scans
  - May be warranted in stable patients with evidence of trauma to further elucidate injuries.
- Ancillary testing and imaging should be done as warranted by the individual circumstance in consultation with the trauma service.

Essential Considerations

Consultations

- Trauma surgery
  - Penetrating neck injuries warrant notification of trauma team or surgeon if available.
- Vascular surgery
- ENT (otolaryngology)
- Anesthesia
  - Be prepared for a potentially difficult airway and consider the use of nasotracheal or awake intubation.
- Neurosurgery or spine service for cervical injuries

DECISION
MAKING

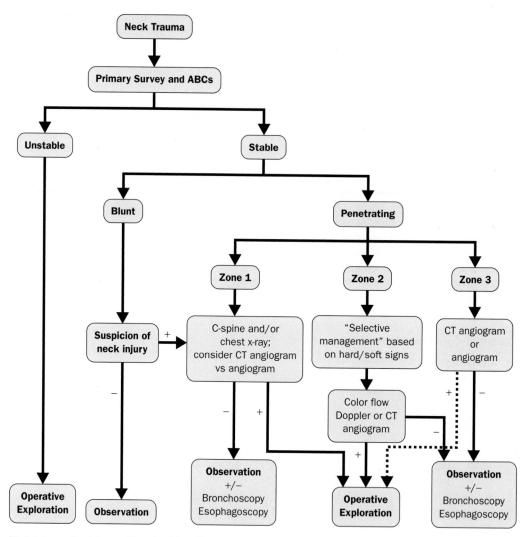

Neck trauma: Decision making algorithm. CT, computed tomography.

39

Penetrating Neck Trauma

Brian Wright

Definition

- Penetrating neck injuries occur when an object or missile projectile violates the platysma layer of the neck and causes injury.
- These injuries are usually caused by missile projectiles such as bullets or sharp objects.

Pathophysiology and Epidemiology

- Penetrating neck injuries account for 5–10% of major trauma.
- There are multiple critical organ systems in close proximity to one another in the neck (Fig. 39.1). Clinicians need to be particularly concerned about injuries to the larynx and trachea, lungs, vascular structures, nervous system, and esophagus.

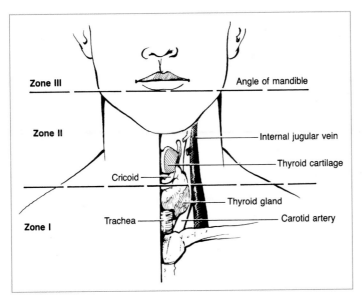

FIGURE 39.1: Anterior view of the neck. Significant structures and the zones of the neck are illustrated. (Reprinted with permission from Harwood-Nuss A, Wolfson AB, et al. *The Clinical Practice of Emergency Medicine*, 3rd ed. Philadelphia: Lippincott Williams & Wilkins, 2001.)

- Even innocuous-appearing neck injuries have the potential to cause either immediate or delayed life-threatening injuries and complications.
- It is important for the clinician to ascertain information about the mechanism of injury. Approximately 50% of gunshot wounds are associated with significant injuries with mortality of 10–15% depending on the firearm. Only 20–30% of stab wounds cause serious injury with an overall mortality of 5%.

- Bleeding from vascular injuries is the leading cause of immediate death and may be apparent on physical examination. Esophageal injuries are the leading cause of delayed mortality and are often not immediately apparent.

Anatomy

- The platysma extends from the upper chest to the mandible. Injuries that do not penetrate the platysma can be considered superficial.
- It is preferable to use the zone system to describe traumatic injuries because the zone system is helpful in guiding management decisions.

Diagnosis

- The physical examination in a patient with penetrating neck trauma can range from a benign examination to subtle injuries to the dramatic presentation of obvious life-threatening injury.
- Patients with penetrating neck trauma will often have multiple injuries. Performing an adequate primary survey while managing airway, breathing, and circulation is of utmost importance.
- Cervical spine immobilization needs to be provided only when there is a blunt mechanism, suspected spinal cord injury has occurred (i.e., projectile trajectory crossing the midline or neurological deficits), or an adequate physical examination cannot be performed because of altered mental status. Spine immobilization can obscure important physical examination findings, so do not use inappropriately.
- It is important to look for "hard" and "soft" signs of injury. The presence of these symptoms will have important management ramifications (Table 39.1).
- Signs and symptoms of an airway or esophageal injury: labored respirations, hemoptysis, hematemesis, blood in oropharynx, dyspnea, dysphonia, dysphagia, subcutaneous air or crepitus, bubbling from wound, and stridor.
- Signs and symptoms of a central nervous system or vascular injury: focal neurological deficits, limb ischemia, hematoma, bleeding, shock, decreased or absent pulse, vascular bruit, or thrill.
- Serial examinations can help determine deterioration in clinical status as well as ongoing hemorrhage.
- There should be a low threshold for obtaining additional imaging studies and/or surgical consultation because of the relatively high associated morbidity and mortality from missed injuries.
- Physical examination is not reliable in ruling out aerodigestive injuries.

TABLE 39.1: The hard signs of penetrating neck trauma

Airway compromise	Circulatory compromise	Active bleeding
Tracheal deviation/stridor	Refractory shock	Expanding hematoma
Need for intubation	Evidence of cerebral stroke	Pulsative hematoma
Subcutaneous emphysema	Vascular bruit	Large hemothorax
Air bubbling in wound	Upper extremity ischemia	

(Reprinted with permission from Bisanzo M, Filbin MR, Bhatia K. *Emergency Management of the Trauma Patient: Cases, Algorithms, Evidence.* Philadelphia: Lippincott Williams & Wilkins, 2007.)

Evaluation and Management (Fig. 39.2)

Airway and Breathing

- The first priority is ensuring the patency of the patient's airway and hemodynamic stability.
- Advanced trauma life support (ATLS) protocols should be followed and the airway should be evaluated and protected if necessary. If there are any deficits in the primary survey, they should be expeditiously addressed. Patients who are unstable (there is evidence of hemorrhagic shock, evolving stroke, expanding hematoma, or an unstable airway) should be intubated, resuscitated, and undergo immediate surgical exploration.
- Clinicians should frequently reassess for changes in airway pathology as certain injuries (expanding hematoma, shock, central nervous system injury) can progress to precipitous airway collapse. Early airway intervention should be considered if there is concern for potential airway compromise or patient transport to an outside institution will occur.
- If a defect in the airway is visualized, the endotracheal tube should be placed distal to the injury to ensure adequate ventilation. Intubation should be performed by an experienced clinician, and care should be taken to avoid converting a partial airway injury into a complete transection with subsequent loss of the airway. Blind intubation attempts should never be performed.
- Anesthesia and surgical backup should be readily available if endotracheal intubation techniques fail.
- If a surgical airway is required, the decision to perform a cricothyroidotomy or tracheostomy will depend on the location of injury. The surgical airway, if possible, should be placed distal to the injury. Cricothyroidotomy can be used if the injury location is known and is above the level of the cricothyroid membrane. If the exact location of injury is unknown, tracheostomy should be performed, with the clinician performing the procedure at least one tracheal ring below the injury when possible to minimize potential complications.
- Surgical complications: Severe bleeding after dissecting into a hematoma, causing a complete transection or laryngotracheal dissociation, and failure to obtain successful airway because of difficult or distorted anatomy.
- In pediatric patients younger than 10 years, surgical cricothyroidotomy is contraindicated because the small cricothyroid membrane and soft poorly calcified larynx make this procedure technically difficult. Tracheostomy or needle cricothyroidotomy with jet ventilation is preferred until the airway can be secured.
- In unstable patients who do not need emergent endotracheal intubation (or stable patients), awake fiberoptic or rapid sequence facilitated fiberoptic techniques can be utilized when available. These techniques should be conducted by experienced clinicians with the proper equipment and monitoring devices available—often in the operating room or bronchoscopy suite. These techniques are limited by time requirements, specialty services, and patient cooperation.
- If the injured patient has signs of respiratory distress, it is important for the clinician to consider potential life-threatening causes like hemothorax, pneumothorax, and tension pneumothorax.

Circulation

- Adequate IV access and monitoring, oxygen and ventilator support when necessary, and fluid and blood product resuscitation should be provided as well as early surgical intervention.
- Control hemorrhage with direct firm pressure. Blind clamping of vessels should be avoided because there is increased risk of injuring nearby structures.

- Wounds should not be probed or examined in the emergency department because clot dislodgement and hemorrhage may occur.
- If there is suspicion for major vascular injury, consider patient placement in Trendelenburg to minimize the risk of venous air embolism (VAE). However, this maneuver may potentially worsen bleeding.
  - VAE can present as cardiac arrest or shock not responding to fluids.
  - If you suspect VAE, place the patient on his or here left side and in Trendelenburg position to try and trap the air in the apex of the right heart and prevent embolization into the pulmonary circulation. If these measures do not work, pericardiocentesis or thoracotomy with needle aspiration may be beneficial.
  - Air embolism can also occur in the arterial system, causing stroke-like symptoms.
- When possible in unilateral injuries, place initial IV access on the contralateral side. Infusing large quantities of crystalloid or blood products on the affected side may dislodge or impair clot formation and lead to further bleeding or extravasation of medication.

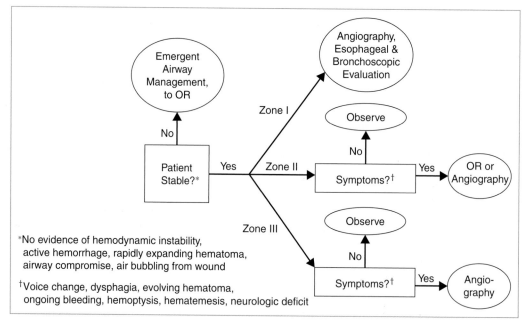

FIGURE 39.2: ED Management of penetrating neck trauma (Reprinted with permission from Wolfson AB, Hendey GW, Ling LJ, et al. *Harwood-Nuss' Clinical Practice of Emergency Medicine*, 5th ed. Philadelphia: Lippincott Williams & Wilkins, 2009.)

Further Care

- If the patient with penetrating neck injury is hemodynamically stable, the clinician should perform a thorough secondary survey to evaluate for other potentially life-threatening injuries and then determine the optimum diagnostic and management strategy given the entire clinical picture.
- The first step in stable patients is to determine whether the wound is superficial or deep. If the platysma is not violated, the wound can be considered superficial and usually no further workup is required. If the platysma is violated, the wound is by definition a deep penetrating neck injury.

- Standard trauma laboratory tests (including a type and screen) should be performed. A chest radiography should be done if pneumothorax is a consideration (Zone I injury).
- After verifying that injury is deep to the platysma, the clinician should evaluate the patient for "hard" and "soft" signs. Patients with "hard" signs usually benefit from surgical exploration. Patients with "soft" signs or no signs of injury can present a diagnostic challenge, and controversy exists over the best way to manage these patients.
- Determine the Zone of injury, as this will determine workup. Depending on the zone of injury, surgery may be delayed pending diagnostic tests. See algorithm in Neck Injury Algorithm and Decision Making chapter; Fig. 39.2.
  - The unstable patient generally is managed in the operating room regardless of the injured zone.
  - **CT-angiography is the recommended initial study of choice to evaluate for vascular injury and may provide information about injuries to additional structures and help delineate the path of the projectile.**
  - Patients with Zone I injuries will likely require "triple evaluation": CT-angiography, bronchoscopy, and esophagoscopy/esophagography.
  - Patients with Zone II injuries should be evaluated by CT-angiography, though some argue that the stable patient with the normal examination can be observed serially. Selective surgical management is now recommended for Zone II injuries and has been shown to be diagnostically equivalent to mandatory exploration. Zone II injuries generally should also have esophageal and laryngeal evaluation, though some sources now advocate testing depending on clinical scenario.
  - Zone III injuries typically need only vascular evaluation and rarely need tracheal or esophageal evaluation.
- Early diagnosis of esophageal injuries is important because delay can lead to mediastinitis and sepsis. **Esophageal injuries are the leading cause of delayed mortality**, especially if there is a delay in diagnosis >24 hours. Broad-spectrum antibiotics are required. Contrast esophagography or esophagoscopy is the gold standard to rule out injury. Computed tomographic imaging modalities may supplant these techniques in the future.
- A thorough neurological examination should be performed to evaluate for signs of ischemia secondary to vascular injury or direct injury to the spinal cord, cranial nerves, or peripheral nerves. In addition, the patient should be questioned about hoarseness, voice changes, or dyspnea as these may be additional signs of nerve deficits.
- Deep penetrating neck injuries may require admission for serial examinations and observation.

Special Considerations

- Penetrating neck trauma can compromise patient's airway, cause respiratory distress, or hemorrhagic shock. Early consultation with trauma surgery, and, when necessary, otolaryngology and anesthesia is recommended. Transfer to a trauma center should be expedited as soon as the patient is clinically stable if local resources do not allow adequate treatment of injury.
- Unstable patients or patients with hard signs require emergent surgical exploration.
- Thorough history and physical examination are important when time permits. Patients with penetrating neck trauma often have other life-threatening injuries that may take precedence. The importance of a thorough secondary survey to evaluate for additional injuries cannot be overstated in the trauma patient.

Best Evidence/Clinical Decision Rules

Can CT determine injury trajectory and essentially rule out significant injury?

"One stop shopping," that is, a single diagnostic test for penetrating neck trauma would be very convenient and save the patient from invasive procedures. Multiple studies have now demonstrated high sensitivity and specificity for the detection of penetrating neck injuries by multidetector row CT-angiography. A normal computed tomographic scan can delineate the injury trajectory and virtually rule out significant injury by demonstrating noninvolvement of vascular, aerodigestive, or nervous structures. Of course, the CT is only as good as the radiologist interpreting the study. Nonetheless, we suspect that multislice CT-angiography will continue to play a larger and larger role in the diagnostic evaluation of penetrating neck trauma.

Suggested Readings

Bell RB, Osborn T, Dierks EJ, et al. Management of penetrating neck injuries: a new paradigm for civilian trauma. *J Oral Maxillofac Surg*. 2007;65:691–705.

Desjardins G, Varon AJ. Airway management for penetrating neck injuries: the Miami experience. *Resucitation*. 2001;48:71–75.

Inaba K, Munera F, McKenney M, et al. Prospective evaluation of screening multislice helical computed tomographic angiography in the initial evaluation of penetrating neck injuries. *J Trauma*. 2006;61(1):144–149.

Mandavia DP, Qualls S, Rokos I. Emergency airway management in penetrating neck injury. *Ann Emerg Med*. 2000;35(3):221–225.

Múnera F, Cohn S, Rivas LA. Penetrating injuries of the neck: use of helical computed tomographic angiography. *J Trauma*. 2005;58:413–418.

Múnera F, Danton G, Rivas LA, Henry RP, Ferrari MG. Multidetector row computed tomography in the management of penetrating neck injuries. *Semin Ultrasound CT MR*. 2009;30(3):195–204.

Newton K, Neck. *Rosen's Emergency Medicine: Concepts and Clinical Practice*. 6th ed. Philadelphia: Mosby, 2006:441–453.

Peralta R, Manrique OJ. Neck Injuries. *The Trauma Handbook of The Massachusetts General Hospital*. New York: Lippincott Williams and Wilkins, 2004:284–295.

Rathlev NK, Medzon R, Bracken ME. Evaluation and management of neck trauma. *Emerg Med Clin North Am*. 2007;25:679–694.

Tisherman SA, Bokhari, Faran, Collier, Bryan, et al. Clinical practice guideline: penetrating zone II neck trauma. *J Trauma*. 2008;64:1392–1405.

40

Blunt Neck Trauma

Darrell Sutijono

Definition/Background

- Blunt injuries to the neck are defined as any injury directly impacting the neck with physical force, excluding those that cause lacerations or penetrate through the skin surface.
- Comprise approximately 5% of all neck trauma, and patients with blunt neck trauma usually have concomitant blunt injuries.
- The neck is a closed anatomical space housing multiple vital contents separated by several fascial planes.
- Injuries to the neck and subsequent complications range from minor to life threatening and can involve airway, neurologic, or vascular compromise.
- Although severe injuries involving the neck are very rare, patients can harbor insidious injuries that necessitate a high index of suspicion to recognize and treat appropriately and expeditiously, as the morbidity of these injuries can be very high.

Pathophysiology

- Mechanisms of injury
  - Motor vehicle accidents are the most common mechanism of injury.
  - Clothesline injuries during motorcycle, all-terrain vehicle, and snowmobile accidents.
  - Direct blows, for example, during sports, assaults, or falling injuries.
  - Occasionally, excessive cervical manipulation (e.g., chiropractic maneuvers).
- Blunt traumatic injuries can be categorized into airway (laryngotracheal), digestive tract (pharyngoesophageal), vascular, and neurologic injuries.
  - Laryngotracheal
    - Rarely, a direct blow to the extended neck against a steering column or dashboard can compress the larynx against the cervical spine, which can lead to asphyxiation if not diagnosed and treated.
    - Fracture of the cricoid cartilage can lead to acute airway obstruction.
  - Pharyngoesophageal
    - A direct blow to the cricoid ring against a steering column or dashboard can compress the esophagus against cervical spine.
    - The cervical esophagus is injured more often than the distal segment.
    - Although their occurrence is rare, these injuries have a high mortality, so a high index of suspicion is necessary as these injuries are the most frequently missed injuries in the neck.
    - Delayed death may result because of infection and inflammation from spillage of orogastric contents into the neck and mediastinum.
  - Vascular
    - Extreme neck hyperextension or hyperflexion with rotation during motor vehicle accidents is the most common mechanism of injury.
      - The affected vasculature is stretched over the cervical spine and a shearing force is applied. This causes a tear in the intimal wall of the vessel, commonly creating a vascular dissection, though an

arteriovenous fistula, arteriocavernous sinus fistula or complete occlusion may occur.

- ◆ Vascular structures may also be lacerated by adjacent bone fractures.
- ◆ The **most frequently injured artery is the internal carotid**, but any vessel may be injured, and any injury can be a nidus for platelet aggregation and subsequent clot formation regardless of the severity of injury. Significant injuries occur in only 1–3% of patients; however, the mortality of these occurrences is as high as 20–30%.
- Neurologic
  - ▷ Neurologic sequelae can be secondary to vascular injury, for example, stroke due to occlusive thromboembolic event or dissection, or due to direct injury to the spinal cord.
  - ▷ Direct injury to the brachial plexus, peripheral nerve roots, and cervical sympathetic chain may also occur.
  - ▷ Vascular injuries are associated with permanent neurological injury in 30–60% of patients.

Diagnosis

- ▪ Physical examination
  - ● Laryngotracheal
    - ▷ Patients may present with dysphonia, aphonia, dyspnea, stridor, or progressive airway obstruction.
    - ▷ Examine for tenderness or ecchymosis over the anterior neck, cervical emphysema, palpable thyroid cartilage disruption, visible neck wounds, or loss of landmarks due to a hematoma.
    - ▷ Pain with tongue movement can be associated with injuries to the epiglottis, hyoid bone, or laryngeal cartilage.
    - ▷ Subglottic injuries usually are not associated with swallowing difficulties or early airway compromise but can present with hemoptysis or persistent air leak from an endotracheal tube.
  - ● Pharyngoesophageal
    - ▷ Patients may present with dysphagia, odynophagia, hematemesis, blood in oro/nasogastric aspirate, dyspnea, dysphonia, stridor, or cough; however, even patients with significant injuries may present with no clinical signs at all.
    - ▷ Examine for crepitus, tenderness over the neck, or tenderness with passive neck movement if cervical spine is cleared.
  - ● Vascular
    - ▷ Carotid injuries typically present with contralateral sensory or motor deficits, and because the sympathetic chain passes along the carotid sheath and through the carotid canal, ipsilateral Horner's syndrome can occur as well.
    - ▷ Vertebral artery injuries typically present with ataxia, vertigo, emesis, or visual field deficits.
    - ▷ A carotid-cavernous sinus fistula may present with orbital pain, decreased vision, diplopia, proptosis, seizures, or epistaxis.
    - ▷ Time from initial injury to presentation of symptoms varies from 1 hour to days; however, symptoms have been noted to occur several weeks after an event.
    - ▷ Certain signs or symptoms (in addition to the standard "hard" and "soft" signs) should elicit an increased suspicion of injury and precipitate immediate further imaging:

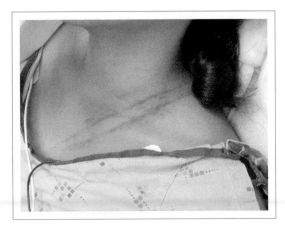

FIGURE 40.1: "Seat belt sign" seen as a patterned hematoma/abrasion of the left side of the neck. (Courtesy of Robert Hendrickson, MD.) Reprinted with permission from Greenberg MI, Hendrickson RG, Silverberg M, et al.: Greenberg's Text-Atlas of Emergency Medicine. Philadelphia: Lippincott Williams & Wilkins, 2005.

- ◆ Ecchymosis to the anterior neck or seat belt sign (Fig. 40.1).
- ◆ Massive epistaxis.
- ◆ Basilar skull fracture, especially with involvement near the petrous bone or the carotid canal, which the internal carotid passes through.
- ◆ Any cervical spine fracture outside of simple spinous process fractures.
- ▶ The presence of a cervicothoracic seat belt sign should prompt further investigation into possible underlying injury. Although there is a fairly low incidence (1–3%) of major underlying injury, it is critical to not miss the diagnosis because the mortality of a missed/delayed diagnosis is as high as 20–30%.
- ▪ Imaging
  - ◦ Laryngotracheal
    - ▶ Plain radiographs of the neck may show extraluminal air, edema, or fracture of cartilaginous laryngeal structures and are recommended as an initial screening tool, but if clinical suspicion is high plain films are not sufficient to definitively rule out injuries.
    - ▶ Computed tomographic (CT) imaging is the modality of choice in a hemodynamically stable patient and is useful for detecting fractures of the hyoid bone, disrupted laryngeal or tracheal cartilages, significant hematomas, or dislocations of cricothyroid or cricoarytenoid joints.
    - ▶ Direct laryngoscopy or flexible nasopharyngoscopy may be used to evaluate laryngeal integrity.
  - ◦ Pharyngoesophageal
    - ▶ Plain radiographs of the neck and chest may show subcutaneous emphysema, retropharyngeal air, or pneumomediastinum if a perforation is present.
    - ▶ The combination of contrast swallow and flexible endoscopy has a sensitivity of 100% in diagnosing esophageal injuries.
    - ▶ CT evaluation of the esophagus is becoming more common but has not yet been accepted as a standard for ruling out esophageal injuries (Fig. 40.2).

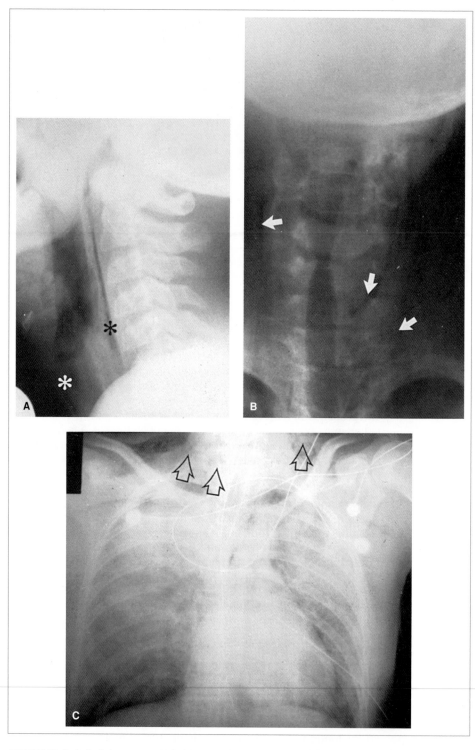

FIGURE 40.2: A–C: Subcutaneous emphysema of neck and chest in a 11-year-old patient. (Reprinted with permission from Fleisher GR, Ludwig S, Henretig FM, et al. *Textbook of Pediatric Emergency Medicine*, 5th ed. Philadelphia: Lippincott Williams & Wilkins, 2005.)

- Vascular
  - ▶ Digital subtraction angiography (DSA) is the gold standard but is invasive, resource intensive, not available in many hospitals, has the risk of complications, and places a trauma patient with potentially multiple injuries in a radiology suite for an extended period of time.
  - ▶ Duplex ultrasound has a sensitivity of 90–95% versus DSA for injuries requiring intervention but can miss nonocclusive injuries with preserved flow and is limited to evaluating the common and external carotids and can thus miss vertebral artery injuries or injuries of the internal carotid at the base of the skull, where most injuries occur.
  - ▶ Magnetic resonance angiography is limited in practicality and has not been shown to be superior to multidetector computed tomography angiography (MD-CTA).
  - ▶ MD-CTA is fast and available at most hospitals, and blunt trauma patients are often already undergoing additional CT imaging; however, the correlation between MD-CTA and DSA is controversial (see Best Evidence below).

Evaluation

- As in all trauma patients, attention must first be given to the airway, with assessment and establishment of a definitive airway in any patient with concerning signs or symptoms such as respiratory distress, expanding neck hematoma, or crepitus.
- Associated injuries with blunt neck trauma are usually of the head and cervical spine, especially in cases of vertebral artery injuries, and thus cervical spine precautions should be taken in all patients.
- Active bleeding should be controlled first with pressure and then surgically if necessary, and any open wounds or bubbling should be covered to prevent the possibility of an air embolus.
- There is no standard screening protocol in the hemodynamically stable patient, and index of suspicion must be correlated to mechanism and/or physical findings.

Management

- Definitive airway protection is the primary focus in management, especially in the hemodynamically unstable patient.
- In-line cervical traction should be used to stabilize the cervical spine during intubation.
- In the case of a tracheal disruption, if the airway can be visualized through a traumatic wound, it may be possible to use a gum-elastic bougie to facilitate intubation directly through the wound.
- Each type of blunt neck injury requires specific considerations during management:
  - Laryngotracheal
    - ▶ In severe injuries, the trachea may only be held together by muscle tone, which would be lost during rapid sequence intubation, and attempts at intubation may lead to soft-tissue intubation.
    - ▶ Options include awake intubation, fiberoptic intubation by an anesthesiologist, or cricothyroidotomy, but if there is severe concern and the patient's clinical status permits, these interventions should be managed in the operating room.
  - Pharyngoesophageal
    - ▶ Administer broad-spectrum antibiotics with anaerobic coverage and consider nasogastric tube placement to reduce amount of spillage of gastric contents.

- Vascular
  - ▶ Management is controversial and often dependent on the institution as well as trauma surgeon. Consultation and treatment should always be made in conjunction with the trauma service.
  - ▶ Surgical options include resection or thrombectomy, whereas interventional radiology may be utilized for embolization or stent placement.
  - ▶ Anticoagulation has been shown to decrease morbidity and mortality, including poor neurological outcome, but many patients have coexisting injuries that may preclude its use.

Special Considerations

- Once stable, patients should be transferred to and managed at a Level I trauma center.
- In alert patients with blunt vascular injuries, caution should be taken in placement of a nasogastric tube, as any retching can dislodge a hematoma.
- Patients with progressive subcutaneous emphysema, difficulty in mechanical ventilation, or uncontrolled hemorrhage, should go to the operating room for definitive surgical exploration and management.

Best Evidence/Clinical Decision Rules

How good is multidetector computed tomography angiography (MD-CTA) compared to the gold standard digital subtraction angiography (DSA) in evaluating blunt vascular injuries?

Malhotra et al. prospectively compared 16-slice CTA versus DSA in 92 hemodynamically stable blunt trauma patients with suspicion of injury and found a sensitivity of 74%, specificity of 84%, positive predictive value (PPV) of 63%, and negative predictive value (NPV) of 90%. However, all the false-negative studies were read during the first half of the study, calling into question improved readings after increased experience of the radiologists. The sensitivity and NPV were 100% over the second half of the study. There have been no major studies thus far comparing 64-slice CT scanners with DSA.

Suggested Readings

Arthurs ZM, Starnes BW. Blunt carotid and vertebral artery injuries. *Injury*. 2008;39: 1232–1241.

Baker WE, Wassermann J. Unsuspected vascular trauma: blunt arterial injuries. *Emerg Med Clin N Am*. 2004;22:1081–1098.

DiPerna CA, Rowe VL, Terramani TT, et al. Clinical importance of the "seat belt sign" in blunt trauma to the neck. *Am Surg*. 2002;68:441–445.

Malhotra AK, Camacho M, Ivatury RR, et al. Computed tomographic angiography for the diagnosis of blunt carotid/vertebral artery injury: a note of caution. *Ann Surg*. 2007;246:632–642; discussion 642–643.

Newton K, Neck. In: Marx JA, Hockberger RS, Walls RM, eds. *Rosen's Emergency Medicine: Concepts and Clinical Practice*. 6th ed. Philadelphia: Mosby, 2006:441–452.

Rathlev NK, Medzon R, Bracken ME. Evaluation and management of neck trauma. *Emerg Med Clin N Am*. 2007;25:679–694.

Rozychi GS, Tremblay L, Feliciano DV, et al. A prospective study for the detection of vascular injury in adult and pediatric patients with cervicothoracic seat belt signs. *J Trauma*. 2002;52:618–624.

41

Strangulation Trauma

Dana Sajed

Definition/Background

- Strangulation is the mechanical disruption of blood flow through the arteries of the neck and/or blockage of air passage through the trachea.
- In children younger than 1 year, strangulation is the fourth most common cause of unintentional injury. Common household implements, such as window cords, sheets, or towels account for a majority of these injuries.
- In adolescents, recent popularity of the "choking-game" has led to a noted increase in the incidence of strangulation injuries and deaths.
- In adult patients, the causes of strangulation injury include assault, self-inflicted/intentional, and seat belt–related injuries.
- Intentional hanging victims often present with strangulation injuries rather than immediate death as a result of improper knot tying.

Pathophysiology

- Hypoxic and ischemic injury plays a key role in neurologic injury and death that follows strangulation.
- Death from strangulation is thought to be provoked by one of four mechanisms:
  - Cardiac dysrhythmia
  - Pressure obstruction of carotid arteries
  - Pressure obstruction of jugular veins
  - Pressure obstruction of larynx
- Cardiac dysrhythmia is instigated by pressure on the carotid artery nerve ganglion causing cardiac arrest. This mechanism (called the carotid body reflex) is very uncommon, as force must be applied over a very localized and specific anatomic area.
- Pressure obstruction of the carotid arteries preventing blood flow to the brain. This mechanism requires significant pressure to obstruct arterial flow in both carotids and is associated with obvious soft-tissue injury.
- Pressure on the jugular veins preventing blood return from the brain, gradually expanding blood in the brain resulting in unconsciousness, depressed respiration, and asphyxia. Even partial obstruction of venous return in all four veins (bilateral external and internal jugulars) diminishes oxygen delivery to the brain, eventually resulting in loss of consciousness.
- Pressure obstruction of the larynx, cutting off air flow to the lungs, producing asphyxia. Often, the strangulation victim initially becomes unconscious as a result of diminished venous return, followed by continued pressure on the larynx, which is the ultimate cause of death.

Diagnosis

- Airway injury may manifest itself by obstruction, subcutaneous emphysema, hematemesis, change in voice, or hypoxia.
- Physical signs such as bruising, lacerations, or abrasion to the neck may develop.

- Pain on palpation of the larynx may indicate laryngeal fracture (Fig. 41.1).
- Respiratory distress is often a late development after prolonged asphyxia or significant laryngeal injury.
- Hypoxia and changes in mental status are typically a late finding and indicative of cerebral ischemia.
- Tardieu spots are mucosal and cutaneous petechiae cephalad to the site of choking and are frequently seen in patients following severe strangulation.

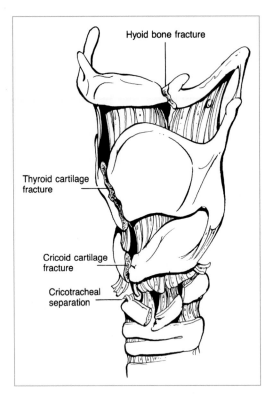

FIGURE 41.1: Types of laryngeal injuries: hyoid bone fracture, thyroid cartilage fracture, cricoid cartilage fracture, and cricotracheal separation. (From Harwood-Nuss A, Wolfson AB, et al. *The Clinical Practice of Emergency Medicine*, 3rd ed. Philadelphia: Lippincott Williams & Wilkins, 2001.)

Evaluation
- Soft-tissue radiographs of the neck should be obtained in nearly all strangulation victims. Fracture of the hyoid bone is a sign of significant soft-tissue injury as well.
- Cervical spine evaluation may also be necessary as many hanging injuries may involve damage to vertebrae as well as soft-tissue structures.
- If suspected, vascular injury to the neck necessitates further evaluation with computed tomography angiography or Doppler sonography.
- Direct fiberoptic laryngoscopy should be obtained in patients who present with signs or symptoms suggestive of tracheolaryngeal injury, as direct visualization will give additional information regarding mucosal injury in the presence or absence of fracture of the larynx, which may be seen on computed tomographic scanning.

Management

- As always, management of the ABCs is paramount.
- Particular care must be taken with airway management in patients with strangulation injury. Orotracheal intubation should be performed by an experienced operator as this method of airway control may lead to iatrogenic complications in patients with fracture of the larynx.
- Some authors recommend emergent tracheotomy as a measure of airway control; however, this is a surgical procedure that requires time, preparation, and an experienced provider (surgeon).
- Cricothyroidotomy can also be considered as a lifesaving option in patients with a totally obstructed airway or severe respiratory distress.

Special Considerations

- Patients with hoarseness of voice, tenderness of the larynx, or subcutaneous emphysema should have direct imaging of the airway.
- Any signs or symptoms of vascular injury necessitates further imaging analysis by Doppler ultrasound, computed tomography or traditional angiography, or magnetic resonance vascular imaging.
- Fracture of the hyoid bone is often associated with concomitant injuries to vascular and airway structures.
- Special care must be taken in airway management in these patients, as injury to the larynx or vocal cords may make traditional orotracheal intubation difficult or impossible.
- Anyone presenting with a self-inflicted injury should be evaluated by a psychiatrist once medically stable.
- Injuries that are the result of assault may require the involvement of local authorities or police to ensure safe disposition of the patient. Protective services for children must be notified in any case of suspected child abuse.

Best Evidence/Clinical Decision Rules

Patients with strangulation injury may not present with signs of significant injury; however, injury may be present in the airway or vascular structures. How can one decide which injuries need to be worked up further?

There are no specific guidelines in the literature about how to evaluate patients with strangulation injury. Soft-tissue neck x-rays should be ordered as a starting point in nearly all strangulation patients. Those with no overt pathology on examination and normal initial screening x-rays should be observed in the emergency department for an extended period and reassessed for symptom emergence prior to discharge.

Suggested Readings

Hawley DA, McClane GE, Strack GB. A review of 300 attempted strangulation cases Part III: injuries in fatal cases. *J Emerg Med*. 2001;21(3):317–322.

McClane GE, Strack GB, Hawley DA. A review of 300 attempted strangulation cases, Part II: clinical evaluation of the surviving victim. *J Emerg Med*. 2001;21:311–315.

Sep D, Thies KC. Strangulation injuries in children. *Resuscitation*. 2007;74(2): 386–391.

Section Editor: Ashley Shreves

42

Chest Trauma: The First 15 Minutes, Algorithm, and Decision Making

Ashley Shreves

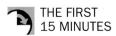 THE FIRST
15 MINUTES

ABCs and Vital Signs

- **Airway:** If stridor or inability to phonate is found, consider and relieve airway obstruction. Rapid sequence intubation should be performed in the patient with an unstable airway.
- **Breathing:** Assess for dyspnea and tachypnea. Continuous pulse oximetry should be initiated to assess for hypoxia. Administer oxygen to hypoxic patients. Auscultate for bilateral breath sounds. Consider needle decompression and/or chest tube placement in patients with unilateral loss of breath sounds and signs of shock.
- **Circulation:** The patient should be placed on the monitor immediately to assess for signs of shock: tachycardia, tachypnea, and hypotension. Large-bore intravenous access should be obtained immediately and isotonic saline and/or blood products administered if hypovolemic shock present.

History

- If an motor vehicle collision (MVC) is the mechanism, careful attention should be paid to speed/impact, as these are important predictors of aortic injury.
- The presence of symptoms such as chest pain and dyspnea should increase suspicion for severe pathology (aortic injury, pneumo/hemothorax); however, the absence of these symptoms, particularly in penetrating chest trauma patients, does not exclude significant injury.

Physical Examination

- Care should be taken in auscultating the chest for breath sounds, specifically apically and in the axilla bilaterally. Unilateral decreased breath sounds are often the only sign of a pneumo/hemothorax. Normal auscultation does not reliably exclude injury in penetrating chest trauma patients.
- Any penetrating thoracoabdominal trauma, especially in the region of the anterior chest wall, suggests the possibility of cardiac injury and tamponade.
- Blunt chest trauma patients with (a) no chest pain, (b) normal vital signs, (c) equal breath sounds on auscultation, and (d) no chest wall tenderness on examination have a <1% incidence of pneumo/hemothorax.

Emergency Interventions

- **Needle decompression and chest tube placement.** In the unstable trauma patient, chest tubes should be performed on the basis of clinically diagnosed pneumo/hemothorax, rather than relying on a radiographic diagnosis.
- **Open thoracotomy**
  - Patients with penetrating chest trauma who have lost vital signs for no longer than 15 minutes should be considered for resuscitative emergency thoracotomy. During this procedure, attention should be focused on rapidly reversible injuries like cardiac lacerations or tamponade. Aortic cross-clamping is performed as a mechanism of increasing cerebral, cardiac, and pulmonary perfusion.
  - Survival rates are highest in patients with penetrating cardiac injuries who present to the emergency department (ED) with vital signs. In such patients, survival rates of up to 35% have been reported in case series. Performing this intervention in blunt trauma patients is much less effective and generally discouraged.
  - Patients with massive hemothoraces (>1,500 cc blood initial output) should go emergently to the operating room for an open thoracotomy.
- **Plain film**
  - Chest radiography (ideally upright) should be performed in all patients presenting with penetrating chest trauma and those with significant blunt trauma.
  - After assessment for pneumo/hemothorax, the mediastinum should be evaluated for any abnormality in appearance as this is a sensitive marker for aortic injury.
- **Bedside ultrasound**
  - This imaging modality is most useful in penetrating chest trauma patients, where detection of fluid in the pericardial space indicates cardiac injury and the possibility of tamponade until proven otherwise.
  - Ultrasound is also reliable (and might be more sensitive than plain film) at detecting pneumo/hemothoraces and can be a supportive tool in the management of these injuries, particularly in the unstable patient.
- **Volume resuscitation.** There is currently debate about the concept of permissive hypotension (and thus minimizing isotonic fluid resuscitation) in patients with penetrating chest trauma. In unstable patients with massive hemothoraces, a cell saver should be sought so that autotransfusion can be performed. Otherwise, current practice dictates transfusion with regular packed red blood cells (PRBCs) in unstable chest trauma patients if initial fluid bolus is unsuccessful at restoring adequate perfusion.

Memorable Pearls

- In patients with chest trauma, the primary survey should focus on identifying immediate, yet quickly reversible life-threatening injuries: tension pneumothorax, massive hemothorax, and cardiac tamponade.
- The chest cavity can hold up to 4 L of blood, so hemorrhagic shock can develop rapidly in patients with isolated chest trauma, particularly penetrating.
- The initial plain film may miss >20% of pneumo/hemothoraces, some of significant size. When these 'occult' injuries are detected via computed tomographic scanning and/or ultrasound, the optimal management strategy is not clear but should likely be guided by the patient's clinical appearance.
- If central line placement is required during resuscitation of a patient with penetrating chest trauma, the line should be placed on the same side as the injury (and potential pneumothorax), unless their is concern that the central vein is injured.

- Although not a rapidly correctable pathology in the ED, aortic injury should be considered early and often in those patients who have significant blunt chest trauma. Of the 15% who survive to reach the hospital, 15% of those patients will die in the first hour. If detected and managed surgically, most patients will survive.

Essential Considerations

Indications for ED Thoracotomy
Penetrating chest trauma
- Loss of pulses at any time with initial vital signs in the field.
- Systolic blood pressure of <70 mm Hg after aggressive fluid resuscitation.

Blunt chest trauma
- Should rarely be performed and generally not recommended.
- Consider for the patient with loss of pulses or systolic blood pressure of <70 mm Hg after aggressive fluid resuscitation AND
  - Initial chest tube output >20 mL/kg of blood, OR
  - Confirmed or highly suspected pericardial effusion, OR
  - Confirmed or highly suspected ongoing intra-abdominal hemorrhage (controversial)

Consultations
General/trauma surgeon
Cardiothoracic surgeon

DECISION
MAKING

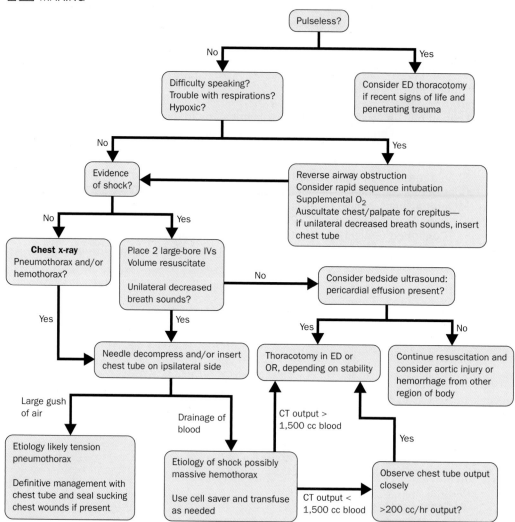

Chest trauma: Decision making algorithm. ED, emergency department; IVs, intravenous; OR, operating room; CT, computed tomography.

Suggested Readings

Bokhari F, Brakenridge S, Nagy K, et al. Prospective evaluation of the sensitivity of physical examination in chest trauma. *J Trauma.* 2002;53:1135–1138.

Keel M, Meier C. Chest injuries—what is new? *Curr Opin Crit Care.* 2007;13:674–679.

Kirkpatrick AW, Ball CG, D'Amours SK, Zygun D. Acute resuscitation of the unstable adult trauma patient: bedside diagnosis and therapy. *Can J Surg.* 2008;51:57–69.

43

Rib and Sternal Fractures

Lucy Willis

Background/Pathophysiology

- Rib fractures are one of the most common chest injuries after blunt trauma. Sternal fractures are less common and usually occur only with high-energy trauma [i.e., motor vehicle collision (MVC)]. Their importance generally lies in the associated complications (Table 43.1).
- Elderly patients and patients with three or more rib fractures have increased morbidity and mortality.
- Fracture of the first rib should raise suspicion of major arterial injury.
- In cases of sternal fracture, as a result of the dissipated energy on the sternum, intrathoracic and mediastinal injury is less common. However, myocardial contusion does occur in up to 5% of these patients.

Diagnosis

- Rib fractures can present with pain, tenderness, bony crepitus, ecchymosis, and pain at the fracture site with bimanual thoracic cage compression.
- Chest x-ray can miss a significant number of rib fractures. They have a sensitivity of approximately 50%.
- Rib series films are helpful in making the diagnosis in patients in whom there is a high suspicion of fracture of ribs 1–2 or 9–12, patients with multiple rib fractures, the elderly, patients with preexisting pulmonary disease, and patients with suspected pathologic fractures.
- Computed tomography (CT) is quite sensitive for identifying rib fractures and associated intrathoracic injury; however, the additional information obtained from CT is not more predictive of mortality/morbidity than the initial supine chest x-ray in stable patients with no clinical concerns other than rib fracture(s).
- Sternal fractures can be seen on a lateral chest x-ray film but more reliably with a dedicated sternal view (Fig. 43.2).

TABLE 43.1: Complications of rib and sternal fractures

Pulmonary contusion
Pneumothorax
Hemothorax
Flail chest
Hepatic or splenic laceration
Pneumonia (delayed)
Atelectasis (delayed)

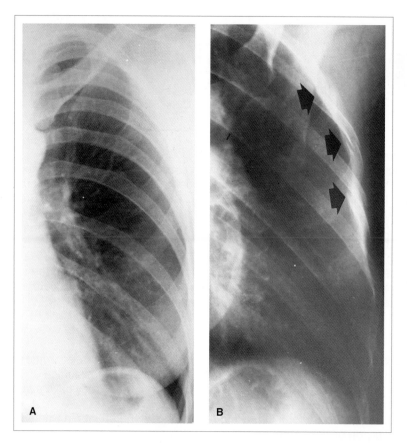

FIGURE 43.1: Minimally displaced, acute, complete fractures in the anterior axillary line of the left upper ribs are not visible in the frontal chest radiograph **(A)** but are clearly evident in the left posterior oblique projection **(B**, arrows). (Reprinted with permission from Harris JH, Harris WH. *The Radiology of Emergency Medicine*, 4th ed. Philadelphia: Lippincott Williams & Wilkins, 2000.)

Evaluation

- Further evaluation should focus on identifying associated injuries.
- Flail chest occurs when three or more adjacent ribs are fractured at two points, allowing paradoxical movement of the flail segment. It is diagnosed by physical examination and visualization of the flail segment moving in the opposite direction from the rest of the chest wall.
- Fracture of the first rib is associated with a 3% rate of arterial injury.
- When the first rib is fractured and one or more of the signs in Table 43.2 is present, a CT angiogram should be ordered.
- Low left-sided rib fractures and low right-sided rib fractures should increase suspicion for splenic and hepatic injuries, respectively.
- Sternal fractures have associated myocardial contusions in approximately 5% of patients. A screening electrocardiogram and serum troponin level should be considered to evaluate for myocardial contusion.

Management

- The management of rib fractures centers on pain control and aggressive pulmonary toilet to prevent atelectasis and pneumonia. While young, healthy

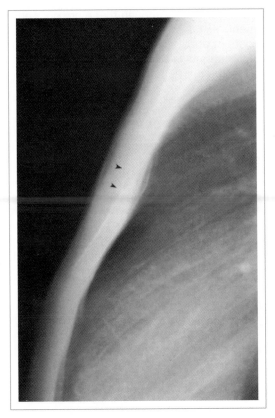

FIGURE 43.2: This patient was wrestling and suffered blunt chest trauma. The sternum is fractured (*arrows*), and there is some presternal and retrosternal soft-tissue swelling. (Reprinted from Swischuk LE. Emergency Imaging of the Acutely Ill or Injured Child. Philadelphia: Lippincott Williams & Wilkins, 2000.)

patients with isolated rib fractures can frequently be discharged with narcotic pain medications, older patients and patients with multiple rib fractures have increased morbidity and mortality and may need to be admitted.
- The mainstay of analgesia for patients with multiple rib fractures is opioid medication. Alternative techniques include intercostal, interpleural, thoracic

TABLE 43.2: Indications for computed tomography angiogram when first rib is fractured

Widened mediastinum
Upper extremity pulse deficit
Posteriorly displaced first rib fracture
Subclavian groove fracture anteriorly
Brachial plexus injury
Expanding hematoma

paravertebral, epidural, and intrathecal blocks, though these are not generally done in the emergency department.

- Management of flail chest consists of analgesia, oxygenation, and selective use of mechanical ventilation in those patients with respiratory compromise.
- Patients with isolated sternal fractures are generally safe for discharge home on oral analgesics.

Best Evidence

Is there any utility in ordering a rib series in the emergency department or is a standard chest radiograph sufficient to evaluate for underlying injury?

In minor blunt chest injury, a standard radiograph is probably sufficient. Davis (2006) suggests that emergency department rib series does not influence the physician treatment plan.

Since three or more consecutive rib fractures correlate with increased morbidity/mortality, rib series should probably be performed if this is suspected clinically and its subsequent diagnosis would result in a change in management (i.e., hospitalization).

Suggested Readings

Brasel KJ, Guse CE, Layde P, Weigelt JA. Rib fractures: relationship with pneumonia and mortality. *Crit Care Med*. 2006;34(6):1642–1646.

Davis S, Affatato A. *Am J Emerg Med*. 2006;24(4):482–486.

Gupta A, Jamshidi M, Rubin JR. Traumatic first rib fracture: is angiography necessary? A review of 730 cases. *Cardiovasc Surg*. 1997;1:48–53.

Karmakar MK Ho AMH. Acute pain management of patients with multiple fractured ribs. *J Trauma*. 2003;54:615–625.

Lee RB, Bass SM, Morris JA Jr, Mackenzie EJ. Three or more rib fractures as an indicator for transfer to a Level I trauma center: a population-based study. *J Trauma*. 1990;30(6):689–694.

Livingston DH, Shogan B, John P, Lavery RF. CT diagnosis of rib fractures and the prediction of acute respiratory failure. *J Trauma*. 2008;64:905–911.

Marx JA, Hockberger RS, Walls RM, Rosen P, Adams J. *Rosen's Emergency Medicine: Concepts and Clinical Practice*. St. Louis: Mosby, 2001.

Shweiki E, Klena J, Wood GC, Indeck M. Assessing the true risk of abdominal solid organ injury in hospitalized rib fracture patients. *J Trauma*. 2001;50:684–688.

Ziegler DW, Agarwal NN. The morbidity and mortality of rib fractures. *J Trauma*. 1994;37(6):975–979.

44

Pneumothorax

Turandot Saul

Definition

- A pneumothorax occurs when air accumulates in the space between the visceral and parietal pleura.
- Tension pneumothorax occurs when air progressively accumulates in the pleural cavity significantly increasing intra-thoracic pressure, shifting the mediastinum and progressively impeding hemodynamics.

Pathophysiology

- Traumatic pneumothorax can occur as a result of penetrating injury, a fractured rib driven inward, or blunt trauma when the force is delivered to the thorax against a closed glottis, causing an increase in intra-alveolar pressure.
- **Closed pneumothorax:** the chest wall is intact and there is no communication with the atmosphere through the chest wall.
- **Open pneumothorax:** the chest wall is penetrated and the pleural space is open to the atmosphere.
- **Tension pneumothorax:** increased intrathoracic pressure shifts the mediastinum, compressing the vena cava and reducing venous return. This leads to decreased cardiac output and shock. Tension pneumothorax can occur in both open and closed pneumothoraces (Figs. 44.1 and 44.2).

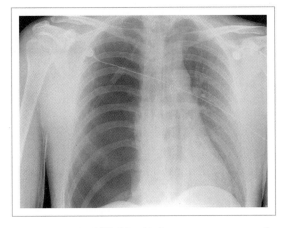

FIGURE 44.1: A 100% right-sided spontaneous pneumothorax. (Courtesy of Robert Hendrickson, MD.)

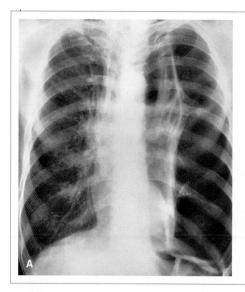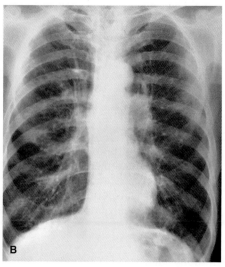

FIGURE 44.2: Spontaneous left tension pneumothorax with displacement of the mediastinal structures to the right **(A)** in a patient with severe chronic obstructive pulmonary disease. Following reexpansion of the left lung **(B)**, the mediastinal structures returned to the midline. (Reprinted with permission from Harris JH, Harris WH. *The Radiology of Emergency Medicine*, 4th ed. Philadelphia: Lippincott Williams & Wilkins, 2000.)

Diagnosis

- Symptoms of pneumothorax include chest pain and shortness of breath, agitation, restlessness, and altered mental status.
- Physical examination findings may include tachycardia, tachypnea, hypotension, and cyanosis. The patient may have decreased or absent breath sounds, hyperresonance to percussion, and decreased chest wall excursion on the affected side. Jugular venous distension, tracheal deviation, pulsus paradoxus, and subcutaneous emphysema may also be present.
- Signs and symptoms do not always correlate with degree of pneumothorax.
- Small pneumothoraces may produce minimal symptoms and are unlikely to be evident on physical examination.
- Definitive diagnosis requires imaging of the chest.
- An upright inspiratory film is the most sensitive type of chest x-ray (CXR). Intrapleural air accumulates at the apex of the lung.
- On the x-ray film, a pleural line can be seen separating the collapsed lung from the air in the pleural space (Fig. 44.3).
- On a film taken with the patient supine, air collects anteriorly and basally. The costophrenic angle may be abnormally deepened and a deep sulcus sign can be seen (Fig. 44.4).
- Theoretically, the lung is more collapsed during expiration; however, expiratory films have not shown to provide added sensitivity.
- Computed tomographic scan approaches 100% sensitivity for pneumothorax although it is not used as the primary method of diagnosis.
- Bedside ultrasound can be used to detect pneumothorax in the supine patient. Findings consistent with pneumothorax include absence of normal pleural sliding and absence of "comet tail" artifacts. The "lung point" may also be visualized demarcating the transition between collapsed and noncollapsed lung.

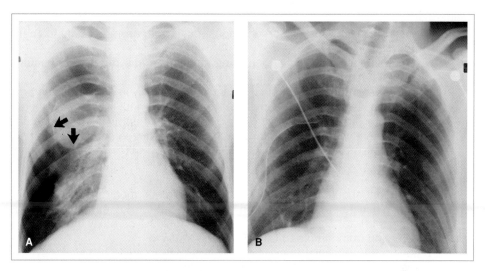

FIGURE 44.3: **A:** Moderate right pneumothorax (arrows) with minimal tension evidenced by very slight displacement of the mediastinal structures to the left in the initial chest radiograph. **B:** After insertion of the right chest tube and reexpansion of the right lung, return of the heart and mediastinal structures to their anatomic position confirms that the original pneumothorax was under tension. (Reprinted with permission from Harris JH, Harris WH. *The Radiology of Emergency Medicine*, 4th ed. Philadelphia: Lippincott Williams & Wilkins, 2000.)

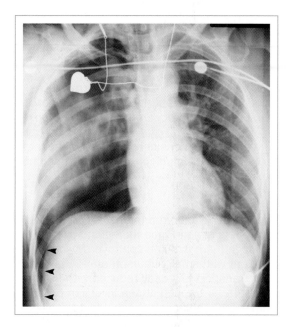

FIGURE 44.4: "Deep sulcus sign" of pneumothorax. In this supine frontal examination of the chest, the most obvious radiographic sign of the right pneumothorax is the abnormal depth and width of the right costophrenic angle (arrowheads) caused by air in the costophrenic pleural space. (Reprinted with permission from Harris JH, Harris WH. *The Radiology of Emergency Medicine*, 4th ed. Philadelphia: Lippincott Williams & Wilkins, 2000.)

Evaluation

- Traumatic pneumothorax presentations range from asymptomatic to complete cardiovascular collapse.
- Evaluation should focus on identifying the signs and symptoms of pneumothorax, as well as other injuries associated with pneumothorax.
- Tension pneumothorax should be diagnosed clinically in the field or on arrival to the emergency department. It should be treated emergently with needle thoracostomy prior to imaging if there is high suspicion or the patient is clinically unstable.
- Every patient with suspicion for pneumothorax requires chest radiography.

Management

- The patient should have cardiac and pulse oximetry monitoring. Supplemental oxygen should be administered to accelerate the rate of intrapleural air absorption.
- Changes in vital signs and clinical status should be carefully monitored for conversion from simple to tension pneumothorax.
- Patients with associated rib fractures should have adequate analgesia to decrease splinting and atelectasis of the lung.
- Reliable patients with small pneumothoraces, minimal symptoms, and no associated rib fractures may be observed for 6 hours with repeat chest radiography. If there is no progression of the pneumothorax, they may be discharged with close follow-up for repeat chest radiography until resolution.
- Significant pneumothorax requires tube thoracostomy. There is some practice discrepancy regarding what constitutes a significant pneumothorax; the decision to place a chest tube is made clinically on the basis of the patient's clinical picture, extent of injuries, and the size of the pneumothorax.
- The chest tube should be placed in the fourth or fifth intercostal space in the anterior midaxillary line with the tip directed posteriorly and toward the apex of the lung. In this position the chest tube can remove both air and fluid.
- A large chest tube, (size 36 French or greater) should be used in trauma patients. Often, there is an associated hemothorax and this will decrease the chance of blood clotting in the tube and inhibiting drainage.
- The chest tube is attached to water-seal drainage to allow for re-expansion of the lung. Patients with displaced rib fractures but no pneumothorax on initial examination should have a chest radiograph repeated in 3 hours to observe for delayed pneumothorax.
- Needle aspiration of intrapleural air can be considered in primary spontaneous pneumothorax but has not been sufficiently studied in traumatic pneumothorax.

Special Considerations

- Patients requiring positive pressure ventilation run the risk of rapidly increasing pneumothorax size. Most experts recommend tube thoracostomy prior to or immediately after intubation, though there is some controversy whether this is necessary for the monitored patient with small pneumothorax.
- Atmospheric pressure during air transport is greatly reduced with increasing altitude, even in pressurized aircraft. Air trapped at sea level can expand to several times the original volume. Tube thoracostomy should be considered even with small pneumothoraces in patients being transported by air.
- Tube thoracostomy should also be considered in patients with small pneumothoraces requiring prolonged ground transport.

Current Concepts/Evidence

What is the Role of Ultrasound in Diagnosing pneumothorax (PTX)?

Supine CXR has a well-documented sensitivity of no higher than ~70% (wide range depending on study). Upright CXR, often difficult to perform in acutely injured patients, has a higher sensitivity of ~80%. Bedside ultrasonography performed by an experienced operator, looking at a single point on each side of the chest (second anterior intercostal space) for lung sliding, has a sensitivity of >90% in many studies. This makes intuitive sense, as free pleural air will usually collect anteriorly in the supine patient. Anterior air will be visible to the sonogram but will have intact lung tissue behind it making it "invisible" to plain radiography. While not routinely done nor the current standard, our experience with bedside thoracic ultrasound (as part of the extended-FAST examination) has shown it to be easily learned and applied. We believe that it will evolve into the standard of care for the acutely injured trauma patient in the near future.

For details on the extended focused assessment with sonography for trauma (or e-FAST) examination, see the Procedures section of this book.

Suggested Readings

Baumann MH. Management of spontaneous pneumothorax. *Clin Chest Med*. 2006; 27(2).

Baumann MH, Strange C, Heffner JE, et al. Management of spontaneous pneumothorax: an American College of Chest Physicians Delphi consensus statement. *Chest*. 2001;119(2):590–602.

Eckstein M, Henderson S. Thoracic trauma. In: Marx JA, ed. *Rosen's Emergency Medicine: Concepts and Clinical Practice*, 6th ed. Philadelphia: Mosby, 2006: 453–486.

Kirsh TD, Mulligan JP. Tube thoracostomy. In: Roberts JR, ed. *Clinical Procedures in Emergency Medicine*, 4th ed. Philadelphia: Saunders, 2004:187–208.

Seow A, Kazeroon i EA, Pernicano PG, Neary M. Comparison of upright inspiratory and expiratory chest radiographs for detecting pneumothoraces. *Am J Roentgenol*. 1996;166:313.

45

Hemothorax

Ann Vorhaben

Definition

- Hemothorax is defined as the accumulation of blood within the pleural cavity.
- There are an average of 300,000 cases of traumatic hemothorax reported in the United States yearly.
- Massive hemothorax is defined as the rapid accumulation of >1,500 mL or one-third of the patient's blood volume in the pleural space.

Pathophysiology

- Hemothorax most commonly results from damage to the chest wall vessels and less frequently from a laceration in the pulmonary parenchyma or an injury of the great vessels.
- Several factors determine an individual's physiologic response to hemothorax: quantity of blood, rapidity of accumulation, mechanism of injury, comorbid conditions, and concomitant injuries.
- As massive amounts of blood accumulate, severe cardiovascular and respiratory compromise occurs. It is important to note that the average 70 kg person can retain up to 4 L of blood in the pleural cavity.
- Rib fractures are common injuries sustained in blunt trauma. Simple rib fractures often result in clinically insignificant hemothoraces which need no further management. As the number of rib fractures approaches four or more, other injuries such as pulmonary contusions or significant blood vessel disruption are more often present.

Diagnosis

- Hemothorax may be suspected in any individual sustaining chest trauma. Abnormal vital signs indicative of hemorrhagic shock suggest possible massive hemothorax.
- Physical examination may show decreased or absent breath sounds on the injured side.
- The upright chest x-ray is the diagnostic test of choice. The accumulation of at least 300 mL of blood in the intrapleural space is required to visualize a hemothorax on chest x-ray film (Fig. 45.1).
- Hemothorax on a supine chest x-ray is less clear and typically appears as a vague haziness unilaterally on the film. As much as 1000 mL of blood may be present in the pleural space without a clear radiographic sign in the supine chest x-ray.
- Chest computed tomography is more sensitive than chest x-ray for detecting hemothoraces but the routine use of computed tomography for such purpose does not usually affect management.

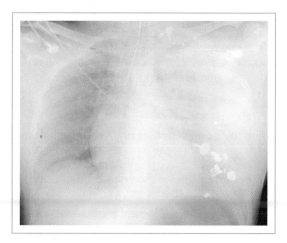

FIGURE 45.1: Gunshot wound to left chest with hemothorax. (Courtesy of Mark Silverberg, MD.)

Evaluation

- Unexplained hypotension in the trauma patient should be assumed to be hemorrhagic shock. Such patients tend to present with pallor, tachycardia, and anxiety. The chest (along with the abdomen and pelvis) is one of the main sources of potential blood loss.
- Listen for decreased breath sounds on the injured chest side.
- Evaluate for signs of respiratory compromise: tachypnea, labored breathing, cyanosis, and hypoxia.
- Examine the chest x-ray film carefully. On a supine film, do not expect the costophrenic angles to be blunted, as the blood will be layering along the entire posterior pleural cavity.

Management

- The primary management of a hemothorax is tube thoracostomy. Most patients with a hemothorax large enough to obscure the costophrenic sulcus should receive this intervention.
- Tube thoracostomy is both therapeutic and diagnostic. It allows re-expansion of the lung tissue and assessment of the degree of hemorrhage and rate of ongoing bleeding.
- A large chest tube (36–42 French; smaller tubes may occlude) should be placed just anterior to the midaxillary line in the fifth intercostal space, directed posteriorly. If a massive hemothorax is present, blood should be collected in a "cell saver" and used for autotransfusion.
- In the setting of a hemopneumothorax, consideration should be made for placing two chest tubes; the tube draining the pneumothorax should be placed in a more anterior and superior position.
- The indications for an emergency thoracotomy are listed in Table 45.1.

TABLE 45.1: Indications for emergent operating room thoracotomy

Immediate drainage >1500 mL (20 mL/kg)
Ongoing drainage >200 mL/hr (3 mL/kg/hr) for 2–4 hr
Continuous blood transfusion needed to maintain hemodynamic stability

Special Considerations

- Empyema and fibrothorax are delayed complications of hemothorax and can be the result of poor early management, specifically inadequate drainage of accumulated blood. A follow-up chest x-ray after tube placement should be assessed for proper tube placement and resolution of hemothorax.

Current Concepts/Evidence

Do prophylactic antibiotics prevent the occurrence of empyema or pneumonia after chest tube placement?

No. In a prospective, randomized, double-blind trial, prophylactic antibiotics (cefazolin) did not significantly affect the incidence of empyema or pneumonia. Duration of tube placement and penetrating injuries were predictive of empyema ($p < 0.05$) and blunt trauma correlated significantly more with pneumonia ($p < 0.05$).

Suggested Readings

Eckstein M, Henderson S. Thoracic trauma. In: Marx JA, ed. *Rosen's Emergency Medicine: Concepts and Clinical Practice*, 6th ed. Mosby: Philadelphia, 2006:453–486.

Kirsh TD, Mulligan JP. Tube thoracostomy. In: Roberts JR, ed. *Clinical Procedures in Emergency Medicine*, 4th ed. Philadelphia: Saunders, 2004:187–208.

Maxwell RA, Campbell DJ, Fabian TC, et al. Use of presumptive antibiotics following tube thoracostomy for traumatic hemopneumothorax in the prevention of empyema and pneumonia—a multi-center trial. *J Trauma*. 2004;57(4):742–748; discussion 748–749.

46

Pulmonary Contusion

Jonathan Kirschner

Definition

- Pulmonary contusion is an injury to the lung parenchyma characterized by alveolar hemorrhage and edema and the loss of normal lung structure and function.
- It is the most common injury identified in blunt chest trauma.
- Nearly 20% of blunt trauma patients with multiple injuries will have pulmonary contusions.
- Acute respiratory distress syndrome (ARDS), atelectasis, and pneumonia are potential complications.
- Mortality is 10–25% and increases to 42% if flail chest is present. Roughly 50% of patients with pulmonary contusions will require mechanical ventilation (Fig. 46.1).

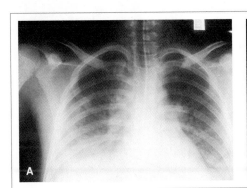 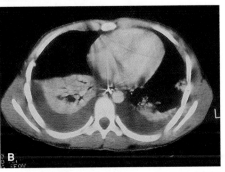

FIGURE 46.1: A 15-year-old child involved in an autopedestrian accident. Vital signs were stable at the scene, but the child had decreased breath sounds bilaterally. **A:** The chest radiograph shows bilateral hemothorax and pulmonary contusions. **B:** Computed tomography confirmed and better delineated hemothorax and pulmonary contusions. (Reprinted with permission from Fleisher GR, Ludwig S, Baskin MN. *Atlas of Pediatric Emergency Medicine*. Philadelphia: Lippincott Williams & Wilkins, 2004.)

Pathophysiology

- Pulmonary contusions occur most commonly via rapid deceleration, such as a motor vehicle collision or fall. Less common mechanisms are blast injury or high-velocity missile.
- Direct bruising of the lung and shearing forces cause alveolar edema and hemorrhage leading to alveolar collapse characterized by:
  - Increased mucus production and decreased mucociliary clearance.
  - Decreased compliance and increased pulmonary vascular resistance result in impaired gas exchange.

Diagnosis

- **Most significant contusions are visible on chest x-ray (CXR).**
- Clinical manifestations include dyspnea, tachypnea, tachycardia, hypoxia, hypotension, and hemoptysis. Auscultation may reveal diminished breath sounds or moist rales.

- Symptoms may be noted on initial presentation or may develop over 24–48 hours.
- Consider pulmonary contusion when rib fractures are present, especially flail chest; however, severe contusions are possible without associated rib fractures as the elastic chest wall transmits forces to the lungs.
- CXR findings range from focal to diffuse opacities that do not necessarily conform to a specific lobe or segment.
- Initial CXR detects pulmonary contusion about one-third of the time and often underestimates the severity. Most significant contusions will be present on CXR within 6 hours of injury.
- Computed tomography is more sensitive in the early phase of pulmonary contusion; however, additional findings generally do not impact clinical management (Fig. 46.2).

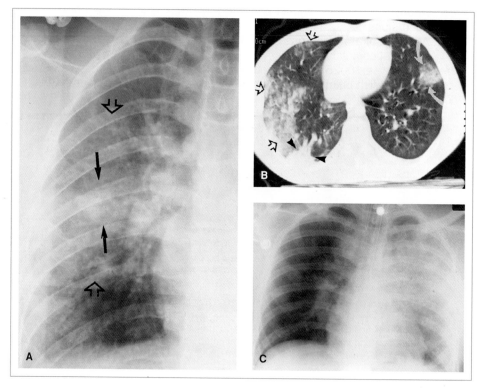

FIGURE 46.2: Mild pulmonary contusion limited to the right midlung zone (open arrows, **A**). Only in the center of the contusion is a smaller, discrete area of focal consolidation (arrows) which could represent an area of more severe contusion or a hematoma. The peripheral location of the pulmonary contusion is shown by computed tomography (CT) (open arrows, **B**). CT also shows that the area of increased density thought to be a focal hematoma on the PA CXR film is actually a focal area of atelectasis (arrowheads) posterior to the contusion. CT also shows a focal contusion of the left lung (curved arrows) not recorded on the CXR film. **C:** Extensive, severe pulmonary contusion involving the area of the majority of the left upper lobe and the atypical segment of the left lower lobe. (Reprinted with permission from Harris JH, Harris WH. *The Radiology of Emergency Medicine*, 4th ed. Philadelphia: Lippincott Williams & Wilkins, 2000.)

Evaluation

- Initial evaluation and stabilization should follow standard trauma management. Greater than 80% of patients with pulmonary contusions have additional injuries.

- Look for related injuries such as rib fractures and maintain a high index of suspicion for both intrathoracic and extrathoracic injuries.
- Serial examinations to assess for progressively increased work of breathing and hypoxia are critical as patients with severe contusions may develop the need for mechanical ventilation.
- A repeat CXR at 6 hours or later generally identifies a delayed pulmonary contusion.

Management
- **The hallmark of pulmonary contusion treatment is supportive care.**
- Pain control for chest wall injury is vital to maintain pulmonary function.
- Fluid resuscitation should be targeted to achieving euvolemia. Fluid overload may worsen pulmonary function, while hypovolemia is associated with ARDS.
- Supplemental oxygen may be required as respiratory function can decline over the initial 24–48 hours.
- Vigorous pulmonary toilet and suctioning may shorten symptom duration.
- Neither prophylactic antibiotics nor steroids are indicated.
- Endotracheal intubation may be necessary and seems to correlate with the volume of contused lung. Intubation should be done only when aggressive supportive care fails, as it is associated with significant morbidity including pneumonia, sepsis, pneumothorax, and longer hospitalization.
- Pulmonary contusions typically resolve over 5–7 days. Pulmonary fibrosis occurs in some patients, which may permanently impair pulmonary function.
- Any patient with pulmonary contusions noted on CXR film should be admitted to monitor respiratory function, as worsening over the next 24 hours is common.

Special Considerations
- Differentiate pulmonary contusion from ARDS or aspiration pneumonitis. **ARDS** is diffuse and onset is delayed 24–72 hours from injury. **Aspiration pneumonitis** will conform to a segment or lobe. **Pulmonary contusions** may cross lobes or segment boundaries.
- Pulmonary contusions are more common in pediatric patients because the chest wall is more flexible and stretches because of external forces transmitting greater force to the lung, whereas the elderly patients with stiff, thin chest walls are prone to rib fractures.
- Elderly patients have much higher morbidity and mortality with pulmonary contusions.

Current Concepts/Evidence
The size of the pulmonary contusion correlates with clinical severity and computed tomographic scan accurately quantifies the extent of the contusion. Should routine computed tomography be performed to aid in management and predict the need for intubation?
One study found that in patients with pulmonary contusion involving more than 20% of the total lung volume, 82% developed ARDS, whereas only 22% developed ARDS if the contusion was less than 20%. In addition, another study reported that all patients with pulmonary contusions more that 28% required intubation compared with no intubations in patients with contusions less than 18%. Prospective studies have shown, however, that chest computed tomography obtained for the sole purpose of assessing the pulmonary contusion does not change management or outcome. **Bottom line:** clinical status is the ultimate determinant for intubation, and computed tomographic findings do not generally influence this assessment.

Suggested Readings

Cohn SM. Pulmonary contusion: review of the clinical entity. *J Trauma*. 1997;42: 973–979.

Eckstein M, Henderson S. Thoracic trauma. In: Marx JA, Hockberger RS, Walls RM, et al, eds. *Rosen's Emergency Medicine: Concepts and Clinical Practice*, 6th ed. Philadelphia: Mosby Elsevier, 2006:453–488.

Miller PR, Croce MA, Bee TK, et al. ARDS after pulmonary contusion: accurate measurement of contusion volume identifies high risk patients. *J Trauma*. 2001; 51:223–230.

Wagner RB, Crawford WO Jr, Schimpf PP, et al. Quantitation and pattern of parenchymal lung injury in blunt chest trauma: diagnostic and therapeutic implications. *J Comput Tomogr*. 1988;12:270–281.

Wanek S, Mayberry JC. Blunt thoracic trauma: flail chest, pulmonary contusion, and blast injury. *Crit Care Clin*. 2004;20:71–81.

47

Pericardial Tamponade

Sonya Seccurro

Definition

- Cardiac tamponade is defined as the critical compression of the heart by the accumulation of blood in the pericardial space (Fig. 47.1).
- Penetrating thoracic trauma, most commonly stab wounds to the midchest, is the primary cause of cardiac tamponade in the trauma patient.
- Blunt thoracic trauma is an uncommon cause of tamponade.

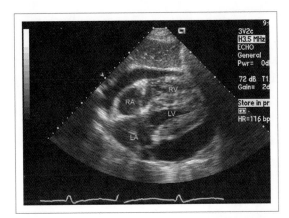

FIGURE 47.1: Subcostal echocardiogram reveals a moderate to large pericardial effusion. Note the effusion surrounding the entire heart, with its greatest dimension lateral to the left ventricular free wall. Fluid is clearly seen surrounding the right atrium (RA) and between the pericardium and right ventricle (RV). LA, left atrium; LV, left ventricle. (Reprinted with permission from Feigenbaum H. *Feigenbaum's Echocardiography*, 6th ed. Philadelphia: Lippincott Williams & Wilkins, 2005.)

Pathophysiology

- The rapid accumulation of blood in the relatively noncompliant pericardial space increases intrapericardial pressure restricting diastolic filling of the right ventricle. Left ventricular filling is ultimately compromised leading to decreased stroke volume and decreased cardiac output.
- Increased heart rate, increased peripheral vascular resistance, and inotropy occur as compensatory mechanisms to restore cardiac output.
- Cardiogenic shock will eventually occur if the tamponade progresses.
- As little as 80 mL of blood in the acute setting may result in a critical reduction of cardiac output.

Diagnosis

- An electrocardiogram may show decreased amplitude or electrical alternans. Some patients may have normal electrocardiograms and still others may present with pulseless electrical activity.

- Chest x-ray may reveal a globular-shaped heart, though this is more commonly seen with chronic accumulation because of medical nontraumatic pathology.
- Echocardiography has emerged as the diagnostic tool of choice to aid in the detection of pericardial fluid as it is noninvasive and available at the bedside. Multiple studies have shown sensitivities of >90% and specificities of >85%. While this modality is operator dependent, our experience has shown this skill to be easily learned by the emergency department (ED) physician with minimal to moderate didactics (Fig. 47.2).
- The subxiphoid pericardial window, a surgical procedure performed under general anesthesia, remains the gold standard for the diagnosis of cardiac injury and pericardial effusion.

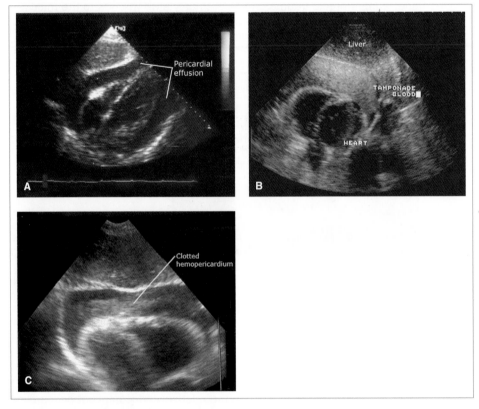

FIGURE 47.2: A: Ultrasound image demonstrating a circumferential pericardial effusion viewed from the subxiphoid transducer position. **B, C:** Images demonstrating clotted hemopericardium. (Reprinted with permission from Cosby KS, Kendall JL. *Practical Guide to Emergency Ultrasound.* Philadelphia: Lippincott Williams & Wilkins, 2005.)

Evaluation

- Unexplained hypotension in the trauma patient should be assumed to be hemorrhagic shock; however, in a patient who is unresponsive to resuscitative efforts, suspicion should be raised for cardiac tamponade.
- **Beck's triad** of distended neck veins, hypotension, and muffled heart tones are "classic" findings but are present in only 40% of patients. Hypovolemic patients may not demonstrate distended neck veins and muffled heart sounds are incredibly difficult to appreciate in a noisy trauma room.

TABLE 47.1: Emergency department management of cardiac tamponade

	Treatment	
Patient condition	**Nontrauma center**	**Trauma center**
Stable	Fluid boluses	Fluid boluses
Unstable	Pericardiocentesis	ED or OR thoracotomy (preferably)
Cardiac arrest	ED thoracotomy or pericardiocentesis	ED thoracotomy

ED, emergency department; OR, operating room.

- Other findings associated with cardiac tamponade include **pulsus paradoxus** (>10 mm Hg drop in blood pressure during inspiration) and **Kussmaul's sign** (increase in jugular venous distention during inspiration).

Management

- Fluid bolus therapy may transiently increase the right atrial filling pressure and increase cardiac output for a brief period as a temporizing measure while preparing for more definitive treatment.
- Most patients with penetrating chest trauma and a bedside ultrasound positive for pericardial fluid should be managed in the operating room for exploration and repair of the pericardium and heart.
- Pericardiocentesis using either an over-the-needle catheter or Seldinger technique is an emergency procedure that can be a lifesaving bridge to definitive operative management.
- ED thoracotomy should be performed in the patient with suspected tamponade who goes into arrest in the ambulance or ED. The pericardium should be incised, blood and clot evacuated, and obvious cardiac injuries repaired (Table 47.1).

Special Considerations

- The presence of a pericardial effusion does not signify tamponade; rather tamponade is a clinical diagnosis that implies some degree of hemodynamic compromise.
- Bedside emergency cardiac ultrasound is a rapid and noninvasive way to assess the pericardial space for effusion and signs of tamponade.
- Since as little as 80 mL of fluid can cause tamponade, a normal cardiac silhouette on chest x-ray does not rule out cardiac tamponade.

Current Concepts/Evidence

What is the demonstrated value of ED cardiac sonography for the patient with tamponade?

One early study suggests that a much earlier time to diagnosis of acute cardiac injury is possible with ultrasound: 42 minutes (no sonography) versus 15 minutes (sonography). Not surprisingly, this translated into a survival benefit: 57% versus 100%. Although the study was small (49 total patients) and retrospective, it clearly demonstrates the power of bedside ultrasonography for diagnosing pericardial effusion.

Plummer D, Brunnette D, Asinger R, Ruiz E. Emergency department echocardiography improves outcome in penetrating cardiac injury. *Ann Em Med*. 1992;21:709–712.

Can emergency medicine (EM) physicians reliably diagnose fluid in the pericardium?
Yes. One recent study had EM physicians with simple training (16-hour sonography course including 5 hours specifically devoted to echocardiography) prospectively evaluate patients at high risk for cardiac effusion (all causes). EM physician ultrasounds were recorded and the studies were subsequently overread by an echocardiologist. Of 478 patients, 103 were deemed to have fluid in the pericardium. EM physician ultrasound interpretations had a sensitivity of 96% and a specificity of 98% in the detection of fluid.

Suggested Readings

Asensio JA, Soto SN, Forno W, et al. Penetrating cardiac injuries: a complex challenge. *Injury*. 2001;32:533–543.

Mandavia DP, Hoffner RJ, Mahaney K, Henderson SO. Bedside echocardiography by emergency physicians. *Ann Emerg Med*. 2001;38(4):377–382.

Rowe BH, ed. *Evidence-Based Emergency Medicine*. West-Sussex, UK: Wiley-Blackwell, 2009:363–372.

Roy CL, Minor MA, Brookhart MA, Choudhry NK. Does this patient with a pericardial effusion have tamponade? *JAMA*. 2007;297(16):1810–1818.

Spodick DH. Pathophysiology of cardiac tamponade. *Chest*. 1998;113:1372–1378.

48

Myocardial Contusion

Sarah Lannum

Definition
- Myocardial contusion, also known as blunt cardiac injury, is caused by severe closed-chest trauma from deceleration injuries, blast injuries, or direct blows.
- The reported incidence in blunt chest trauma is variable; when a significant mechanism exists the incidence is probably ~10%.
- The right ventricle is the most commonly injured area of the heart secondary to its vulnerable location beneath the sternum.
- Clinically important sequelae include life-threatening arrhythmias and cardiac failure.

Pathophysiology
- The myocardium is injured when blunt force compresses it within the thoracic cage. Physiologic changes such as intramyocardial hemorrhage, edema, and myocardial necrosis may occur.
- Complications include coronary artery laceration, acute valvular dysfunction, ventricular dysfunction with congestive heart failure, and most commonly, arrhythmia.

Diagnosis
- Identifying the patient with myocardial contusion remains a diagnostic challenge. There is no gold standard for making this diagnosis. **Clinical suspicion along with electrocardiogram (ECG), cardiac enzymes, and echocardiogram may aid in making the diagnosis.**
- Patients who sustain a myocardial contusion usually have external evidence of chest trauma and complain of chest pain.
- ECG abnormalities, which occur in 40–85% of patients with a myocardial contusion, include signs of myocardial injury (ST elevation and Q waves), nonspecific ST and T wave changes, conduction disorders, and arrhythmias (supraventricular dysrhythmias, atrial fibrillation, and ventricular fibrillation/tachycardia).
- Troponin is a useful diagnostic test for myocardial contusion as it is highly sensitive and specific for myocardial injury and is released only after disruption of myocardial cell membrane. The lapse in time between chest wall trauma and detectable elevation of troponin in the blood has not been determined, so a similar approach to acute myocardial infarction patients is advocated.
- Evidence suggests that the combination of a normal ECG and troponin (done at arrival, 4 and 8 hours) has a very high negative predictive value for ruling out myocardial contusion of consequence and its subsequent complications.
- Performing an echocardiogram in patients with suspected myocardial contusion may be useful as contused heart muscle will have a similar appearance to infarcted tissue and subtle wall motion abnormalities can be detected.

Echocardiogram can also show valvular lesions and possible septal rupture. Transesophageal echo is superior to transthoracic for evaluation but is generally difficult to obtain in a trauma patient in the initial emergency department setting.

Evaluation

- The patient with blunt trauma and concern for myocardial contusion is at risk for other chest injuries: pneumothorax, hemothorax, pulmonary contusion, and rib and sternal fractures. The physical examination should begin by focusing on identifying or ruling out these injuries.
- Findings suggestive of significant chest injury include jugular venous distention (JVD), tachypnea, ecchymosis, "seat belt sign" (imprint of the seat belt on the skin), palpable crepitus, clinically evident rib and sternal fractures, and distant heart sounds.
- An upright chest x-ray should be the first step in any workup of a patient with chest trauma.

Management

- Patients who sustain myocardial contusions are usually victims of multisystem trauma and should immediately be assessed clinically to determine whether they are hemodynamically stable. Unstable patients need a full trauma workup and admission.
- Consider consultations from cardiology and trauma surgery, especially for those patients who are admitted. Patients should be admitted for observation to a monitored setting as arrhythmias are the most common and dangerous sequelae.
- Most arrhythmias will occur within 24–48 hours of admission. Ventricular fibrillation is the most common cause of death.
- Serial normal ECGs and troponins at arrival and at 6–8 hours appear to rule out clinically significant myocardial contusion. Patients who meet such criteria can probably be safely discharged home.

Special Considerations

Risk factors for clinically significant blunt chest trauma:

- Age older than 50 years
- Frontal impact
- Multiple rib fractures
- Multisystem trauma (including chest trauma)
- History of cardiac disease

Current Concepts/Evidence

Should all patients with significant blunt chest injury undergo routine echocardiography?

The current consensus opinion is no.

Karalis et al. (1994) prospectively evaluated 105 consecutive patients with severe blunt chest trauma (Abbreviated Injury Scale of ≥2) with routine transthoracic echocardiograms (TTE). Transesophageal echocardiography was performed when TTE was suboptimal. Myocardial contusions were detected in 24 patients, an additional seven contusions were found on transesophageal echocardiography that were missed on TTE. Cardiac events occurred in 8 of 31 patients with contusions versus 2 of 74 patients

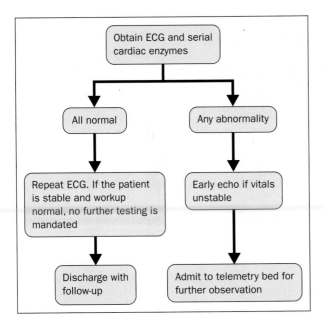

FIGURE 48.1: Algorithm for management of blunt chest trauma patients with suspected myocardial contusion.

with normal echocardiograms. The echocardiograms added value only to patients with hemodynamic instability or arrhythmias and had minimal prognostic use; the authors recommend routine echocardiography only for these groups (Fig. 48.1).

Suggested Readings

Bansal MK, Maraj S, Chewaproug D, Amanullah A. Myocardial contusion injury: redefining the diagnostic algorithm. *Emerg Med J.* 2005;22:465–469.

Jackson L, Stewart A. Best evidence topics: use of troponin for the diagnosis of myocardial contusion after blunt chest trauma. *Emerg Med J.* 2005;22:193–195.

Karalis DG, Victor MF, Davis GA, et al. The role of echocardiography in blunt chest trauma: a transthoracic and transesophageal echocardiographic study. *J Trauma.* 1994;36:53–58.

Maenza RL, Seaberg D, D'Amico F. A meta-analysis of blunt cardiac trauma. *Am J Emerg Med.* 1996;14:237–241.

Miller PR, Croce MA, Bee TK, et al. ARDS after pulmonary contusion: accurate measurement of contusion volume identifies high risk patients. *J Trauma.* 2001;51:223–230.

Salim A, Velmahos GC, Jindal A. Clinically significant blunt cardiac trauma: role of serum troponin levels combined with electrocardiographic findings. *J Trauma.* 2001;50:237–243.

Sybrandy KC, Cramer MJM, Burgersdijk C. Diagnosing cardiac contusion: old wisdom and new insights. *Heart.* 2003;89:485–489.

Wagner RB, Crawford WO Jr, Schimpf PP, et al. Quantitation and pattern of parenchymal lung injury in blunt chest trauma: diagnostic and therapeutic implications. *J Comput Tomogr.* 1988;12:270–281.

49

Aortic Trauma

May Li

Definition

- Aortic injury is usually the result of blunt trauma, often after sudden deceleration as in a high-speed motor vehicle collision (MVC) or fall from significant height.
- In blunt trauma, the descending thoracic aorta is the most commonly injured segment.

Epidemiology

- Blunt aortic injury accounts for 16% of MVC deaths and is second only to head injury as the cause of death in MVCs.
- For blunt aortic injuries, the most common crash impact is head-on (72%), followed by side impact (24%) and rear impact (4%).
- Up to 85% of aortic injury patients die before reaching the hospital. Of the 15% who reach the hospital, 15% die in the first hour and 30% in the first 6 hours.
- The majority of patients who reach the hospital alive survive if prompt diagnosis and treatment occur.

Pathophysiology

- Eighty percent to 85% of aortic tears occur in the descending aorta at the isthmus— the junction between the fixed and mobile parts of the aorta just distal to the left subclavian artery. Traditional theories postulate that sudden deceleration causes the mobile aortic arch to lurch forward and tear away from the tethered descending aorta.
- When rupture occurs, the usual result is immediate death. In surviving patients, the tear is usually partial (of the intima and media, but not the adventitia). Clotting within the remaining wall and formation of pseudoaneurysm may tamponade further bleeding.

Diagnosis

- Common symptoms are nonspecific: chest pain, back pain, dyspnea, and cough.
- Signs of aortic injury are uncommon (isolated upper or lower extremity hypertension or widened pulse pressure) or nonspecific (generalized hypertension or precordial systolic murmur).
- Acute coarctation syndrome, combination of upper extremity hypertension with concurrent absent or diminished lower extremity pulses, may be present.
- Patients with aortic injury usually present with multiple fractures or injuries, a high index of suspicion is necessary to make the diagnosis.
- Aortography remains the gold standard in identifying aortic injury. However, its invasiveness and need for special services make it impractical in most emergency departments.

TABLE 49.1: Traumatic aortic injury chest x-ray findings

Widened mediastinum
Pleural apical cap
Abnormality of the aortic arch
Loss of the aortopulmonary window (e.g., obscuring of the aortic knob)
Tracheal shift to the right
Left paraspinal line widening (without fracture)
Deviation of the nasogastric tube to the right
Widened paratracheal stripe
Upper rib fractures

- Chest x-ray (CXR) is valuable as a screening tool. On CXR, subjective assessment of a **widened mediastinum** (rather than adherence to strict criteria about diameter) is a sensitive (but nonspecific) marker for aortic injury. Table 49.1 lists the other less common findings that suggest a possible aortic injury (Fig. 49.1).

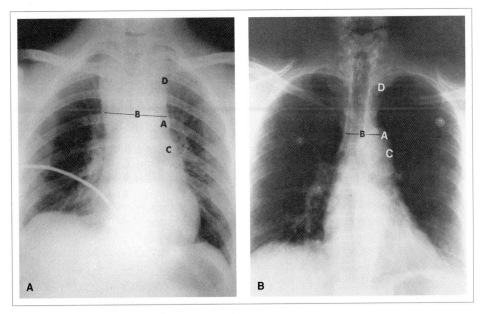

FIGURE 49.1: Upright posteroanterior chest radiographs of a 20-year-old man involved as a driver in a head-on motor vehicle collision (A) compared with that of a normal person (B). The first radiograph has several abnormalities suggestive of a great vessel disruption. (A) Loss of detail of aortic knob with blurring of the aortic outline. (B) Widened mediastinum (mediastinal width to chest width ratio >0.28). (C) Opacification of the clear space between the aorta and pulmonary artery (aortopulmonary window). (D) Obliteration of the medial aspect of the left upper field. The aortogram revealed rupture of the aortic arch. (Radiographs courtesy of the Department of Radiology, St. Luke's Hospital, Milwaukee, WI.) (Reprinted with permission from Wolfson AB, Hendey GW, Ling LJ, et al. *Harwood-Nuss' Clinical Practice of Emergency Medicine,* 5th ed. Philadelphia: Lippincott Williams & Wilkins, 2009.)

- Helical computed tomography of the thorax has a high sensitivity (83–100%) and specificity (54–100%) in identifying aortic injury. It has become the test of choice for making this diagnosis and should be performed in all patients with mechanisms that evoke a high index of suspicion for aortic injury and in those with suspicious findings on CXR film (Fig. 49.2).

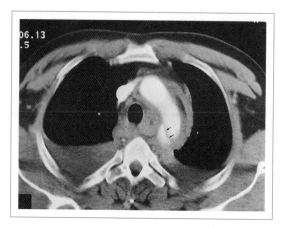

FIGURE 49.2: Computed tomographic image at the level of the aortic knob demonstrates an intimal flap in the descending aorta (arrows). Notice the mediastinal widening from unopacified blood. (Reprinted with permission from Daffner RH. *Clinical Radiology: The Essentials,* 3rd ed. Philadelphia: Lippincott Williams & Wilkins, 2007.)

Management

- Once the diagnosis of severe aortic injury is made, immediate consultation with vascular or trauma surgeon is required as operative repair is indicated. In patients with multisystem injuries (e.g., intracranial bleeding, intra-abdominal or pelvic exsanguination, or severe lung injury), a delayed approach to aortic repair (while addressing the other life-threatening injuries) has been successful.
- If aortic repair is delayed, a regimen of beta-blockers and antihypertensives might help decrease shearing forces on the partially torn aortic wall. Esmolol with or without nitroprusside is usually preferred because these short-acting medications can be quickly turned off if hypotension occurs.
- There are several surgical repair techniques; however, endovascular grafting is an increasingly popular approach that is minimally invasive. Studies comparing efficacy to open thoracotomy are limited.

Special Considerations

- Patients can have "minimal aortic injury," which usually refers to a situation in which the patient is stable but there are various findings on computed tomographic (CT) scan:
  - Small intimal flap without periaortic hematoma
  - Small pseudoaneurysm
- The optimal management of these patients is unknown. Most sources advocate observation, as emergent surgery is usually not warranted.

Best Evidence

Many centers are now "pan-scanning" (head/spine/chest/abdomen/pelvis CT imaging) trauma patients with significant mechanisms. Is there evidence to support CT scan of the chest of patients with normal CXRs?

There is no clear evidence to tell us which patients mandate chest CT imaging. Clearly, all trauma patients with a significant mechanism of injury and an abnormal CXR should receive chest computed tomography angiography; mechanism and suspicion for injury currently guide the use of computed tomography in patients with normal CXRs.

More than 90% of patients with aortic injury have abnormal CXRs (usually manifesting as mediastinal abnormalities such as widening, loss of the aortopulmonary window, or blunting of the aortic knob). Unfortunately, the CXR will miss some aortic injuries and other studies have shown that up to 5% of patients with aortic injury have completely normal initial CXRs.

Suggested Readings

Mirvis SE, Shanmuganathan K. Diagnosis of blunt traumatic aortic injury 2007: still a nemesis. *Eur J Rad.* 2007;64:27–40.

Neschis DG, Scalea TM, Flinn WR, Griffith BP. Blunt aortic injury. *N Engl J Med.* 2008;359:1708–1716.

O'Conor CE. Diagnosing traumatic rupture of the thoracic aorta in the emergency department. *Emerg Med J.* 2004;21:414–419.

Raptopolous V, Sheiman RG, Phillips DA, et al. Traumatic aortic tear: screening with chest CT. *Radiology.* 1992;182:667–673.

Takagi H, Kawai N, Umemoto T. A meta-analysis of comparative studies of endovascular versus open repair for blunt thoracic aortic injury. *J Thorac Cardiovasc Surg.* 2008;135:1392–1394.

50

Diaphragmatic Trauma

Lisa Fort

Definition/Background
- There is a spectrum of traumatic diaphragm injuries, the most severe of which is diaphragmatic rupture in which the contents of the abdominal cavity herniate into the pleural space.
- Seventy-five percent of diaphragmatic injuries are due to blunt trauma, usually associated with motor vehicle accidents and less frequently via falls and crush injuries. Approximately 1% of patients with significant blunt abdominal trauma have diaphragmatic injury.
- Penetrating trauma has a higher incidence of injury. Fifteen percent of lower thoracic stab wounds and 46% of lower thoracic gunshot wound are associated with diaphragmatic injury.
- Left-sided injuries are more common (>66%), because the stabilizing attachments are stronger on the right and the liver exerts a protective effect.
- Children, however, have equal rates of rupture per side, likely due to the laxity of liver attachments.
- The diagnosis of diaphragmatic injury is often delayed. About 40% are made preoperatively, 40% discovered on surgical exploration, and 15% of diagnoses are delayed.
- The mortality is 17% when diagnosed in the acute phase, mostly due to pulmonary complications.

Pathophysiology
- The diaphragm is an essential respiratory muscle and also functions as a dome-shaped septum to divide the abdominal and thoracic organs. Cervical motor roots C3, C4, and C5 control the diaphragm. Contraction drops intrathoracic pressure and facilitates chest wall expansion, allowing air to rush into the lungs during inspiration.
- Diaphragmatic rupture has physiologic consequences on the respiratory, circulatory, and digestive systems.
  - Respiratory distress or dyspnea is caused by insufficient expansion of the chest wall via pressure equalization and direct compression of lung by herniated contents.
  - Circulatory collapse via cardiac tamponade is possible if herniated contents involve the pericardium.
  - Bowel may become strangulated and even perforate in a tear in the diaphragm causing obstruction or sepsis.

Diagnosis
- No imaging modality approaches 100% sensitivity. Accordingly, many injuries are missed in the acute phase. The vague and inconsistent clinical presentation adds to the diagnostic dilemma. Ultimately, if there is a high index of suspicion for this injury and imaging modalities are inconclusive, injury must be excluded via exploratory laparoscopy or laparotomy.

190

- Chest radiography
  - Approximately 35% of ruptured diaphragms can be diagnosed from the initial chest radiograph.
  - Classic findings include soft-tissue opacification which may have the radiographic appearance of gas, bowel pattern, or pneumothorax once the bowel is perforated.
  - If a nasogastric tube has been placed it may be identified in the chest if the stomach has herniated.
  - Compression atelectasis of the lower lobe of the lung may be seen.
  - Mediastinal shift in the absence of pneumothorax is sometimes seen, as well as an elevated diaphragm or irregularity of the diaphragmatic outline.
  - Associated injuries may obscure the findings, and herniation at the costophrenic angle is often misinterpreted as a hemothorax or pneumothorax, leading to chest tube placement into the herniated organs.
  - In delayed or missed presentations, the stomach may appear to be a subphrenic abscess, and a herniated kidney may appear as an intrathoracic mass (Figs. 50.1 and 50.2).

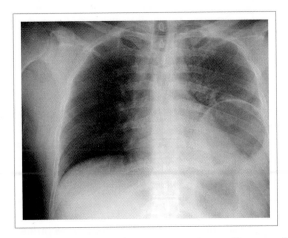

FIGURE 50.1: Rupture of the left hemidiaphragm. Chest x-ray film demonstrates an "elevated left hemidiaphragm" but the line may actually be the fundus of the stomach projecting through the diaphragmatic tear. (Reprinted with permission from Greenberg MI, Hendrickson RG, Silverberg M, et al. *Greenberg's Text-Atlas of Emergency Medicine*. Philadelphia: Lippincott Williams & Wilkins, 2005.)

- Fluoroscopy/barium studies
  - Often useful to interpret in conjunction with the initial chest x-ray, especially if the case is suspicious for diaphragmatic rupture.
- Computed tomography (CT) with contrast
  - CT is the most useful and reliable tool for detecting traumatic diaphragm injuries.
  - It can used to detect up to 78% of left-sided and 50% of right-sided injuries. If the patient is relatively stable, the studies can be performed and interpreted quickly (Table 50.1).
  - Associated injuries are also easily evaluated with CT, as are indirect signs of herniation such as abnormal liver position.

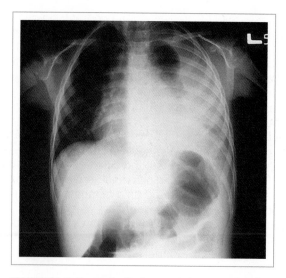

FIGURE 50.2: Traumatic diaphragmatic hernia. This 5-year-old boy was on a snowmobile when it crashed into a tree. He was tachypneic, but his breath sounds were reportedly normal. The chest radiograph shows a left-sided diaphragmatic hernia. (Reprinted with permission from Fleisher GR, Ludwig S, Baskin MN. *Atlas of Pediatric Emergency Medicine*. Philadelphia: Lippincott Williams & Wilkins, 2004.)

Evaluation

- Grimes suggested a classification system that divides diaphragmatic injuries into acute, latent, and obstructive phases.
  - *Acute phase*—begins with the injury and associated injuries and ends with apparent recovery from initial injuries.
    - ▶ Clinical features may include abdominal pain, respiratory distress, and cardiac dysfunction/tamponade.
    - ▶ Delayed diagnosis of diaphragm injury is more frequent in unstable patients and those with multiple associated injuries.
  - *Latent phase*—when visceral compression or herniation becomes involved in the injury.
    - ▶ Clinical features include upper gastrointestinal discomfort, epigastric pain, left upper quadrant or chest pain, referred pain in the left shoulder, dyspnea, orthopnea, and decreased breath sounds. These symptoms may prompt additional workup and diagnosis.

TABLE 50.1: Computed tomography findings of diaphragmatic injury

Diaphragmatic discontinuity
Intrathoracic herniation of organs
"Collar sign"—constriction of abdominal viscera
Avulsions or hemiavulsions
Omental herniation

- *Obstructive phase*—indicative of visceral obstruction or ischemia.
    - ▷ Clinical features include nausea and vomiting, severe unrelenting abdominal pain, respiratory distress, fever, and septic shock.
    - ▷ Borchardt's triad of retching, inability to pass nasogastric tube (NGT), and abdominal pain may be present.
    - ▷ Chest x-ray findings at this point may show mediastinal shift (Fig. 50.3).

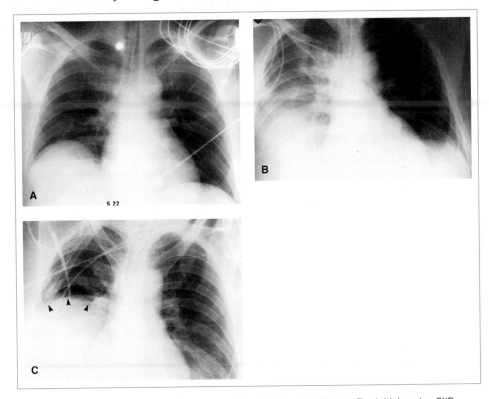

FIGURE 50.3: Missed acute traumatic rupture of the right hemidiaphragm. The initial supine CXR film **(A)** of a patient involved in a major motor vehicle collision obtained in the emergency center was interpreted as showing only elevation of the right hemidiaphragm—the patient was unconscious and had no broken right ribs or other physical signs of blunt right thoracoabdominal trauma. The posttrauma supine CXR film obtained 24 hours later was interpreted as showing right lower lobe consolidation, possible pulmonary contusion, and right upper lobe aspiration pneumonitis. The diagnosis of acute traumatic rupture of the right hemidiaphragm was suggested on the supine CXR film obtained on the third posttrauma day **(B)** based on the greater degree of elevation of the right hemidiaphragm (arrowheads) in **(C)** compared with its position in **(A)**. At laparotomy, the right hemidiaphragm represented the dome of the liver herniated through a large diaphragmatic tear. (Reprinted with permission from Harris JH, Harris WH. *The Radiology of Emergency Medicine*, 4th ed. Philadelphia: Lippincott Williams & Wilkins, 2000.)

Management
- Initial resuscitation should be directed toward patient stabilization, primary and secondary survey, airway management, fluid resuscitation, and hemostasis.
- **Diaphragm injuries rarely occur without associated injuries.** The most common of these include pelvic fracture in up to 40%, splenic rupture in 25%, liver laceration in 25%, and thoracic aortic tear in 5–10%.
- The mainstay of treatment for diaphragmatic injury is surgical repair, and the injury is most often repaired via laparotomy.

Special Considerations

- Most diaphragmatic injuries occur in the setting of the severely injured patient. Initial emergency department care should focus on resuscitation and identifying immediate life-threatening injuries.
- Given this prerogative and the difficulty in diagnosis, it is not surprising that this injury is frequently missed. Diaphragmatic injury has significant morbidity, so a high index of suspicion should be maintained in those patients with a significant traumatic mechanism.

Best Evidence/Clinical Decision Rules

Current surgical trends in the management of blunt trauma are towards a decreased use of laparotomy in the hemodynamically stable patient. It follows that we will continue to miss diaphragmatic injuries, possibly now at an even higher rate. Should we be advocating for more laparascopies, or at least in certain specific scenarios?

There is no strong evidence to guide us in this area, making this problem all the more taxing. One small study from 1995 evaluated 133 patients with trauma (blunt and penetrating) who were hemodynamically stable and with clinically suspected abdominal injuries. 4 were found to have diaphragm injuries that were repaired intra-operatively. The cost of laparoscopy and its attendant risks will continue to reserve its indication and use for patients with high clinical suspicion for injury.

Suggested Readings

Grimes OF. Traumatic injuries of the diaphragm. Diaphragmatic hernia. *Am J Surg.* 1974;128(2):175–181.

Hanby WB. *The Case Reports and Autopsy Records of Ambroise Paré.* Springfield, IL: Thomas, 1968:50–51.

Schneider CF. Traumatic diaphragmatic hernia. *Am J Surg.* 1956;91:290–294.

Shah R, Sabanathan S, Mearns AJ, Choudhury AK. Traumatic rupture of the diaphragm. *Ann Thorac Surg.* 1995;60:1444–1449.

Smith RS, Ery WR, Morabito DJ, et al. Therapeutic laparoscopy in trauma. *Am J Surg.* 1995;170:632–637.

Section Editor: Leon Sanchez

51 Abdominal Trauma: The First 15 Minutes, Algorithm, and Decision Making

Erin R. Horn

The mechanism of injury, location of injury, and hemodynamic status of the patient determine the priority and the best method of abdominal assessment. Abdominal trauma can be usually split among blunt and penetrating injuries, with penetrating being further subdivided into stab wounds (SW) and gunshot wounds (GSW). **The care of these patients is often confounded by distracting injuries, intoxication or altered mental status, and lack of historical information.**

Blunt Abdominal Trauma

 THE FIRST
15 MINUTES

ABCs
- Check vital signs and determine stability.
- Follow ATLS guidelines and Blunt Abdominal Trauma Algorithm.

History
Most often results from motor vehicle collision and when combined with pedestrian versus auto accidents, accounts for approximately 75% of cases of blunt abdominal trauma (BAT). The remaining 25% comprises direct abdominal blows and falls.

Although often lacking, historical information may help guide management. If the trauma resulted from a motor vehicle collision, an attempt should be made to discern information regarding fatalities at the scene, vehicle type and velocity, use of seat belts and air bags, location within the vehicle, and damage to the vehicle.

Physical Examination
- All patients with BAT should be assumed to have significant abdominal injury as the accuracy of physical examination for diagnosing injury is between 55% and 65%.
- Intra-abdominal injury should be suspected in patients with altered mental status and significant extra-abdominal injuries.
- Hypotension from BAT most often results from injury to solid organs, especially the spleen, but often the liver or the kidney. It is also important to evaluate extra-abdominal sources of hemorrhage: scalp laceration, thoracic injury, long bone fracture, and in infants, severe head injury.

- In hemodynamically stable patients who are alert and without distracting injury, **abdominal pain, tenderness, and peritoneal signs are the most reliable findings and are found in approximately 90% of patients with visceral injury.**
- Abdominal wall ecchymosis, often called the "seat belt sign" indicates intra-abdominal injury in one-third of patients. Abdominal distention and decreased bowel sounds should prompt further exploration.

Laboratory Testing

- Mostly of limited use in the management of a BAT patient. Should be considered adjunct to care only.
- A blood type and cross match should be ordered if anticipating transfusion.
- Baseline hematocrit may be useful but rarely alters care. Can use serial hematocrits to assess ongoing hemorrhage.
- Base deficit or elevated serum lactate is a marker for hemorrhagic shock and should be obtained in the severely injured trauma patient. However, this data must be interpreted within the context of the current clinical picture as laboratory values often lag behind clinical improvement.
- Obtain a pregnancy test in all women of childbearing age.
- Further testing should be clinically correlated to the specific patient, that is, obtaining a coagulation panel for patients taking warfarin.

Emergency Interventions

- Hemodynamic status must be determined immediately. This is followed by ascertaining the need for immediate operative care. This assessment should be performed concurrently with resuscitation methods including two large-bore peripheral intravenous lines (IVs) and crystalloid infusion followed by blood products if necessary.
- Focused assessment with sonography for trauma (FAST) is the preferred diagnostic test over diagnostic peritoneal lavage (DPL) to triage unstable patients with BAT. FAST is quick, noninvasive, cheap, and can be performed at the bedside. It has reasonable sensitivity (65–95%) for detecting as little as 100 mL of intraperitoneal fluid. **A negative FAST does not rule out intra-abdominal injury and further diagnostic testing is required.**
- DPL which can be simplified to just a diagnostic peritoneal tap (DPT) is especially useful for identifying hollow viscus injury which will not typically be seen on a FAST examination. If 10 mL or more of blood is aspirated, an emergency laparotomy may be warranted.
- With the advent of the multidetector helical computed tomographic (CT) scanner, abdominal imaging has improved in speed and resolution. The benefits include the ability to define organ (spleen, liver, kidney) injury and thus, the potential for nonoperative management, as well concomitant assessment of the retroperitoneum and vertebral column. Computed tomography alone cannot reliably exclude injury to hollow viscus, diaphragm, or pancreas. In addition, the computed tomography is limited to use in hemodynamically stable patients.
- Plain radiographs may help determine the presence of extra-abdominal injury in the chest or pelvis, that is, pneumothorax, hemothorax, severe diaphragmatic rupture, or pelvic fractures.

Memorable Pearls

- Patients with pelvic fracture and hemoperitoneum requiring laparotomy may need temporary pelvic stabilization (sheet wrap or T-pod) until a more definitive external pelvic fixator can be placed in the operating room.

- Closed head injury can often complicate BAT. If a patient has lateralizing signs as well as hemodynamic instability, a burr hole can be placed concurrently with laparotomy in the operating room. A resuscitated patient without lateralizing signs can have a head CT scan concurrently with the abdominal CT scan.

 DECISION
MAKING

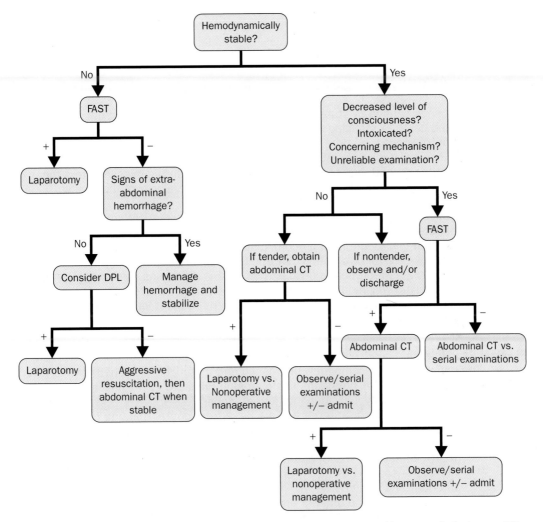

Blunt abdominal trauma: Decision making algorithm. FAST, focused assessment with sonography for trauma; DPL, diagnostic peritoneal lavage; CT, computed tomography.

Penetrating Abdominal Trauma

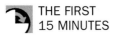
THE FIRST
15 MINUTES

ABCs
- Check vital signs and determine stability.
- Follow ATLS guidelines and either the Gunshot or Stab Wound Algorithm.

History
- Penetrating abdominal trauma (PAT) includes both stabbing and GSW. GSW, though three times less prevalent than SW, cause more than 90% of the mortality from PAT. GSWs cause greater tissue damage due to their higher velocity and force.
- The wounds caused by stabbing are determined by the instrument used and its path and depth. A stabbing implement tends to injure only the tissues through which it traverses.
- GSWs can inflict injury to intraperitoneal structures despite traversing an entirely extraperitoneal path due to energy waves created when the missile enters the body. The injury pattern of a GSW is dependent upon velocity of the missile as well as its path.
- The titles "low velocity" (i.e., SW) and "high velocity" (i.e., GSW) may be more appropriate given the number of different weapons used in today's crimes and the fact that injury pattern is predominantly dependent upon the velocity of the missile; however, for convention, SW and GSW will be employed.
- Shotgun wounds represent a special type of GSW. Shotguns have longer barrels and use pellets which decrease rapidly in velocity and disperse with distance. Overall, shotguns result in fewer mortalities with the most lethal shotgun wounds occurring at a distance of <2.7 meters (<3 yards).

Physical Examination
- The patient must be completely undressed and thoroughly examined for injury. **Wounds to the axilla, perineum, scalp, or skin folds are easily missed.**
- The abdominal cavity is divided into four anatomic zones:
  - Anterior abdomen: anterior axillary lines from costal margins to groin creases.
  - Thoracoabdominal area: the superior margin is bound by the nipple line (fourth intercostal space) anteriorly to the tips of the scapulae (seventh intercostal space) posteriorly and extends to the inferior costal margin anteriorly and posteriorly.
  - Flanks: between the anterior and posterior axillary lines from the inferior costal margins to the iliac crests.
  - Back: area between the posterior axillary lines from the tips of the scapulae to the iliac crests.
- The organ most commonly injured with SWs is the liver. With GSWs, the small bowel is most commonly injured.

Emergency Interventions
- Regardless of the type of PAT, immediate laparotomy is indicated for either hemodynamic instability or peritoneal signs on physical examination.

■   The most important principle of PAT, whether SW or GSW, is determining the presence of peritoneal violation and resulting intraperitoneal injury, which thus determines a need for laparotomy. The method for evaluating for violation differs somewhat between the two injury mechanisms.

■   Implement-in-situ, evisceration, and gastrointestinal bleeds associated with abdominal wounds are included as indications for surgical intervention as there is a high incidence of associated intra-abdominal injury (newer studies are beginning to challenge this idea).

■   If the implement-in-situ is in a patient with severe comorbidities or a pregnant patient, then laparotomy should be avoided if possible.

Stab Wounds

■   Peritoneal violation occurs in up to 70% of SWs, but only one-fourth to one-third of these will require operative management.

■   A combination of local wound exploration (LWE), CT, DPL, laparoscopy, and ultrasound may be able to select the stable patient without signs of peritonitis or evisceration for nonoperative management.

■   LWE can be performed at the bedside to evaluate a SW's depth and tract. LWE does not entail blind probing with fingers or cotton swabs but rather uses blunt and sharp dissection to determine whether the tract ends before the violation of the abdominal fascia. If the tract does not violate the peritoneum, the patient can be discharged after appropriate wound care. If termination of the tract cannot be clearly visualized further testing should ensue.

■   CT scan is a noninvasive method to determine peritoneal penetration and visceral injury and can also help plan both operative and nonoperative management. Newer studies suggest that only IV contrast is needed and that oral and rectal contrast be reserved for patients with potential colorectal injuries (i.e., stab wound to flank). As with BAT, a high suspicion for diaphragmatic, pancreatic, or bowel injuries should prompt further investigation despite a negative CT scan.

■   Ultrasound's role is continuing to evolve. A positive FAST may indicate injury but a negative FAST does not exclude an injury. In addition to looking for intraperitoneal fluid, in the future, bedside ultrasound may also be used to determine fascial violation.

■   DPL, although invasive, remains a sensitive way to obtain information regarding solid organ injury as well as bowel and diaphragmatic injury. There is some debate over the red blood cell count that should be used as the threshold for detecting injury.
  •   General agreement is that aspiration of 10 mL of blood or >10,000 red blood cell counts per high-powered field indicates visceral injury.
  •   A reduced range of 5,000–10,000 should be used when evaluating thoracoabdominal wounds as this increases the likelihood of identifying a bowel or diaphragmatic injury.

■   Direct laparoscopy has been proposed as a screening tool for evaluating the depth of the wound tract and inspecting the diaphragm. There is still controversy surrounding this method.

Gunshot Wounds

■   GSW to the abdomen requires laparotomy with few exceptions. Eighty-five percent of anterior GSWs penetrate the peritoneum and 95% require repair of an intra-abdominal injury.

■   Hemodynamic instability, peritoneal signs, and evisceration should prompt immediate laparotomy.

- LWE in GSWs is less helpful than in SWs as the missiles often destroy tissue making the tract hard to follow.
- If the event of a tangential abdominal GSW or unlikely peritoneal penetration, LWE, CT scan, and DPL can be considered to determine the need for laparotomy.
- CT scan is used to determine trajectory, organ injury, and can identify patients with injuries optimal for nonoperative management. Sensitivity and specificity is high even when IV contrast is used alone, but the addition of oral contrast may allow for better visualization of hollow viscus injuries.

 DECISION MAKING

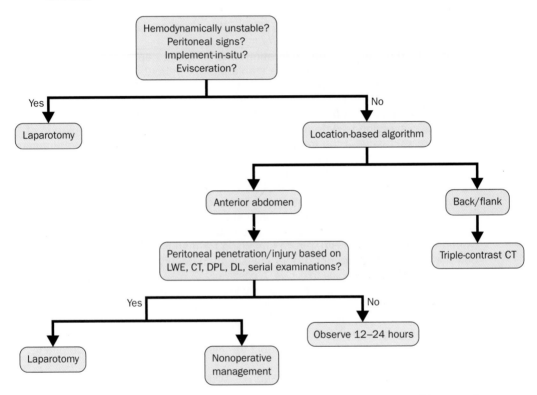

Abdominal/back stab wounds: Decision making algorithm. LWE, local wound exploration; CT, computed tomography; DPL, diagnostic peritoneal lavage; DL, direct laparoscopy.

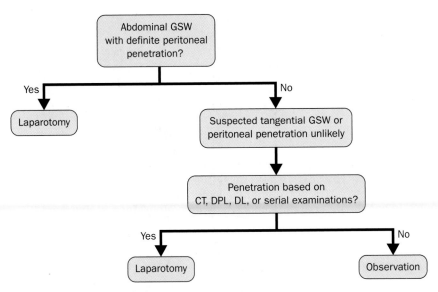

Abdominal gunshot wounds: Decision making algorithm. GSW, gunshot wounds; CT, computed tomography; DPL, diagnostic peritoneal lavage; DL, direct laparoscopy.

Memorable Pearls

- Flank, back, and thoracoabdominal wounds often involve more than one anatomic space and can be difficult to manage. If the patient is stable, CT scan is usually the best way to evaluate these patients.
- Two orthogonal plain radiographs with radio-opaque markers on any wounds can help elucidate the trajectory of the missile. If there are an odd number of wounds, x-ray film should also reveal the location of the missile.

52

Liver Trauma

Russell Evan Berger

Definition

- More than 75% of blunt liver trauma results from motor vehicle accidents, whereas an additional 15% results from falls. Direct blows to the abdomen represent approximately 10% of blunt abdominal trauma.
- Liver trauma is common. In patients undergoing laparotomy for a stab wound, 40% will have injury to the liver. In patients undergoing laparotomy for a gunshot wound, 30% will have injury to the liver.
- In addition, abdominal injuries from gunshot wounds account for 90% of the mortality associated with these injuries.
- Furthermore, hepatic trauma occurs in approximately 5% of all admissions from emergency departments.

Pathophysiology

- Blunt force applied along the anterior abdominal wall may compress the liver against the more rigid posterior thoracic cage or vertebral column, resulting in crushing of compressed tissue.
- In addition, deceleration injuries in which the liver continues to move after the body has stopped can produce tearing of the liver from its attachment to the diaphragm and lacerations of the liver capsule.
- Patients with hepatitis have softer, larger livers increasing their risk of hepatic injury from trauma. Elderly and alcoholic patients have lax abdominal walls allowing more compressive force to be applied to their abdominal viscera (Table 52.1).
- Morbidity and mortality of liver trauma is correlated with hemorrhagic shock and infectious complications following surgery.

Diagnosis

- **The liver is the most frequently injured intra-abdominal organ.**
- Liver trauma should be suspected in any trauma patient who complains of right upper quadrant (RUQ) pain or right shoulder pain.
- Patients with abdominal visceral injury present with local or generalized abdominal tenderness in 90% of cases.
- Definitive diagnosis requires intravenous (IV) contrast abdominal computed tomography (CT).

TABLE 52.1: High risk for liver trauma

Elderly
Alcoholics
Patients with hepatitis

TABLE 52.2: American Association for the Surgery of Trauma hepatic computed tomography injury grading scale

Grade 1	Laceration <1 cm deep Subcapsular hematoma <1 cm deep
Grade 2	Laceration 1–3 cm deep Subcapsular or central hematoma 1–3 cm diameter
Grade 3	Laceration 3–10 cm deep Subcapsular or central hematoma 3–10 cm diameter
Grade 4	Laceration >10 cm deep Subcapsular or central hematoma >10 cm diameter
Grade 5	Bilobar tissue maceration or devascularization
Grade 6	Hepatic avulsion

- On computed tomographic imaging, active extravasation of blood may be appreciated as contrast pooling or a "blush."
- Hemodynamically unstable patients should have empiric laparotomy.
- In some trauma centers, hypotension defined as systolic blood pressure of 90–120 mm Hg that is fluid responsive constitutes hemodynamic stability.

Evaluation
- If the patient is hemodynamically stable, perform rapid abdominal CT with IV contrast.
- Liver injuries are graded from 1 to 6 in terms of severity by the AAST (American Association for the Surgery of Trauma; Table 52.2).
- An abdominal computed tomographic scan with adequate IV contrast misses between 0.2% and 5% of intra-abdominal injuries.
- Missed injuries most commonly are diaphragmatic and hollow viscous injuries.

Management
- Follow ATLS guidelines for initial stabilization with the goal being to ensure hemodynamic stability.
  - Large-bore IV access should rapidly be obtained.
  - Serial hematocrits and coagulation studies are essential.
  - Blood should be made available for rapid transfusion.
- Trauma surgical consultation is a helpful adjunct to the emergency physician (EP). Hemodynamically unstable patients need emergent laparotomy to control hemorrhage.
- Operative versus nonoperative management of stable patients is based predominantly on computed tomographic findings.
  - Grade 1 or grade 2 injuries are considered minor and represent 80–90% of cases. Nonoperative management is the rule.
  - Grade 6 injuries are considered incompatible with survival (although case reports have noted occasional survival).
- The vast majority of liver trauma can be safely managed nonoperatively.
- As many as 67% of exploratory laparotomies for blunt trauma are nontherapeutic; therefore, nonoperative treatment is associated with decreased hospital stays and decreased transfusion requirements.

- Delayed bleeding from liver injuries happens <2% of the time; most liver injuries heal within 6 weeks. Fifty to eighty percent of liver injuries stop bleeding spontaneously.
- In cases of missed hepatic injury, angiography and percutaneous drainage can be effectively employed.
- Individuals with high-grade injuries should be admitted to the intensive care unit for continuous monitoring.

Special Considerations

- With shotgun wounds to the abdomen, all foreign bodies must be removed to prevent infection.
- On rare occasions, missiles to the liver may migrate into the hepatic vein and embolize.

Best Evidence/Clinical Decision Rules

Why is the threshold lower to operate on splenic injuries compared with liver injuries?

The goal of an operation is to stop hemorrhaging. The spleen can be easily removed whereas the liver has to be packed or cauterized (lobar resection is rarely performed). Angiography with embolization is another alternative to surgery.

Is nonoperative management of liver injuries safe?

In hemodynamically stable patients, studies have demonstrated that nonoperative management is safe and successful regardless of grade of liver injury. No single criterion can predict which patients will fail nonoperative management and require laparotomy.

Suggested Readings

Carrillo EH, Richardson JD. The current management of hepatic trauma. *Adv Surg.* 2001;35:39–59.

Cushing BM, Clark DE, Cobean R, Schenarts PJ, Rutstein LA. Blunt and penetrating trauma—has anything changed? *Surg Clin North Am.* 1997;77(6):1321–1332.

Fabian TC. Infection in penetrating abdominal trauma: risk factors and preventive antibiotics. *Am Surg.* 2002;68(1):29–35.

Feliciano DV, Rozycki GS. Hepatic trauma. *Scand J Surg.* 2002;91(1):72–79.

Fingerhut A, Trunkey D. Surgical management of liver injuries in adults—current indications and pitfalls of operative and non-operative policies: a review. *Eur J Surg.* 2000;166(9):676–686.

Franklin GA, Casos SR. Current advances in the surgical approach to abdominal trauma. *Injury.* 2006;37(12):1143–1156.

Galvan DA, Peitzman AB. Failure of nonoperative management of abdominal solid organ injuries. *Curr Opin Crit Care.* 2006;12(6):590–594.

Knudson MM, Maull KI. Nonoperative management of solid organ injuries. Past, present, and future. *Surg Clin North Am.* 1999;79(6):1357–1371.

Lee SK, Carrillo EH. Advances and changes in the management of liver injuries. *Am Surg.* 2007;73(3):201–206.

Ochsner MG. Factors of failure for nonoperative management of blunt liver and splenic injuries. *World J Surg.* 2001;25(11):1393–1396.

Parks RW, Chrysos E, Diamond T. Management of liver trauma.[see comment]. *Br J Surg.* 1999;86(9):1121–1135.

Schroeppel TJ, Croce MA. Diagnosis and management of blunt abdominal solid organ injury. *Curr Opin Crit Care.* 2007;13(4):399–404.

Schwab CW. Selection of nonoperative management candidates. *World J Surg.* 2001;25(11):1389–1392.

Trunkey DD. Hepatic trauma: contemporary management. *Surg Clin North Am.* 2004;84(2):437–450.

Vargo D, Sorenson J, Barton R. Repair of a grade VI hepatic injury: case report and literature review. *J Trauma.* 2002;53(5):823–824.

Velmahos GC, Toutouzas KG, Radin R, Chan L, Demetriades D. Nonoperative treatment of blunt injury to solid abdominal organs: a prospective study. *Arch Surg.* 2003;138(8):844–851.

53

Splenic Trauma

Andrea Dugas

Definition

- Splenic injury can result from either penetrating or blunt trauma to the abdomen or left lower chest.
- Blunt splenic injury from compression or deceleration forces is more common than penetrating injury.
- Injury patterns include subcapsular hematomas, laceration, devascularization, or a completely shattered spleen.

Pathophysiology

- **The spleen and liver are the two the most commonly injured abdominal organs in blunt trauma.**
- Because of anatomical proximity, splenic injuries may also be associated with diaphragmatic, pancreatic, or bowel injury.
- Bleeding is the initial concern in splenic injury.

Diagnosis

- Patients may report left upper quadrant or lower chest pain or referred pain to the left shoulder (Kehr sign).
- Physical examination is insensitive but may reveal left lower rib or left upper quadrant tenderness or bruising, or peritoneal signs.
- Evaluate for rib fractures, as 25% of patients with left lower rib fractures (ribs 9–12) will have a splenic injury.
- Disruption of the spleen may be seen on a focused assessment with sonography for trauma (FAST) examination; however, this test is not sensitive for splenic injury.
- Both computed tomography (CT) and FAST examination can show intraperitoneal blood which is commonly from splenic injury.
- Splenic injury is often graded by severity (Table 53.1) on the basis of either CT or postoperative specimen.

TABLE 53.1: Splenic computed tomographic Injury grading scale

Grade 1	Laceration <1 cm deep Subcapsular hematoma <1 cm deep
Grade 2	Laceration 1–3 cm deep Subcapsular or central hematoma 1–3 cm diameter
Grade 3	Laceration >3 cm deep Subcapsular or central hematoma >50% surface area
Grade 4	Laceration involving segmental/hilar vessels Major devascularization (>25% of spleen)
Grade 5	Completely shattered spleen Hilar vascular injury that devascularizes spleen

- CT is the main mechanism of diagnosing splenic injury
  - Although sensitive for detecting splenic injury, there is poor correlation between the grade of injury seen on CT and the grade of injury seen operatively.
  - **Oral contrast is not helpful for diagnosing splenic injury by CT; however, intravenous contrast is and may show a splenic blush—a sign of contrast extravasation and active bleeding.**

Evaluation

- Follow the guidelines of ATLS and secure the ABCs.
- If the patient is hypotensive with signs of blood in the abdomen based on FAST or diagnostic peritoneal lavage, the patient should go to the operating room. Liver and spleen are the most likely sources of hemorrhage.
- In a hemodynamically stable patient, facilitate rapid CT to diagnose potential injuries.
- Suspicion for splenic injury should be high in any patient with left upper quadrant or left lower chest tenderness or bruising.

Management

- Any hemodynamically unstable patient with blunt abdominal trauma and a positive FAST or diagnostic peritoneal lavage should go to the operating room.
- Patients with penetrating trauma to the spleen should go to the operating room for exploration and diagnosis of associated injuries.
- In a hemodynamically stable patient with isolated splenic injury, the patient may be managed operatively or nonoperatively with observation or embolization.
- Operative management includes exploratory laparotomy to evaluate the degree of injury and potential associated injuries, splenorrhaphy, or splenectomy depending on the location and degree of injury.
- Nonoperative management includes admission to an intensive care unit for close monitoring along with serial hematocrits and abdominal examinations.
  - Hemodynamic instability, rapidly decreasing hematocrit, and peritoneal signs are all indications of failed nonoperative management and the patient should be taken rapidly to the operating room or angiography suite for embolization.
  - The grade of splenic injury on CT is predictive of the success rate of nonoperative management (Table 53.2).
- An estimated 40–60% of adults with splenic injury are managed nonoperatively, of which approximately 20% fail nonoperative management (Table 53.3).

Special Considerations

- Angiography and embolectomy have been shown to improve the success rate of nonoperative management and can be considered in hemodynamically stable patients with persistent tachycardia despite fluids, splenic blush on CT, higher grade of splenic injury based on CT, or decreasing hematocrit.

TABLE 53.2: Failure of Nonoperative Management of Splenic Injury by Grade

	Grades				
	I	II	III	IV	V
Percent failure of nonoperative management	5	10	20	33	75

TABLE 53.3: Risk factors that predict failed nonoperative management

| Large hemoperitoneum |
| Multiple injuries |
| Comorbid disease |
| Anticoagulation |
| Portal hypertension |
| Presence of a splenic blush on computed tomography |

- There is conflicting data on whether patients older than 55 years have higher failure rates of nonoperative management.
- Nonoperative management is not without risk as some studies show as high as 13% mortality, often due to missed injuries such as bowel or pancreas, or formation of a pseudoaneurysm.
- The success rate of nonoperative management is higher in children, likely due to a thicker splenic capsule and firmer parenchyma.

Best Evidence/Clinical Decision Rules

Which patients should be selected for nonoperative management?

Nonoperative management should be considered only in a hemodynamically stable patient at a facility that can offer appropriate monitoring, which includes an intensive care unit, as well immediate access to a CT scanner, a surgeon, and an operating room. If selected, the patient will require hemodynamic monitoring as well as serial hematocrits and abdominal examinations. This necessitates that the patient is alert enough to provide a reliable examination. Additional considerations such as age, comorbidities, presence of a splenic blush on CT, grade of splenic injury, amount of hemoperitoneum, and other injuries should also be considered.

Angiography with splenic embolization has been demonstrated to be a successful alternative to surgery. It has raised the success rate of nonoperative management in multiple studies and at multiple institutions where it is available.

Suggested Readings

Haan JM, Bochicchio GV, Kramer N, Scalea TM. Nonoperative management of blunt splenic injury: a 5-year experience. *J Trauma*. 2005;58(3):492–498.

Jacoby RC, Wisner DH. Injury to the spleen. In: Feliciano DV, Mattox KL, Moore EE, eds. *Trauma*. 6th ed. New York: McGraw-Hill, Medical Pub. Division, 2008:661–680.

Mileski MJ. Injuries to the liver and spleen. In: Flint L, Meredith JW, Schwab CW, Trunkey DD, Rue LW, Taheri PA, eds. *Trauma: Contemporary Principles and Therapy*. Philadelphia: Lippincott Williams & Wilkins, 2008:433–441.

Mirvis SE, Whitley NO, Gens DR. Blunt splenic trauma in adults: CT-based classification and correlation with prognosis and treatment. *Radiology*. 1989;171(1):33–39.

Moore EE, Cogbill TH, Jurkovich GJ, Shackford SR, Malangoni MA, Champion HR. Organ injury scaling: spleen and liver (1994 revision). *J Trauma.* 1995;38(3):323–324.

Peitzman AB, Harbrecht BG, Rivera L, Heil B; Eastern Association for the Surgery of Trauma Multiinstitutional Trials Workgroup. Failure of observation of blunt splenic injury in adults: variability in practice and adverse consequences. *J Am Coll Surg.* 2005;201(2):179–187.

Definition

- Bowel injuries can be divided into three major groups:
  - Perforations
  - Bowel wall hematomas
  - Mesentery injuries
- **Bowel perforations** are defined as disruption of the bowel wall integrity such that intestinal contents are free to exit the bowel into the peritoneal space.
- **Bowel wall hematomas** occur primarily from blunt traumatic mechanisms. The compression of bowel between the spine and an external object such as a steering wheel or seat belt can cause bruising and injury to the bowel wall. A bowel wall hematoma occurs when this hemorrhage is contained within the bowel wall.
- **Mesentery injuries** can be caused by both penetrating and blunt trauma. Penetrating injuries to the mesentery can injure mesenteric vessels resulting in hemorrhage. Blunt trauma acceleration/deceleration forces shear the mesentery from its attachment to bowel leading to vessel laceration and avulsion injuries.

Pathophysiology

- Both penetrating and blunt traumatic mechanisms are capable of causing bowel perforations. The mechanism of penetrating bowel perforation is self-explanatory. Blunt traumatic mechanisms exert external compression forces (via objects like the seat belt or steering wheel) through the abdominal wall and on to potentially closed loops of bowel. This creates high intraluminal pressures and can cause subsequent perforation. Blunt traumatic mechanisms also cause bowel perforation as a result of acceleration/deceleration forces shearing bowel from attachment sites at the ligament of Treitz and ileocecal valve.
- Bowel perforations result in movement of bowel contents into the peritoneal cavity. Within 6–8 hours an inflammatory reaction to the bowel contents will occur, causing symptoms and signs of peritonitis including abdominal pain, tenderness, nausea, vomiting, and fever.
- Bowel wall hematomas can cause obstruction of the bowel lumen due to the enlarging hematoma. Luminal obstruction will result in nausea with vomiting as well as abdominal pain.
- Mesenteric vascular injuries and avulsions can result in decreased blood supply to the involved area of bowel. If the collateral circulation is not adequate, the bowel will become ischemic and necrotic.
- **Morbidity and mortality from bowel injuries is correlated with delayed diagnosis and intervention.**

Diagnosis

- When working up a trauma patient one must maintain a high degree of suspicion for bowel injury to minimize missed and delayed diagnoses.

- Bowel injuries should be suspected in any trauma patient complaining of abdominal pain, nausea, vomiting, or abdominal tenderness on physical examination.
- Bowel trauma should be assumed until proven otherwise in certain cases:
  - Mechanisms commonly associated with bowel injuries including motor vehicle accidents with lap belt restraints (without shoulder harness) and bicycle accidents with handlebar direct trauma injuries.
  - Findings commonly associated with bowel injuries including abdominal bruising (see Fig. 54.1 demonstrating the seat belt sign) and Chance fractures of the lumbar spine.
  - Traumatic pancreatic injuries should raise the possibility of duodenal involvement given the close anatomic relationship between the two organs.

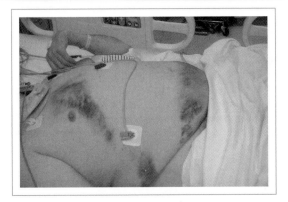

FIGURE 54.1: Ecchymosis across the anterior chest and abdomen of a patient using a three-point safety restraint. This physical examination finding is known as a *seat-belt* sign, and is associated with flexion-distraction fractures of the spine and blunt small bowel injury following motor vehicle collision. Photo courtesy of Bruce Ham, MD (Oregon Health and Science University). (Reprinted with permission from Flint L, Meredith JW, Schwab CW, et al. *Trauma: Contemporary Principles and Therapy.* Philadelphia: Lippincott Williams & Wilkins, 2008.)

- Definitive diagnosis requires imaging of the abdomen with computed tomography (CT).
  - Computed tomographic scan is reported to be up to 95% sensitive for bowel injuries.
  - Findings suspicious for bowel or mesentery injury include unexplained peritoneal fluid or air collections, mesentery or bowel wall thickening, mesenteric stranding, bowel wall defects, evidence of bowel wall infarct, and focal bowel wall hematomas.
- Diagnostic peritoneal lavage (DPL) is of use if positive (gross enteric contents aspirated, positive Gram's stain, or lavage with >500 white blood cells/mm^3 or >100,000 red blood cells/mm^3). If negative, DPL is of limited use as signs of peritonitis can take up to 8 hours to develop. In addition, DPL is of no use for diagnosis of duodenal injury given the retroperitoneal location of the duodenum (Table 54.1).

Evaluation
- Evaluate for external signs of intra-abdominal injury such as abdominal wall bruising (e.g., "seat belt sign").

TABLE 54.1: Interpretation and appropriate action based on lavage findings

Findings	Interpretation	Action
>500 WBC	Positive	Laparotomy
>100,000 RBC	Positive	Laparotomy
20,000–100,000 RBC	Indeterminate	Consider further imaging; correlate clinically
Gross enteric contents	Positive	Laparotomy

RBC, red blood cell; WBC, white blood cell. (Reprinted and modified with permission from Shah K, Mason C. *Essential Emergency Procedures.* Philadelphia: Lippincott Williams & Wilkins, 2007.)

- Evaluate for signs of developing peritonitis such as fever, abdominal tenderness, rebound or guarding.
- Facilitate rapid computed tomographic scan to identify intra-abdominal injuries.
- Consider observation and serial physical examinations in high-risk patients.
- Plain radiographs are of limited use in detecting bowel injuries. Free air beneath the diaphragm should raise suspicion for a perforation; however, only 25–50% of bowel injuries have pneumoperitoneum detectable on plain film.
- Upper gastrointestinal contrast study is of limited use except for detecting or following duodenal hematoma.

Management

- Bowel perforations require immediate operative intervention. **Preoperative antibiotics covering bowel flora are essential to decrease postoperative risk of infection.** The goals of operative management are control of hemorrhage, control of contamination by bowel contents, systematic identification of injuries, and subsequent repair of injuries.
- Bowel wall hematomas are preferably treated nonoperatively. The goal of management is for the bowel to rest while the hematoma resorbs and the obstruction resolves. This requires nasogastric (NG) tube suction and total parenteral nutrition. Repeat imaging should be performed at 5- to 7-day intervals. If extensive progression occurs, perforation develops, or the obstruction does not resolve within 14 days, operative intervention is indicated.
- Mesenteric injuries often cause a significant amount of bleeding requiring operative intervention to control hemorrhage. Extensive mesenteric injuries and avulsions put bowel at risk for ischemia; bowel viability and blood supply must be assessed intraoperatively.

Special Considerations

- **Tension pneumoperitoneum** is a rare complication of bowel perforation in which a large amount of air extravasates into the peritoneal cavity and causes increased pressure and abdominal distension with subsequent shortness of breath and circulatory collapse. Treatment requires emergent decompression of the abdominal cavity with a chest tube.
- Children are at increased risk for bowel injury resulting from blunt trauma due to thinner, less muscular abdominal walls. In addition, in children the seat belt,

particularly the lap component, is often not correctly positioned across the iliac crests. This improper placement increases translation of blunt forces directly to the abdomen. Using proper car and booster seats helps remedy these increased risks.

- Bowel injuries related to lap belts are decreasing with the widespread use of lap belts combined with a shoulder harness. This serves to transmit forces over a larger area of the body.
- Child abuse should be suspected when signs of upper abdominal trauma are detected without an appropriate mechanism.

Best Evidence/Clinical Decision Rules

Does a negative computed tomography scan rule out bowel injury?

Multidetector CT scan is reported to be as high as 95% sensitive for bowel and mesentery injuries, with specificities between 94% and 100%. The range in reported sensitivities is related to multiple factors including radiologist expertise, the CT scanner technology, the severity of injuries, and the use or lack of use of oral contrast material. Bowel injuries are more easily detected when the injuries are more severe, and when oral contrast material is used. However, because of time constraints, most trauma centers do not use oral contrast on initial trauma CT, and thus sensitivity is likely closer to 80–90%. Although CT scan is the definitive study of choice for abdominal trauma, including for bowel injury, a negative scan does not absolutely rule out bowel and mesenteric injuries. Thus, when suspicion for bowel injury is high, such as in patients with abdominal wall bruising or with abdominal pain, an equivocal or negative CT is not adequate. The patient should be observed with serial examinations performed for 12–24 hours postinjury to detect symptoms and signs of bowel injury such as developing peritonitis or obstruction. In the current era of increased reliance on the CT scan and conservative/nonoperative management of solid organ abdominal injuries, it is especially important to maintain a high degree of suspicion for bowel injury. Bowel and mesentery injuries previously identified only in the operating room may be initially missed, with the potential for late development of peritonitis and bowel obstruction resulting in increased morbidity and mortality for the patient.

Suggested Readings

Brofman N, Atri M, Hanson JM, et al. Evaluation of bowel and mesenteric blunt trauma with multidetector CT. *Radiographics*. 2006;26(4):1119–1131.

Ferrera PC, Marx J, Colucciello SA, et al. *Trauma Management: An Emergency Medicine Approach*. St. Louis, MO, Mosby, 2001:296–304.

Flint L, Meredith JW, Schwab CW, et al. *Trauma: Contemporary Principles and Therapy*. Philadelphia, PA, Lippincott, Williams & Wilkins, 2008;40:425–429, 42:443–449.

Holmes JF, Offerman SR, Chang CH, et al. Performance of helical computed tomography without oral contrast for the detection of gastrointestinal injuries. *Ann Emerg Med*. 2004;43(1):120–128.

Shatz DV, Kirton OC, McKenney MG, et al. *Manual of Trauma and Emergency Surgery*. Philadelphia, PA, WB Saunders Company, 2000:132–135, 150–152.

Stuhlfaut JW, Soto JA, Lucey BC, et al. Blunt abdominal trauma: performance of CT without oral contrast material. *Radiology*. 2004;233:689–694.

55 Pancreatic Trauma

Francis J. O'Connell

Definition
- Pancreatic injury is uncommon, accounting for <1% of trauma and between 1% and 12% of abdominal trauma.
- Pancreatic injuries are graded by an organ injury scale (Table 55.1).

Pathophysiology
- The pancreas is a retroperitoneal organ located in the upper abdomen shielded posteriorly by the spine, musculature of the back and other retroperitoneal organs and anteriorly by the abdominal muscles, omentum, and bowel.
- In the United States, penetrating trauma accounts for a large percentage of pancreatic injuries; however, in Europe and Australia blunt trauma is a more common cause of pancreatic injuries.
- **In cases of penetrating trauma it is rare to have isolated pancreatic injury.** Pancreatic injury is most often associated with liver; stomach; and vascular, duodenal, colonic, and kidney injury.
- In blunt trauma almost 50% of pancreatic trauma is isolated in nature.

Diagnosis
- Gross abdominal injury or tenderness involving the upper abdominal quadrants in the presence of a positive FAST, free air under the diaphragm, or an elevated amylase or lipase is highly suspicious for pancreatic injury.
- Positive computed tomographic findings: visible injuries to pancreas or fluid between the splenic vein and the pancreas (suggestive of pancreatic trauma).

Evaluation
- There is no one test that has both excellent sensitivity and specificity to screen patients for pancreatic injury in the emergency department.
- Computed tomography is capable of screening patients for most abdominal pathology; however, literature from 1998 and 2009 suggests that it is far from perfect to use as a screening modality for pancreatic injury. The other evaluation

TABLE 55.1: Pancreas injury grading scale

Grade I	Superficial laceration/minor contusion without ductal injury
Grade II	Major laceration/major contusion without ductal injury or tissue loss
Grade III	Distal transection or parenchymal/duct injury
Grade IV	Proximal transection or parenchymal injury involving ampulla
Grade V	Massive disruption of pancreatic head

tools for diagnosing pancreatic injury are nonspecific for pancreatic injury but are useful in detecting abdominal trauma which is often associated with pancreatic trauma.
- Nonspecific tests.
  - Abdominal examination—the presence of exit/entry wounds or discrete tenderness to palpation may be helpful.
  - FAST examination—the presence of blood in dependent areas is sensitive for intra-abdominal injury.
  - Upright chest radiograph—presence of free air indicates hollow viscous injury.
  - Amylase and lipase—while lipase is a more sensitive marker for acute pancreatitis, its role in pancreatic trauma is not well understood and the ubiquity of amylase in the upper gastrointestinal tract makes it an insensitive marker of pancreatic injury; however, rises in either in the presence of other positive findings may guide a more focused workup.
- Endoscopic retrograde cholangiopancreatography (ERCP) and magnetic resonance cholangiopancreatography (MRCP)
  - Sensitivity and specificity that approach 100% for assessing pancreatic injury, but neither can be performed in emergent circumstances.
  - Can be performed after the patient is stabilized to assess for a pancreatic injury if clinical suspicion remains high.
- Laparotomy (if indicated) with direct inspection of the pancreas is ideal.
  - If other trauma warrants emergent exploration of the abdomen, inspect the pancreas for trauma, especially when projectile injury or trauma to nearby organs is present.
  - Intraoperative pancreatic ductogram with cholangiogram is an option if unable to completely visualize the pancreas.

Management
- Surgical consultation.
- Identify and correct any coagulopathies.
- The grade of pancreatic injury dictates operative versus nonoperative intervention (Table 55.2).

Special Considerations
- Care should be taken in evaluating patients with slow impact abdominal blunt force trauma, patients with negative FAST examinations, intoxicated patients, and very young and elderly patients because pancreatic injury can be easily missed.
- In absence of negative findings on computed tomography, laboratory tests, or even laparotomy the patient can be observed and if suspicion persists a nonemergent ERCP/MRCP can be performed.

TABLE 55.2: Operative versus nonoperative intervention scale

Grades	Management
I	Conservative management/drainage
II	Conservative management/debridement with/without drainage
III	Distal pancreatectomy with/without splenectomy
IV and V	Pancreatoduodenectomy (consider damage control hemorrhage control, packing, laparotomy, placement of drains with a delayed closure)

Best Evidence/Clinical Decision Rules

Is there a role for octreotide in pancreatic injury?

Octreotide, a somatostatin analogue that is a potent inhibitor of pancreatic exocrine function, has shown to decrease pancreas-related morbidity following major pancreatic resection in patients with pancreatic **neoplasm** and acute severe **pancreatitis**. It was theorized that giving octreotide following pancreatic **injury** would reduce mortality and morbidity by limiting exocrine secretion; however, no study has shown octreotide to be overwhelmingly beneficial. In fact, some studies suggest that the administration of octreotide in the setting of pancreatic trauma can lead to more complications.

Suggested Readings

Akhrass R, Kim K, Brandt C. Computed tomography: an unreliable indicator of pancreatic trauma. *Am Surg.* 1996;62:647–651.

Akhrass R, Yaffe MB, Brandt CP, et al. Pancreatic trauma: a ten-year multi-institutional experience. *Am Surg.* 1997;63:598–604.

Amirata E, Livingston DH, Elcavage J. Octreotide acetate decreases pancreatic complications after pancreatic trauma. *Am J Surg.* 1994;168:345–347.

Bradley EL, Young PR, Chang MC, et al. Diagnosis and initial management of blunt pancreatic trauma. *Ann Surg.* 1998;227:861–869.

Brooks A, Shukla A, Beckingham I. Pancreatic trauma. *Trauma.* 2003;5:1–8.

Brooks KBA. Pancreatic trauma—injuries to the pancreas and pancreatic duct. *Eur J Surg.* 2000;166:4–12.

Harun T, Madanur M, Bartlett A, et al. Pancreatic trauma—12-year experience from a tertiary care center. *Pancreas.* 2009;38(2):113–116.

Moore EE, Cogbill TH, Malangoni MA, et al. Organ injury scaling, II: pancreas, duodenum, small bowel, colon, and rectum. *J Trauma.* 1990;30:1427–1429.

Nwariaku FE, Terracina A, Mileski WJ, et al. Is octreotide beneficial following pancreatic injury? *Am J Surg.* 1995;170(6):582–585.

Patel SV, Spencer JA, el-Hasani S, et al. Imaging of pancreatic trauma. *Br J Radiol.* 1998;71:985–990.

Smith RC, Southwell-Keely J, Chesher D. Should serum pancreatic lipase replace serum amylase as a biomarker of acute pancreatitis? *ANZ J Surg.* 2005;75(6):399–404.

Takishima T, Sugimoto K, Hirata M, et al. Serum amylase level on admission in the diagnosis of blunt injury to the pancreas: its significance and limitations. *Ann Surg.* 1997;226:70–76.

Udekwu PO, Gurkin B, Oller DW. The use of computed tomography in blunt abdominal injuries. *Am Surg.* 1996;62:56–59.

Vasquez JC, Coimbra R, Hoyt DB, et al. Management of penetrating pancreatic trauma: an 11-year experience of a level-1 trauma center. *Injury.* 2001;32:753–759.

Young PR, Meredith JW, Baker CC, et al. Pancreatic injuries resulting from penetrating trauma: a multi-institution review. *Am Surg.* 1998;64:838–844.

Section Editor: Kaushal Shah

56 Pelvic Trauma: The First 15 Minutes, Algorithm, and Decision Making

Kaushal Shah

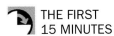 THE FIRST
15 MINUTES

ABCs
- Check vital signs and determine stability.
- Follow ATLS guidelines and Severe Pelvic Trauma Algorithm.

History
- Motor vehicle collisions account for the vast majority of pelvic fractures.

Physical Examination
- If there is instability with pelvic manual compression, do not manipulate the pelvis further other than for pelvic stabilization. Repeat examinations should be discouraged to prevent further hemorrhage.
- High risk for urethral injury. Carefully check for blood at the penile meatus and ecchymosis of perineum/scrotum. If either is present, do not attempt to pass a Foley catheter.
- One of the few instances when a rectal examination might be useful in trauma.
  - Gross rectal bleeding suggests rectal/colon injury.
  - Poor sphincter tone suggests spinal injury.
  - "High-riding prostate" is a theoretical finding for possible urethral injury.

Emergency Interventions
- **Hemorrhage** is the most significant complication of pelvic trauma with almost 50% mortality when the patient is hypotensive on presentation. Order blood products (packed red blood cells and fresh frozen plasma [FFP]) immediately.
  - Two large-bore peripheral intravenous lines (IVs) are necessary.
  - If central line is being placed, a cordis in the internal jugular or subclavian vein is ideal; avoid the femoral vein.
  - Resuscitate with 2 L of fluid followed by packed red blood cells and fresh frozen plasma, if necessary.
- **Plain film** of the pelvis is critical to determine the type/mechanism of injury, which will dictate the method of treatment and stabilization.

TABLE 56.1: Young/Burgess Classification—based on pattern of injury

	Lateral compression	Anterior-posterior compression	Vertical shear
Grade I	Crush injury to sacrum	Diastasis of pubic symphysis only	Vertical fracture through anterior and posterior pelvis with superior displacement of hemipelvis
Grade II	Iliac wing injury	Widened sacroiliac joint with anterior ligament disruption	
Grade III	Either I or II plus external rotation of contralateral pelvis	Sacroiliac joint, anterior and posterior ligament disruption	

- **Pelvic stabilization** (pelvic sheet wrap, commercially available TPOD, external fixation) should be considered in all unstable "open book" pelvic injuries.
  - Helps control venous bleeds (particularly from the presacral venous plexus) but does not cease arterial bleeding.
- **Identify associated injuries.** Severe pelvic fractures often have concomitant intra-abdominal, urethral, and bladder injuries.
- **Angiography with embolization** should be considered for persistent hypotension or hemorrhage when all other sources of bleeding are controlled or ruled out.

Memorable Pearls

- On plain film, follow the edge of the posterior and anterior pelvic rings closely to identify disruptions.
- If pelvic instability is noted, do not perform/allow repeated examinations as this will only worsen hemorrhage.
- Abdomen trumps pelvis. If there is a suspicion of intra-abdominal injury (e.g., abdominal focused assessment with sonography for trauma [FAST] examination is positive and patient is unstable), patient needs laparotomy prior to angiography.
- Genitourinary (GU) tract evaluation with dye should not be performed prior to pelvic angiography because extravasation of dye will obscure visualization of arterial bleeding.
- If performing a diagnostic peritoneal lavage, use open, supraumbilical approach.

Essential Considerations

Know the anatomy and the common classification systems (Tables 56.1 and 56.2).

Consultations

- Trauma surgeon/team
- Orthopedic surgeon
- Interventional radiologist

TABLE 56.2: Tile Classification—based on radiographic signs

A	Stable	No pelvic ring disruption
B	Rotationally unstable Vertically stable	B1—open book with symphysis pubis displacement B2—double rami and sacral fractures
C	Rotationally unstable Vertically unstable	Vertical displacement of hemipelvis

DECISION
MAKING

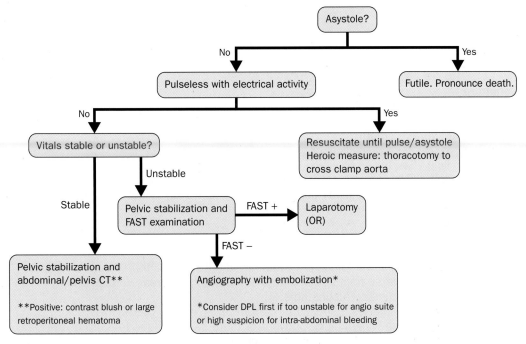

Severe pelvic trauma: Decision making algorithm. FAST, focused assessment with sonography for trauma; OR, operating room; CT, computed tomography; DPL, diagnostic peritoneal lavage.

Definition

- Lateral compression injuries are the result of broadside impact with forces concentrated toward the side of the pelvis (e.g., pedestrian struck or side impact motor vehicle crash).
- Young/Burgess Classification.
  - Type I-Sacral compression fracture on the side of impact.
  - Type II-Pelvic wing "stove-in" fracture on the side of impact.
  - Type III-Sacroiliac injury on the side of impact plus contralateral external rotation pelvis injury.

Pathophysiology

- In sacral injuries, the forces are transmitted either in the transverse or vertical planes. Transverse fractures are considered stable whereas vertical shear fractures are considered unstable.
- In pelvic wing injuries, usually the fracture fragment is rotated inward with a portion of the wing hinging outward or there is an oblique fracture of the posterior ileum extending from the sacroiliac joint. Although the iliac fragment may be unstable, the weightbearing stability of the pelvis is preserved.
- In type III injuries, the lateral forces cause an anterior/superior displacement of the ipsilateral portion of the hemipelvis, while causing external rotation of the anterior pelvis on the contralateral side. This generally results in a double pubic ramus fracture. Due to transmitted forces, there may also be a fracture of the sacrum with ligamentous disruption of the ileum. **Type III injuries are considered unstable.**
- Fractures involving the ipsilateral pubic ramus are usually stable but if there is associated disruption of the sacroiliac complex then they are classified as unstable.
- Lateral compression injuries can also cause pubic rami fractures on the side of injury.
- Life-threatening hemorrhage may accompany any type of pelvic fracture.
- Due to the forces needed to generate lateral compression fractures, the potential for associated injuries is increased Fig. 57.1. These injuries are usually minimal but may include bowel, sacral nerves, and/or the urogenital system.

Diagnosis

- On physical examination, there may be signs of ecchymosis, abrasions, hematomas, bleeding, and pelvic/leg asymmetry. Focal tenderness to palpation, instability with gentle lateral pressure on the iliac wings, and difficulty with active and passive range of motion of the hip are associated with a fractured pelvis.
- **Imaging is essential for definitive diagnosis.** Although the standard trauma film will adequately assess significant pelvic injuries in most cases (Fig. 57.2),

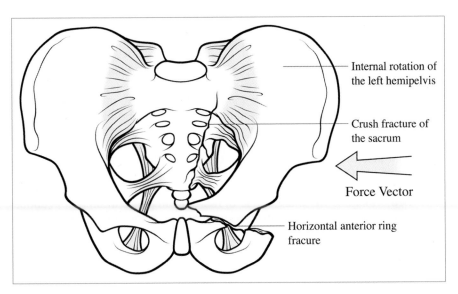

Internal rotation of
the left hemipelvis

Crush fracture of
the sacrum

Force Vector

Horizontal anterior ring
fracure

FIGURE 57.1: Lateral compression injury. The causative force vector is delivered from the side, crushing the affected hemipelvis inward. Lateral compression injuries typically reduce pelvic volume. Instability is variable. (Reprinted with permission from Wolfson AB, Hendey GW, Ling LJ, et al: *Harwood-Nuss' Clinical Practice of Emergency Medicine*, 5th ed. Philadelphia: Lippincott Williams & Wilkins, 2009.)

computed tomographic (CT) scan is superior at assessing the posterior aspect of the pelvis. Specifically, injuries involving the sacrum, sacroiliac joints, and posterior ilium can be missed on plain film. In the hemodynamically stable trauma patient, CT is indicated and can be used to assess for accompanying injuries.

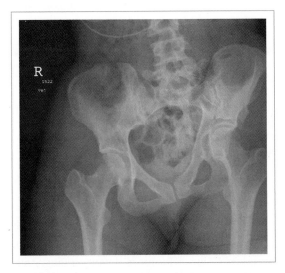

FIGURE 57.2: AP plain film of a severe lateral compression injury. The left hemipelvis is crushed inwards. (Reprinted with permission from Wolfson AB, Hendey GW, Ling LJ, et al: *Harwood-Nuss' Clinical Practice of Emergency Medicine*, 5th ed. Philadelphia: Lippincott Williams & Wilkins, 2009.)

Evaluation
- In acute trauma, attention to airway, breathing, and circulation/hemorrhage is the primary focus.
- Suspect pelvic fracture in all cases of serious or multiple trauma.
- Radiologic evaluation is essential for definitive diagnosis. The standard trauma AP pelvis film is generally sufficient for initial identification of pelvic ring fractures.
- In the hemodynamically stable patient, CT scan may be of value in determining full extent of bony and vascular injury.
- **In pelvic trauma there is a high incidence of associated injuries; therefore, special attention should be paid to the rectal and urogenital examinations.** Also due to the location of the sacral nerve plexus, lower extremity neurological examination is indicated.
- As hemorrhage is the main cause of mortality in pelvic trauma, it is critical to assess hemodynamic stability and identify ongoing bleeding in the chest, abdomen, and long bones. If no clear source of hemorrhage is identified and patient remains unstable, suspicion for primary pelvic hemorrhage should be high.
- Order a pregnancy test in any woman of childbearing age as there are significant implications in the gravid patient.
- If the pelvis is determined to be unstable on physical examination, repeated examinations by various members of the trauma team should be avoided to prevent worsening of the injury.

Management
- Institute aggressive resuscitation with crystalloid and blood products, if needed.
- The hemodynamically unstable patient with a positive focused assessment with sonography for trauma (FAST) or diagnostic peritoneal lavage requires immediate laparotomy.
  - Diagnostic peritoneal lavage, if performed, should be via an open, supraumbilical approach.
- In the setting of pelvic fractures with hemodynamic compromise due to bleeding pelvic vessels, therapeutic angiography with embolization is often necessary and the process to mobilize resources needed for interventional radiology should be initiated as soon as possible.
- If the patient is hemodynamically stable, evaluation via computed tomography is indicated.
- Sheets or compressive devices in lateral pelvic injuries should be used with caution; the goal is only to stabilize the pelvis as excessive compression can cause further injury and bleeding.
- External fixators will not control bleeding if there is a posterior pelvic disruption.
- Early consultation with surgery and orthopedics is recommended.
- Patients with simple or isolated stable fractures can be managed conservatively and may not require hospital admission.

Special Considerations
- Significant pelvic trauma should be managed at a Level I trauma center.
- Always obtain an AP x-ray film of the pelvis when history/mechanism suggests pelvic injury or in an unconscious trauma patient.
- With lateral compression forces, a posterior pelvic injury/fracture may be missed on a plain film. Consider obtaining a CT scan for more definitive diagnosis.
- In pelvic trauma with hypotension, suspect and address sources of bleeding in the chest, intra-/extraperitoneum, or long bones. If no identifiable source of hemorrhage, suspect pelvic hemorrhage and activate interventional radiology for angiography.

Best Evidence/Clinical Decision Rules

Are patients with major ligamentous injury (lateral compression fracture type III, anteroposterior compression type II and III, and vertical shear patterns) more likely to require angiographic embolization compared with nonmajor ligamentous injury?

When comparing all pelvic fractures, certainly those with major ligamentous injury are more likely to require embolization; however, if we compare pelvic fractures among patients presenting with a blood pressure <90 mm Hg, the fracture pattern does not always predict the need for urgent embolization.

What are the indications for angiographic embolization in patients with pelvic fractures?

- Hemodynamic instability (despite fluid resuscitation) and FAST examination negative.
- Contrast blush on pelvic CT scan.
- Large retroperitoneal hematoma on CT scan.
- Expanding retroperitoneal hematoma on sequential CT scans.
- Persistent hemodynamic instability after placement of external fixator and/or laparotomy.
- Prolonged transfusion requirement (>3 units/24 hr) or clinical signs of ongoing hemorrhage.

Suggested Readings

Goslings JC, van Delden OM. Angiography and embolisation to control bleeding after blunt injury to the abdomen or pelvis. *Ned Tijdschr Geneeskd.* 2007;151(6): 345–352.

Hamill J, Holden A, Paice R, Civil I. Pelvic fracture pattern predicts pelvic arterial haemorrhage. *Aust N Z J Surg.* 2000;70(5):338–343.

Sarin EL, Moore JB, Moore EE, et al. Pelvic fracture pattern does not always predict the need for urgent embolization. *J Trauma.* 2005;58(5):973–977.

58

Anterior-Posterior Compression Pelvic Trauma

Mária Némethy

Definition

- Anterior-posterior (AP) compression injuries result from force delivered to the pelvis either from the front (e.g., front-on motor vehicle collisions) or from the back (e.g., pedestrian struck from behind).

Pathophysiology

- Force is applied along the anterior and/or posterior iliac spines or through the femur, causing widening of the pelvis (Fig. 58.1).
- AP compression injuries tend to disrupt the anterior pelvis, with ligamentous injury being common. Concomitant fractures of the pubic rami are also frequently seen.
- Widening of the pelvis leads to pelvic instability and increased pelvic volume and is generally associated with injury to the sacral venous plexus. The risk of severe hemorrhage is consequently very high, with associated mortality of 20–50%.
- A 3-cm widening of the pubic symphysis will effectively double the normal pelvic volume. The retroperitoneum can accommodate up to 4 L of blood; this capacity is further increased in pelvic ring injuries.
- Neurologic and urologic sequelae are also common, along with gait abnormalities and chronic back pain.

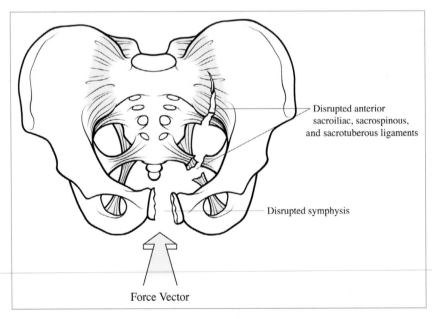

Disrupted anterior sacroiliac, sacrospinous, and sacrotuberous ligaments

Disrupted symphysis

Force Vector

FIGURE 58.1: AP compression injury. The causative force vector is delivered from the front (or back), causing the pelvic ring to "open like a book." These injuries are mechanically unstable, and associated with increases in pelvic volume. (Reprinted with permission from Wolfson AB, Hendey GW, Ling LJ, et al. *Harwood-Nuss' Clinical Practice of Emergency Medicine,* 5th ed. Philadelphia: Lippincott Williams & Wilkins, 2009.)

TABLE 58.1: **Young-Burgess Classification: Anteroposterior compression**

Type	Symphyseal diastasis	SI Joint widening	Ligaments affected	Stability
I	<2.5 cm	Slight	Stretched but intact	Stable
II	>2.5 cm	Moderate	Disruption of anterior ligaments; posterior ligaments intact	Rotationally unstable; vertically stable
III	>2.5 cm	Complete	Complete disruption of anterior and posterior ligaments	Rotationally and vertically unstable

SI, sacro-iliac.

Classification

AP compression injuries are graded according to the Young-Burges Classification scale (Table 58.1).

Diagnosis

- Suspect pelvic fracture in all cases of serious or multiple trauma.
- Physical examination findings suggestive of pelvic injury.
  - Rotation of iliac crests
  - Leg-length discrepancy
  - Perineal or pelvic edema, ecchymoses, or deformities
  - Irregularity, tenderness, or crepitus at iliac crests or pubic symphysis
  - Blood at urethral meatus
  - Gross blood on rectal examination
  - High-riding prostate
  - Peripheral neurovascular deficits
- **Imaging is essential for definitive diagnosis.** Although the standard trauma film will adequately assess significant pelvic injuries in most cases, computed tomographic scan is superior at assessing the posterior aspect of the pelvis. Specifically, injuries involving the sacrum, sacroiliac joints, and posterior ilium can be missed on plain film. In the hemodynamically stable trauma patient, computed tomography is indicated and can be used to assess for accompanying injuries (Fig. 58.2).

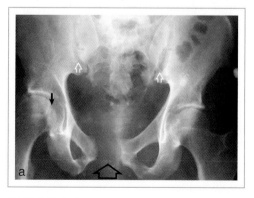

FIGURE 58.2: Open-book pelvic ring disruption with pure lateral rotation of each hemipelvis. The pubic symphysis is separated (open black arrow). Each sacroiliac joint is slightly widened (open white arrows), as is confirmed by computed tomography. (Reprinted with permission from Harris JH, Harris WH. *The Radiology of Emergency Medicine,* 4th ed. Philadelphia: Lippincott Williams & Wilkins, 2000.)

Evaluation

- In acute trauma, attention to airway, breathing, and circulation/hemorrhage is the primary focus.
- Suspect pelvic fracture in all cases of serious or multiple trauma.
- Radiologic evaluation is essential for definitive diagnosis. The standard trauma AP pelvis film is generally sufficient for initial identification of pelvic ring fractures.
- In the hemodynamically stable patient, CT scan may be of value in determining full extent of bony and vascular injury.
- **In pelvic trauma there is a high incidence of associated injuries; therefore, special attention should be paid to the rectal and urogenital examinations.** Also due to the location of the sacral nerve plexus, lower extremity neurological examination is indicated.
- As hemorrhage is the main cause of mortality in pelvic trauma, it is critical to assess hemodynamic stability and identify ongoing bleeding in the chest, abdomen, and long bones. If no clear source of hemorrhage is identified and patient remains unstable, suspicion for primary pelvic hemorrhage should be high.
- Order a pregnancy test in any woman of childbearing age as there are significant implications in the gravid patient.
- If the pelvis is determined to be unstable on physical examination, repeated examinations by various members of the trauma team should be avoided to prevent worsening of the injury.

Management

- Resuscitative efforts per advanced trauma life support (ATLS) protocol.
- Correct hemodynamic instability. This may require large volumes of intravenous crystalloid and blood products.
- Evaluate for other sources of bleeding: focused assessment with sonography for trauma (FAST), diagnostic peritoneal lavage.
  - Evidence of intra-abdominal free fluid is an indication for emergent laparotomy prior to pelvic repair.
  - Diagnostic peritoneal lavage, if performed, should be via an open, supraumbilical approach.
- Suspect pelvic injury/hemorrhage in patients with high fluid requirements, particularly if no intra-abdominal or thoracic source is found.
  - If pelvic hemorrhage is suspected, consider stabilization of pelvis in the emergency department and emergent angiography with embolization via interventional radiology.
- Stabilization of the pelvis in the emergency department.
  - Primary goal is early reduction of pelvic volume, which decreases hemorrhage through tamponade and clot formation, thereby improving mortality.
  - Noninvasive methods are preferred.
  - Circumferential wrapping of the pelvis with a sheet is an easy and inexpensive option. Commercially available pelvic binders including the trauma pelvic orthotic device (T-POD) are also an excellent option.
  - Other methods of stabilization, more complicated and less commonly used, include military anti-shock trousers (MAST) trousers, spica casting, application of a posterior C-clamp, or external fixation.
- Operative management.
  - Gold standard of definitive management remains open reduction with internal fixation (ORIF).
- Avoid hypothermia. Use warmed fluids when possible.

Special Considerations

- Significant pelvic trauma should be managed at a Level I trauma center.
- Always obtain an AP x-ray film of the pelvis when history/mechanism suggests pelvic injury or in an unconscious trauma patient.
- In pelvic trauma with hypotension, suspect and address sources of bleeding in the chest, intra-/extraperitoneum, or long bones. If no identifiable source of hemorrhage, suspect pelvic hemorrhage and activate interventional radiology for angiography.

Best Evidence/Clinical Decision Rules

Is circumferential wrapping of the pelvis with a sheet effective?

There are a growing number of published case reports supporting the use of circumferential sheeting in early management of unstable open-book pelvic ring injuries (see Suggested Readings). These reports emphasize the rapidity and ease of applying the pelvic sheet wrap, as well as the low cost of materials needed. All of the patients demonstrated rapid and dramatic improvement in vital signs following pelvic binding, supporting the technique's efficacy. Follow-up radiographs indicate significant reduction of the pelvic ring and symphyseal opening. With the exception of one death secondary to brain injury, all of the cited patients survived to discharge.

Suggested Readings

Bottlang M, et al. Noninvasive reduction of open-book pelvic fractures by circumferential compression. *J Orthop Trauma.* 2002;16:367–373.

Gibbs M, Tibbles C. Pelvic fractures. In: Wolfson A, ed. *Clinical Practice of Emergency Medicine.* Philadelphia: Lippincott Williams & Wilkins, 2005:1070–1078.

Harris JH. Pelvis, acetabulum, and hips. In: Harris J, Harris W, eds. *The Radiology of Emergency Medicine.* Philadelphia: Lippincott Williams & Wilkins, 2000:725–814.

Nunn T, et al. Immediate application of improvised pelvic binder as first step in extended resuscitation from life-threatening hypovolaemic shock in conscious patients with unstable pelvic injuries. *Injury.* 2007;38:125–128.

Routt MLC Jr, et al. Circumferential pelvic antishock sheeting: a temporary resuscitation aid. *J Orthop Trauma.* 2002;16:45–48.

Simpson T, et al. Stabilization of pelvic ring disruptions with a circumferential sheet. *J Trauma.* 2002;52:158–161.

Vermeulen B, et al. Prehospital stabilization of pelvic dislocations: a new strap belt to provide temporary hemodynamic stabilization. *Swiss Surg.* 1999;5:43–46.

59

Vertical Shear Pelvic Trauma

Kaushal Shah

Definition

- Vertical shear injury is when force is delivered to the pelvis vertically either from below (e.g., fall from height) or from above (e.g., heavy object falls on back or shoulders).
- Malgaigne fracture is a fracture/dislocation of the hemipelvis; it is characterized by disruption of the pubic symphysis or 2–4 pubic rami fractures (anterior ring fracture) AND disruption of the ipsilateral sacroiliac joint (posterior ring fracture).

Pathophysiology

- The most common mechanisms of vertical shear injury are fall from a height and head-on motor vehicle collisions in which the passenger has legs extended. The force is delivered vertically usually impacting one hemipelvis more than the other.
- Because there is often disruption of the ligaments and the pelvis is widened, the result is pelvic instability and increased pelvic volume (Fig. 59.1). The hemodynamic consequences are often severe with hypotension and mortality as high as 20%.
- Associated neurologic and urologic injuries are common.

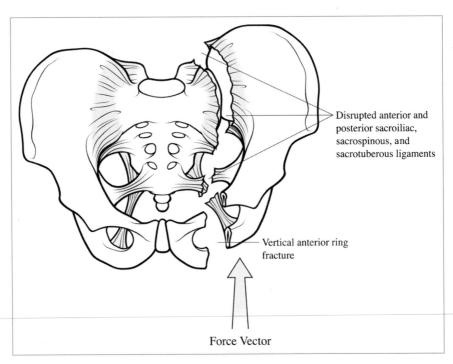

Disrupted anterior and posterior sacroiliac, sacrospinous, and sacrotuberous ligaments

Vertical anterior ring fracture

Force Vector

FIGURE 59.1: Vertical shear injury. The causative force is transmitted up the ipsilateral femur, driving the affected hemipelvis upwards. Vertical shear injuries are extremely unstable and associated with increases in pelvic volume. (Reprinted with permission from Wolfson AB, Hendey GW, Ling LJ, et al. *Harwood-Nuss' Clinical Practice of Emergency Medicine*, 5th ed. Philadelphia: Lippincott Williams & Wilkins, 2009.)

Diagnosis

- Pelvic fracture can be suspected on physical examination if (a) instability is noted with gentle downward and lateral pressure on the iliac wings or (b) there is inability of an awake patient to actively flex the hip (90% sensitivity and 95% specificity for pelvic fracture).
- Definitive diagnosis requires imaging of the pelvis (Fig. 59.2). The standard trauma AP pelvis film will readily identify significant vertical shear injuries, such as Malgaigne fractures (anterior and posterior ring fractures with dislocation of hemipelvis).
  - Anterior ring fracture—unilateral ischiopubic rami fracture or widening of the pubic symphysis.
  - Posterior ring fracture—ipsilateral sacral, iliac, or sacroiliac joint fracture.

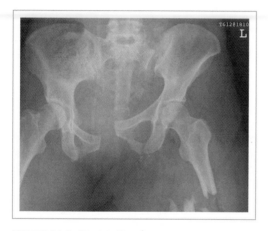

FIGURE 59.2: AP plain film of vertical shear injury with symphysis diastasis and upward-migration of the left hemipelvis. (Reprinted with permission from Wolfson AB, Hendey GW, Ling LJ, et al. *Harwood-Nuss' Clinical Practice of Emergency Medicine*, 5th ed. Philadelphia: Lippincott Williams & Wilkins, 2009.)

Evaluation

- In the acute trauma scenario, further imaging of the fracture/dislocation pattern is not necessary. The high mortality associated with Malgaigne fractures is due to hemorrhage and associated injuries.
- Evaluation should focus on identifying associated injuries.
  - Rectal examination revealing gross blood suggests bowel injury/laceration, possibly as a result of a pelvic fracture fragment.
  - Bladder and urethra are at high risk of injury given their location in the pelvis.
  - Foley catheter placement should be deferred if there is blood at the penile meatus, ecchymosis of the perineum/scrotum, or high-riding prostate on rectal examination.
  - Bimanual pelvic examination may reveal lacerations (rare).
  - Lower extremity neurologic examination is essential because lumbosacral plexus injuries are present in almost 50% of patients with posterior pelvis disruptions.

Management

- Given the significant force required to create a Malgaigne fracture, the predominant source of hemorrhage should be identified as soon as possible.
  - Intra-abdominal hemorrhage (positive FAST or diagnostic peritoneal lavage) requires immediate laparotomy.

- Therapeutic angiography with embolization is often necessary in "unstable" pelvic fractures, such as Malgaigne fractures.
- Suspect the need for aggressive resuscitation in patients with Malgaigne fractures. The "trauma triad of death" needs to be considered.
  - Acidosis—Check the serum lactate and base deficit but patient will likely require a blood transfusion (Malgaigne fractures require on average 6–7 units of packed red blood cells).
  - Hypothermia—Warm fluids and blood products are preferable.
  - Coagulopathy—Order and initiateresh frozen plasma (FFP) administration early.
- Reducing pelvic volume is a critical step in managing pelvic hemorrhage; however, this should not be performed in patients with vertical displacement of the hemipelvis. The "book" will not close evenly and may exacerbate the pelvic bleeding.
- External fixators cannot control hemorrhage in Malgaigne fractures because of the posterior disruption. These should not be placed during emergency resuscitation.

Special Considerations
- Vertical shear injuries need to be managed at a Level I trauma center. Initiate a timely transfer.
- With the widespread availability of ultrasound at the bedside, diagnostic peritoneal lavage (DPL) should be performed only in unstable patients with a high suspicion for intra-abdominal injury. Otherwise, patients should go directly to angiography.
- If a DPL is performed, it should be an "open" procedure with a supraumbilical approach.

Best Evidence/Clinical Decision Rules

Patients with significant vertical shear pelvic trauma often have significant associated injuries. How do you decide which injury should be addressed first?

The goal of trauma resuscitation is to identify and control the source of hemorrhage. If the patient is hypotensive, the blood is in the chest, abdomen, pelvis, long bones, or left in the street. Consider the source to be the pelvis when everything else is ruled out: chest x-ray film does not demonstrate hemothorax; FAST is negative; no long bone fractures on examination; and no history of significant prehospital bleeding. Given that control of pelvic hemorrhage requires angiography by interventional radiologists outside of the emergency department and intensive care unit, management of abdomen and chest hemorrhage trumps pelvic bleeding.

Suggested Readings
Gibbs M, Tibbles C. Pelvic fractures. In: Wolfson A, ed. *Clinical Practice of Emergency Medicine*. Philadelphia: Lippincott Williams & Wilkins, 2005:1070–1078.

Harris JH. Pelvis, acetabulum, and hips. In: Harris J, Harris W, eds. *The Radiology of Emergency Medicine*. Philadelphia: Lippincott Williams & Wilkins, 2000:725–814.

Section Editor: Ari Lipsky

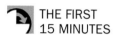

60

Genitourinary Trauma: The First 15 Minutes, Algorithm, and Decision Making

Pranav Shetty and Clinton J. Coil

THE FIRST 15 MINUTES

ABCs and Vital Signs

■ Follow ATLS protocols and Genitourinary Trauma algorithm.

History

■ Injuries to the external genitalia (penis, scrotum, testes, labia, vagina) and urinary tract (urethra, bladder, ureter, and kidney) are primarily caused by blunt trauma, such as motor vehicle collisions, falls, straddle injuries, and sexual activity.

■ Less commonly, penetrating trauma such as gunshot and stab wounds can also cause serious injury.

Physical Examination

■ A careful examination of the genitourinary system is an important part of the secondary survey. Signs of renal, urethral, and external genitalia trauma are listed in Table 60.1.

■ Gross or microscopic hematuria can indicate injury anywhere along the urinary tract.

TABLE 60.1: Signs of injury to the kidney, urethra, and external genitalia

Injury	Signs
External genitalia	Swelling, redness, and/or bruising
Urethra	Blood at meatus Hematoma/ecchymosis to penis/perineum/scrotum "High-riding" or boggy prostate Evidence of pelvic fracture
Renal	Flank tenderness Flank hematoma/ecchymosis Penetrating flank wound

Emergency Interventions

- Evaluation of genitourinary trauma progresses in a retrograde fashion: urethra, bladder, and kidney.
- A Foley catheter must not be placed if there are signs of urethral injury. In addition, if Foley catheter placement is difficult or unsuccessful, urethral injury should be suspected. A **retrograde urethrogram** must be performed prior to further attempts at Foley catheter placement.
- In the case of gross hematuria alone, or microscopic hematuria in the presence of a pelvic fracture, evaluation of bladder integrity should be performed with **retrograde cystography**.
- If upper urinary tract injury is suspected, evaluation of the kidneys and ureters should occur using a **computed tomographic (CT) scan** or intravenous pyelogram.
- In the special setting of penile amputation, the severed penis should be cleaned, wrapped in sterile saline gauze, and placed in a bag which is then placed on ice in preparation for possible reattachment.

Memorable Pearls

- Urethral injury is almost exclusively seen in male patients. Female patients rarely sustain urethral injury due to its short course and increased mobility.
- Clamping the Foley catheter prior to CT scan and taking care to avoid spilling contrast on the patient or bedding can make interpretation of studies easier.
- Injury to the kidney or ureter should be suspected if nearby structures are injured, such as fractures of a lower rib or lumbar vertebra, or injury to the liver or spleen.

Essential Considerations

- In most cases, genitourinary trauma is not life-threatening. As with any trauma patient, evaluation and management of the ABCs and life-threatening injuries take precedence.
- Renal vascular injury with massive hemorrhage is one exception to the above rule. This should be suspected in a patient with unexplained hypotension, possibly with gross or microscopic hematuria.
- The evaluation of genitourinary trauma normally progresses in a retrograde fashion so as to rule out distal injuries prior to the evaluation of more proximal injuries.

Consultations

- Trauma surgery
- Urology

DECISION
MAKING

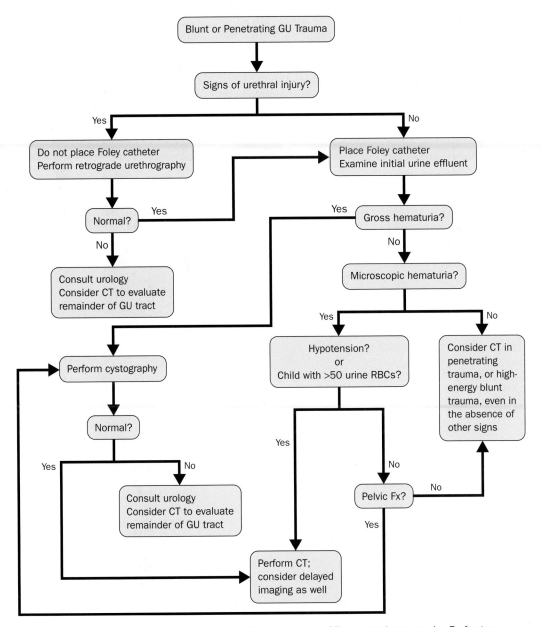

Genitourinary trauma: Decision making algorithm. GU, genitourinary; CT, computed tomography; Fx, fracture; RBCs, red blood cells.

Suggested Readings

Dreitlein DA, Suner S, Basler J. Genitourinary trauma. *Emerg Med Clin North Am.* 2001;19(3):569–590.

Schneider R. Genitourinary procedures. In: *Clinical Procedures in Emergency Medicine,* 4th ed. Mosby Elsevier, 2004:1001–1024.

Schneider R. Genitourinary system. In: Marx J, et al., eds. *Rosen's Emergency Medicine: Concepts and Clinical Practice.* 6th ed. Mosby, 2006:514–536.

Tibbles CD. Genitourinary trauma. In: Wolfson AB, ed. *Harwood-Nuss' Clinical Practice of Emergency Medicine,* 5th ed. Lippincott Williams & Wilkins, 2009:238–243.

Wessells H, Long L. Penile and genital injuries. *Urol Clin North Am.* 2006;33(1): 117–126.

61   Urethral Trauma
                                        Casey Buitenhuys

Definition
- Traumatic urethral injuries are more common in the male population given the longer length of the male urethra.
- The male urethra is divided into the proximal and distal segments by the urogenital diaphragm. The anterior urethra can be further divided into the membranous and prostatic segments.

Pathophysiology
- Shearing forces associated with pelvic fractures cause most injuries to the posterior urethra, whereas straddle injuries or penetrating trauma causes most anterior urethral injuries.
- During high-force mechanisms causing trauma to the bony pelvis, any significant displacement of the anterior pelvis can cause disruption of the posterior urethra.
- Straddle injuries can disrupt the anterior urethra by compressing the urethra between a hard object and the symphysis pubis. This injury is most commonly seen in bicycle accidents, skateboard accidents, and other falls onto the perineum.
- The location of trauma during penetrating mechanisms is variable. Typical causes include selfmutilation, stab wounds, foreign body insertion, and bullet wounds.

Diagnosis
- The diagnosis of urethral injuries should be prioritized after the initial resuscitation of life-threatening injuries.
- Signs of possible urethral trauma are listed in Table 61.1.
- A urinalysis should be performed to look for gross hematuria.
- Any signs of potential urethral trauma should preclude the passage of a urethral catheter prior to imaging to exclude a urethral tear.

TABLE 61.1: Signs of possible urethral trauma

Unstable pelvis or pelvic pain with stress
Hematoma of the perineum, scrotum, or anterior-inferior abdominal wall
Blood at the urethral meatus
Gross hematuria
Microscopic hematuria in the setting of shock
Prostate that is difficult to palpate, boggy, high rising, or that cannot be palpated
Inability to spontaneously void

- Passage of a Foley catheter can convert a partial urethral tear into a complete urethral tear.
- A retrograde urethrogram should be performed to look for a urethral tear (see Chapter "Retrograde Urethrogram" for details).
  - A retrograde urethrogram is performed by instilling 10 mL of undiluted contrast into the urethra and taking a plain radiograph of the pelvis.
  - Anterior tears will demonstrate extravasation below the urogenital diaphragm, whereas posterior tears will demonstrate extravasation above the urogenital diaphragm.

Evaluation
- Follow ATLS protocol and manage life-threatening injuries appropriately first.
- Any evaluation of urethral injury should be done after mandatory resuscitative and operative measures have been completed.
- When there are signs of possible urethral trauma, a retrograde urethrogram should be performed prior to passage of any catheter. The radiological test of choice for urethral injury is a retrograde urethrogram.
- If there are no signs of a urethral injury, a Foley catheter may be placed.

Management
- Management of urethral injuries should proceed after stabilization of life-threatening injuries.
- If there are no signs of urethral trauma, the passage of clear urine or successful placement of a Foley catheter with return of clear urine makes urethral trauma extremely unlikely.
- For all suspected urethral tears, a retrograde urethrogram should be performed.
  - A urethrogram that is negative for extravasation excludes a urethral tear.
  - If a partial tear is seen on urethrogram, a urologist should be consulted immediately. A single attempt at passage of a 12F or 14F coude catheter may be made after a partial tear is determined. If there is any resistance to passage, there should be no further attempts.
  - If a complete urethral tear is seen on urethrogram, a urologist should be consulted immediately and a diverting suprapubic cystostomy should be considered (performed in conjunction with the consultant).

Special Considerations
- Passage of a urinary catheter in the unstable trauma patient is not contraindicated and is unlikely to convert a partial urethral tear into a complete tear.
- Before placement of a suprapubic cystostomy, consultation with a urologist is advised. Many anterior urethral injuries can be repaired primarily without a diverting cystostomy.

Suggested Readings
Bent C, Iyngkaran T, Power N, et al. Urological injuries following trauma. *Clin Radiol.* 2008;63:1361–1371.
Brewer ME, Wilmoth RJ, Enderson BL, Daley BJ. Prospective comparison of microscopic and gross hematuria as predictors of bladder injury in blunt trauma. *Urology.* 2007;69:1086–1089.

Coburn M. Genitourinary trauma. In: Feliciano DV, Mattox KL, Moore EE, eds. *Trauma*, 6th ed. New York: McGraw-Hill, 2008.

Schneider RE. Genitourinary system. In: Marx JA et al, eds. *Rosen's Emergency Medicine*, 6th ed. Philadelphia: Mosby, 2006:514–536.

Wessells H. Injuries to the urogenital tract. In: Souba WW et al, eds. *ACS Surgery: Principles and Practice*. New York: WebMD Professional Publishing, 2009.

Bladder Trauma

Neil Patel and Amy Kaji

Definition

- The adult empty bladder is relatively protected by the bony pelvis. However, when distended, it may rise up to the level of the umbilicus, exposing the bladder to blunt and penetrating trauma.
- Bladder injuries range from minor contusions to complete perforation.
- Bladder contusions are partial thickness injuries to the bladder wall without perforation.
- Bladder perforation can be either extraperitoneal or intraperitoneal:
  - Extraperitoneal bladder perforation is frequently associated with fractures of the anterior pelvic ring with laceration of the bladder by a fracture fragment.
  - Intraperitoneal bladder perforation usually occurs from blunt force to a distended bladder at the anatomically weak dome of the bladder.

Pathophysiology

- After the kidney, the bladder is the second most commonly injured organ in the setting of genitourinary trauma.
- Blunt trauma accounts for the majority of bladder injuries.
- **The majority of bladder ruptures and perforations are associated with pelvic fractures.**
- Bladder perforation usually requires a significant mechanism of injury as reflected by the relatively high associated mortality (22–44%) and its association with other intraabdominal, genitourinary, and skeletal injuries.

Diagnosis

- Bladder injuries should be clinically suspected in any trauma patient with gross hematuria (98% sensitive), inability or difficulty voiding, or significant lower abdominal pain and tenderness.
  - The majority of bladder injuries with or without pelvic fractures present with either gross or microscopic hematuria (≥25 red blood cells/high power field (HPF)).
- Definitive diagnosis requires imaging of the bladder via either a conventional or computed tomographic (CT) retrograde cystogram:
  - Conventional retrograde cystogram
    - Obtain a baseline KUB film.
    - After approximately 400 mL (amount for those younger than 11 years: [age + 2] × 30) of 10% water-soluble contrast is instilled into the bladder via a Foley catheter, clamp the catheter.
    - Obtain an AP view of the contrast-filled bladder and then unclamp the Foley catheter.
    - After evacuation of all contrast material from the bladder, obtain a postevacuation film to check for posterior bladder wall perforation.

▷   *Extraperitoneal perforation* will demonstrate extravasated contrast material limited to the pelvic region, whereas *intraperitoneal perforation* will demonstrate contrast enhancement of intraperitoneal organs.
- CT retrograde cystogram
  - ▷ After retrograde instillation of 400 mL of 10% water-soluble contrast via a Foley catheter, clamp the catheter.
  - ▷ Obtain a standard computed tomography of the abdomen and pelvis and then unclamp the Foley.
- Note the importance of forcefully distending the bladder, as false-negative retrograde cystograms most commonly result from inadequate distension of the bladder from insufficient contrast instillation (Figs. 62.1 and 62.2).

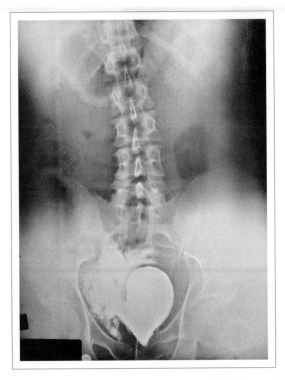

FIGURE 62.1: Cystogram with extraperitoneal bladder rupture (Reprinted with permission from Wolfson AB, Hendey GW, Ling LJ, et al. *Harwood-Nuss' Clinical Practice of Emergency Medicine,* 5th ed. Philadelphia: Lippincott Williams & Wilkins, 2009.)

Evaluation
- Evaluation of bladder trauma is generally not time-sensitive or critical but evaluation of associated injuries is very important given the significant mechanism required to produce bladder perforation; assess and address all life-threatening injuries first.
- **Evaluation of the genitourinary tract should proceed in a retrograde fashion.**
  - Urethral injury must first be ruled out clinically or via a retrograde urethrogram before placement of a Foley catheter to facilitate evaluation for bladder injury.
  - The AP pelvis film should be examined for evidence of a pelvic fracture.

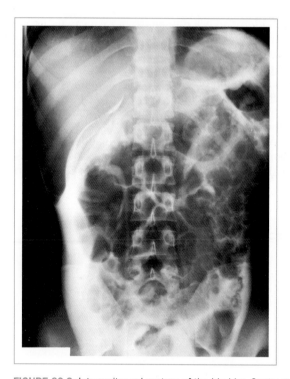

FIGURE 62.2: Intraperitoneal rupture of the bladder. Contrast medium is seen between loops of intestine. The sharp definition of the lateral margins of the contrast medium in the paracolic gutters and outlining the surfaces of the liver and the relative homogeneity of the collections of contrast as well as the sharp definitions of the contrast outlining loops of bowel are absolutely characteristic of intraperitoneal bladder rupture. (Reprinted with permission from Harris JH, Harris WH. *The Radiology of Emergency Medicine,* 4th ed. Philadelphia: Lippincott Williams & Wilkins, 2000.)

- A FAST scan may help identify intraperitoneal injury, but ultrasound cannot reliably distinguish blood from urine.
- Patients with suspected concomitant bladder and intra-abdominal injury requiring computed tomography of the abdomen/pelvis should have the CT retrograde cystogram performed prior to injection of intravenous contrast.

Management
- Patients with bladder contusions or superficial lacerations without perforation may be managed expectantly with or without Foley catheter placement.
- Most cases of *extraperitoneal bladder perforation* can be *managed nonsurgically* with continuous Foley catheter drainage for 1–2 weeks to allow spontaneous healing.
  - If the bladder perforation involves the bladder neck or proximal urethra, consideration should be given to primary surgical repair, given the risk of long-term urinary incontinence with these injuries.
  - Patients undergoing abdominal surgery for other injuries may also be candidates for primary surgical repair, if the perforation site is readily accessible.
- *Intraperitoneal bladder perforation requires surgical repair* after more life-threatening injuries have been addressed.

Special Considerations

- In children, the bladder is largely within the abdominal cavity, making the bladder more vulnerable to injury and intraperitoneal perforation more common.
- For retrograde cystograms and CT retrograde cystograms in children up to age 11, the amount of water-soluble contrast that should be instilled is calculated in milliliters as follows: (age + 2) × 30.
- In patients with pelvic fractures and suspected bladder injury, avoid excessive movement of the patient during diagnostic maneuvers to prevent rebleeding by displacing a possible retropubic hematoma.
- **Bladder injuries are rarely life-threatening and priority should therefore be given to the diagnosis and management of associated injuries with a potential for greater morbidity and mortality.**

Best Evidence/Clinical Decision Rules

When can I clinically exclude significant bladder injury?

The evidence suggests that bladder perforation can be reliably excluded in trauma patients with grossly clear urine in the absence of a pelvic fracture. Conversely, the presence of gross hematuria with or without a pelvic fracture or microscopic hematuria (≥25 RBCs/HPF) with a pelvic fracture mandates further diagnostic investigation for a bladder injury.

Suggested Readings

Deck AJ, et al. Computerized tomography cystography for the diagnosis of traumatic bladder rupture. *J Urol*. 2000;164:43.

McAninch JW. Injuries to the genitourinary tract. In: Tanagho EA, McAninch JW, eds. *General Urology*. Norwalk, Conn: Appleton & Lange, 1999.

Schneider RE. Genitourinary system. In: Marx JA, et al, eds. *Rosen's Emergency Medicine*. Philadelphia: Mosby, 2006:514–536.

Tibbles CD. Genitourinary trauma. In: Wolfson AB, ed. *Harwood-Nuss' Clinical Practice of Emergency Medicine*. 5th ed. Philadelphia: Lippincott Williams & Wilkins, 2009:238–243.

Definition/Pathophysiology

- The kidneys are located in the retroperitoneal space along T10 through L4 spine levels. Although they are supported by arteries, veins, adipose tissue, and Gerota fascia, they are not fixed and move with the diaphragm.
- The kidneys receive one-quarter of the body's cardiac output.
- Renal trauma often occurs concomitantly with abdominal, thoraco-lumbar, and/or pelvic injuries. In the United States, 80% of renal injuries are due to blunt trauma and 20% are due to penetrating trauma.
- The American Association for the Surgery of Trauma Organ Injury Scale is the most widely used anatomic scheme for classifying kidney injuries (Table 63.1; Fig. 63.1). Its usefulness in predicting morbidity for blunt and penetrating injuries and mortality for blunt trauma has been validated in multiple studies.

Diagnosis

History

- Renal injury must be considered with any blunt or penetrating trauma to the lower thorax, abdomen, or pelvis.

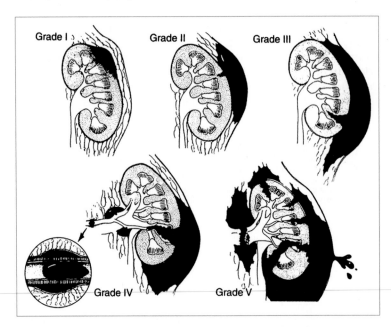

FIGURE 63.1: Artist's rendering of the American Association for the Surgery of Trauma organ injury severity scale for the kidney. (Reprinted with permission from Santucci RA, McAninch JW, Safir M, et al. Validation of the American Association for the Surgery of Trauma organ injury severity scale for the kidney. *J Trauma.* 2001;50(2):195–200.)

TABLE 63.1: Kidney injury scale

I	Contusion	Microscopic or gross hematuria; urologic studies normal
	Hematoma	Subcapsular, nonexpanding without parenchymal laceration
II	Hematoma	Nonexpanding perirenal hematoma confined to the renal retroperitoneum
	Laceration	<1 cm parenchymal depth of renal cortex without urinary extravasation
III	Laceration	>1 cm parenchymal depth of renal cortex without collecting system rupture or urinary extravasation
IV	Laceration	Parenchymal laceration extending through the renal cortex, medulla, and collecting system
V	Vascular	Main renal artery or vein injury with contained hemorrhage
	Laceration	Completely shattered kidney
	Vascular	Avulsion of renal hilum that devascularizes kidney

Reprinted with permission from Moore EE, Shackford SR, Pachter HL, et al. Organ injury scaling: spleen, liver, and kidney. *J Trauma*. 1989;29:1664.

- Associated pain is often described as a dull ache; other symptoms may include nausea and vomiting. The patient may have or develop a paralytic ileus.

Physical Examination
- In general, the **physical examination of the kidneys in the setting of trauma has limited utility.**
- Clinical signs and symptoms such as flank pain, ecchymoses, lower rib fractures, and hematuria are helpful, but *their absence does not exclude significant renovascular injury*.

Evaluation
- Consider renal injury in any trauma patient with a plausible mechanism.
- If renal injury is suspected in a *stable* trauma patient, computed tomographic (CT) scan should be obtained for further characterization of the injury (Fig. 63.2).

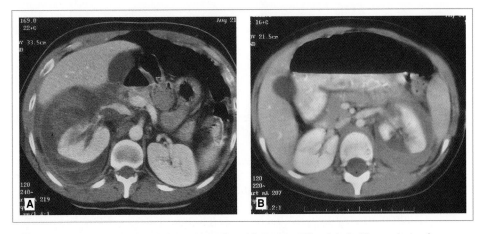

FIGURE 63.2: **(A, B)** Renal lacerations with perirenal hematoma (Reprinted with permission from Wolfson AB, Hendey GW, Ling LJ, et al. *Harwood-Nuss' Clinical Practice of Emergency Medicine*, 5th ed. Philadelphia: Lippincott Williams & Wilkins, 2009.

TABLE 63.2: Imaging modalities for evaluating renal injuries

Modality	Advantages	Disadvantages	Recommended uses
Computed tomographic scan with intravenous contrast	Most comprehensive diagnostic tool available. Readily available at most institutions. Simultaneous evaluation for other nonrenal injuries	May miss or incompletely characterize some vascular injuries. Commonly misses ureteral injuries. Requires intravenous contrast for adequate sensitivity	Imaging modality of choice in any hemodynamically stable patient. *Delayed follow-up CT*: if the initial CT shows deep parenchymal laceration or large perirenal fluid collection, the scan may be repeated in 3–5 minutes to obtain excretory phase images
Ultrasound	Easy visualization of perinephric hematomas	Poor sensitivity (22%) for evaluating renal parenchyma or collecting system injuries. Cannot distinguish between extravasated blood and urine	Worthwhile in patients with indications for FAST examination (blunt trauma to the abdomen) but should not be used as the definitive modality in patients in whom one suspects renal or other solid organ injury
Intravenous pyelogram. Involves flat plate abdominal x-ray 10 minutes after an intravenous contrast injection; both kidneys and ureters should be visualized	Quick, bedside examination that demonstrates basic function of both kidneys (useful in a critical patient to establish the presence of one functional kidney to decide whether nephrectomy of the injured kidney is possible)	Nonspecific findings often necessitate additional studies	Unstable patients who cannot go for CT or who are already in the operating room
Angiography	Gold standard for vascular pedicle injuries. Angiography with transcatheter embolization is becoming the standard of care in patients with vascular injuries	Less sensitive than CT for vascular contrast extravasation and characterizing injuries. Invasive and not readily available at most institutions	Rarely used. Can be employed for evaluation and transcatheter noninvasive treatment of vascular complications (fistulas, aneurysms)

CT, computed tomography; FAST, focused assessment with sonography for trauma.

- Currently, most centers rarely use modalities other than computed tomography. Table 63.2 summarizes other radiographic methods of evaluating the genitourinary system; indications are listed in Table 63.3.
- Hemodynamically stable adults with blunt trauma, microscopic hematuria, no shock (systolic blood pressure <90 mm Hg) in the field or in the emergency department, and no other indication for imaging or admission can be safely discharged.
- Children are more vulnerable to renal injuries than adults due to their relatively pliable thorax and underdeveloped abdominal musculature. Based on analysis of current practice guidelines, Table 63.4 summarizes the commonly used indications for obtaining a CT scan of the abdomen and pelvis in children.

TABLE 63.3: Indications for renal imaging in adults

Blunt trauma and gross hematuria

Penetrating injury and any degree of hematuria

Significant deceleration injury in a stable patient

Microscopic hematuria (>5 RBCs/HPF) and hypotension (SBP <90 mm Hg)

Microscopic hematuria (>5 RBCs/HPF) associated with other injuries, especially abdominal trauma

RBCs, red blood cells; HPF, high power field; SBP, systolic blood pressure.

- If the sole indication for imaging is to evaluate the kidneys in a child with blunt trauma without symptoms or hematuria, the clinician may opt to delay computed tomography and observe the child. In other words, isolated blunt renal injury without symptoms, examination findings, or hematuria is rare.
- A low threshold for investigation and imaging is appropriate for possible renal injury, as symptoms, physical examination, and indirect tests such as urinalysis may be nonspecific, insensitive, or misleading.
- Renal injury is often identified when the CT scan was obtained to evaluate other organ injuries (Fig. 63.3).

Management
- As in any trauma, prioritization of injuries is paramount. Resuscitation is tailored to the patient's clinical presentation (stable vs. unstable, blunt vs. penetrating).
- Per ATLS guidelines, unstable patients with blunt or penetrating trauma should be brought to the operating room for exploration without the delay involved in imaging studies; the possible exception to this is bedside imaging such as FAST or one-shot intravenous pyelogram (IVP) to aid in surgical approach.
- Unless there is extensive devitalized tissue, active hemorrhage, significant injury to the collecting system, or ureteral disruption, **even severe renal injuries are increasingly managed by nonoperative measures** (Table 63.5).
- Exsanguination into the retroperitoneum is the most dreaded complication from renal injury.
- An **injured kidney can tolerate only 4 to 6 hours of warm ischemia**; precious time may be lost if the evaluation is not focused and expeditious.
- A patient with renal trauma needs close monitoring. Hemodynamic instability necessitates a change in course of management, such as angiography with transcatheter embolization or surgical control of the hemorrhage.

TABLE 63.4: Indications for renal imaging in children

Blunt trauma with *significant* microscopic hematuria (>50 RBCs/HPF)

Significant deceleration injury in a stable patient

Penetrating trauma in a hemodynamically stable patient

RBCs, red blood cells; HPF, high power field.

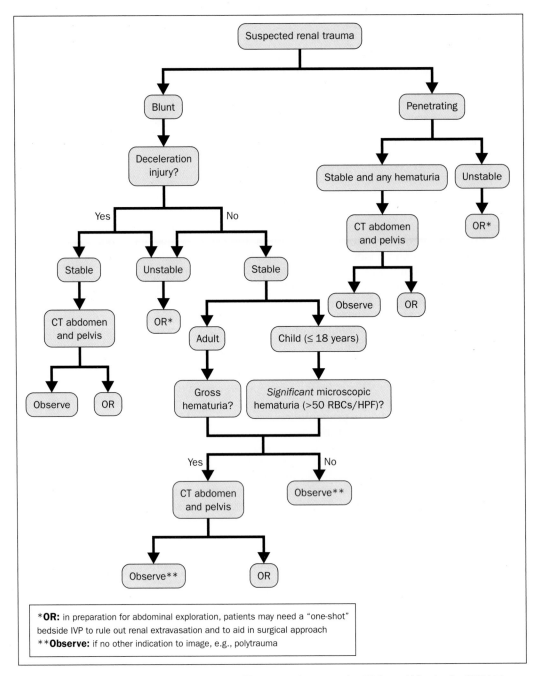

FIGURE 63.3: Suspected renal trauma algorithm. CT, computed tomography; RBCs; red blood cells; HPF, high power field; IVP, intravenous pyelogram.

TABLE 63.5: Kidney injury grade-based management

Grades 1–3	Nonoperative expectant management
Grade 4	Case-specific
Grade 5	Operative repair or nephrectomy

Pearls

- Renal injuries rarely occur in isolation.
- Absence of hematuria does not necessarily exclude renal injury.
- The degree of hematuria does not correlate with the severity of injury.
- The patient's age, mechanism of injury, vital signs, and clinical status guide evaluation and management.

Best Evidence/Clinical Decision Rules

Grade I-III renal injuries should be managed expectantly with serial examinations and reimaging as necessary. What acute and long-term sequelae are these patients at risk for?

Acute complications include expanding urinoma or hematoma and ileus. Eventually, patients may develop *Page kidney*. Chronic hypertension after renal trauma was first described by Irwin Page in 1939. Parenchymal damage by hematoma compression or segmental devitalization causes increased renin secretion, which results in chronic hypertension. This may take months to years to develop. Close follow-up is recommended.

Suggested Readings

Bent C, Iyngkaran T, Power N, et al. Urological injuries following trauma. *Clin Radio.* 2008;63:1361–1371.

Kuan JK, Wright JL, Nathens AB, et al. American Association for the Surgery of Trauma Organ Injury Scale for kidney injuries predicts nephrectomy, dialysis, and death in patients with blunt injury and nephrectomy for penetrating injuries. *J Trauma.* 2006;60:351–356.

Mee SL, McAninch JW, Robinson AL, et al. Radiographic assessment of renal trauma: a 10-year prospective study of patient selection. *J Urol.* 1989;141:1095–1098.

Perez-Brayfield MR, Gatti JM, Smith EA, et al. Blunt traumatic hematuria in children. Is a simplified algorithm justified? *J Urol.* 2002;167:2543–2546.

Rogers CG, Knight V, MacUra KJ, et al. High-grade renal injuries in children—is conservative management possible? *Urology.* 2004;64:574–579.

Santucci RA, McAninch JW, Safir M, et al. Validation of the American Association for the Surgery of Trauma organ injury severity scale for the kidney. *J Trauma.* 2001;50:195–200.

Shariat SF, Roehrborn CG, Karakiewicz PI, et al. Evidence-based validation of the predictive value of the American Association for the Surgery of Trauma kidney injury scale. *J Trauma.* 2007;62:933–939.

Smith JK, Kenney PJ. Imaging of renal trauma. *Radiol Clin North Am.* 2003;41:1019–1035.

Stein JP, Kaji DM, Eastham J, et al. Blunt renal trauma in the pediatric population: indications for radiographic evaluation. *Urology.* 1994;44:406–410.

Penile Trauma

Herbert C. Duber

Definition

- Penile trauma is a broad category of injuries that includes, but is not limited to, amputation, fracture, entrapment, and strangulation injuries.
- **Amputation:** Complete or partial severing of the penis. Complete transection comprises severing both the corpora cavernosa and the urethra.
- **Fracture:** Tunica albuginea thins from 2 mm to 0.25–0.5 mm when erect. Decreased thickness makes the tunica more vulnerable to direct trauma and an abnormal bending of the penis can result in tearing of the tunica and traumatic rupture of the underlying corpus cavernosum. Although one corpus cavernosum is usually injured, both may be involved.
- **Strangulation:** An object placed around the penis which leads to venous and subsequent arterial flow obstruction.

Pathophysiology

- The bulk of the penis consists of two corpora cavernosa and one corpus spongiosum. The corpora cavernosa are larger and located on the dorsal aspect of the penis. The corpus spongiosum is located ventrally, surrounds the urethra, and expands distally to form the glans. The tunica albuginea is a dense fibrous tissue that encases each of the three corpora.
- Vascular supply of the penis consists of two dorsal penile arteries and one small artery in each of the corpora. There is a single dorsal vein that drains most of the penis.

Diagnosis

- Amputation
  - Diagnosis is self-evident.
  - Mechanism of injury should be elucidated as human bite injuries place patient at increased risk of infection and often present late secondary to embarrassment.
- Fracture (Fig. 64.1)
  - Signs include localized pain, hematoma, and detumescence.
  - Penis is abnormally curved, commonly taking on an "S" shape.
  - Usually occurs during vigorous intercourse, and often accompanied by a snapping or popping sound.
- Strangulation (Fig. 64.2)
  - Distal swelling with proximal penile ring, hair tourniquet, or other circumferential obstruction.

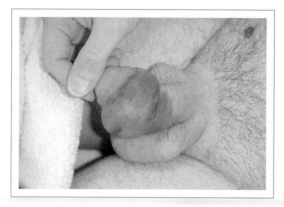

FIGURE 64.1: **A:** Penile fracture. Note swelling, deformity, and ecchymosis. (Courtesy of Donald Sallee, MD.) (Reprinted with permission from Greenberg MI, Hendrickson RG, Silverberg M, et al. *Greenberg's Text-Atlas of Emergency Medicine*. Philadelphia: Lippincott Williams & Wilkins, 2005.)

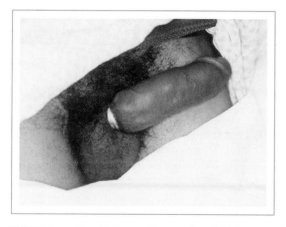

FIGURE 64.2: Constricting penile ring. (Copyright James R. Roberts, MD.) (Reprinted with permission from Greenberg MI, Hendrickson RG, Silverberg M, et al. *Greenberg's Text-Atlas of Emergency Medicine*. Philadelphia: Lippincott Williams & Wilkins, 2005.)

Evaluation

- No imaging or laboratory studies are indicated for most isolated penile injuries.
- Severe penile injury is often associated with urethral injury. If urethral injury is considered, urinanalysis should be ordered to evaluate for hematuria and retrograde urethrogram is the study of choice.
- Penile fracture is usually a clinical diagnosis. However, in equivocal cases diagnostic cavernosography or magnetic resonance imaging can be performed.
- In cases of strangulation, look closely for offending object. Often difficult to see hair or string tourniquets which are common in younger children.

Management

- Amputations
  - Emergent urologic consult for primary reanastomosis or local reshaping.
  - Reanastomosis is possible within 6 hours of amputation.

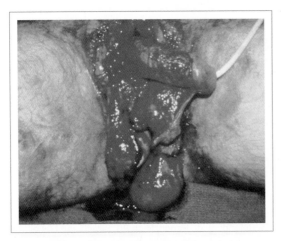

FIGURE 64.3: Genital degloving injury. (Courtesy of Lewis J. Kaplan, MD.) (Reprinted with permission from Greenberg MI, Hendrickson RG, Silverberg M, et al. *Greenberg's Text-Atlas of Emergency Medicine*. Philadelphia: Lippincott Williams & Wilkins, 2005.)

- A recovered distal penis should be treated like an amputated finger—place in a sealed bag and then put on ice/cold saline.
- Degloving injury (Fig. 64.3)
    - Emergent urologic consult.
    - Commonly treated by either a urologist or a plastic surgeon in the operating room.
- Entrapment
    - Entrapment with a zipper is best handled by cutting the median bar of the zipper with a bone or wire cutter. This allows the upper and lower shields of the zipper to separate, releasing the skin with minimal injury (Fig. 64.4).

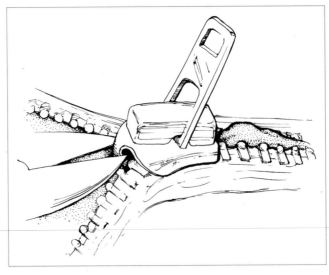

FIGURE 64.4: Penile zipper injury. A wire cutter may be used to cut the median bar of the zipper, releasing the two sides of the zipper and freeing the penis. (Reprinted with permission from Fleisher GR, Ludwig S, Henretig FM, et al. *Textbook of Pediatric Emergency Medicine*, 5th ed. Philadelphia: Lippincott Williams & Wilkins, 2005.)

- Fracture
  - Most are treated surgically—evacuation of penile hematoma, torn tunica albuginea sutured, and pressure dressing applied.
  - Occasional nonoperative management entails bed rest, ice packs for 24–48 hours followed by local heat, and pressure dressing.
- Hemorrhage
  - Direct pressure.
  - If unsuccessful can use a Penrose drain at the base of the penis as a tourniquet until urosurgical consultation is available. Should not be used for extended periods.
- Lacerations
  - Superficial lacerations can be repaired with 4–0 chromic or vicryl (absorbable) suture.
- Strangulation
  - Remove the offending device.
  - Ring cutters or the "string technique" may be used to remove rings.
  - Softer tourniquets (hair, thread, etc.) may be cut but often difficult to locate secondary to edema.

Special Considerations

- Penile fractures
  - Surgical management generally associated with better outcomes.
  - Ten percent of penile fractures result in permanent deformity, suboptimal coitus, or impaired erections (especially if treated nonoperatively).
- Penile strangulation (in children)
  - Look closely for a hair tourniquet. These are often difficult to see secondary to surrounding edema.
  - If the tourniquet has been in place for an extended period of time, urethra and dorsal nerve supply to the penis may be involved. Consider retrograde urethrogram to evaluate urethra and ultrasonography (Doppler) to confirm distal penile arterial blood supply.

Best Evidence/Clinical Decision Rules

Is penile strangulation in children concerning for abuse?

The answer to this question is unclear. Within the pediatric literature there is some disagreement as to whether or not the so called "tourniquet syndrome" is most commonly a form of intentional abuse or accident. While several cases of documented abuse have been reported (including intentional wrapping of the penis to prevent bed-wetting), the assumption that all cases of tourniquet syndrome represent abuse is not generally accepted. When tourniquet syndrome in young children is present, abuse should be considered but need not always be concluded.

Suggested Readings

Coburn M. Genitourinary trauma. In: Feliciano DV, Mattox KL, Moore EE, eds. *Trauma*, 6th ed. New York: McGraw-Hill, 2008.

Garcia CT. Genitourinary trauma. In: Fleisher GR, Ludwig S, Henretig FM, eds. *Textbook of Pediatric Emergency Medicine*, 5th ed. Philadelphia: Lippincott Williams & Wilkins, 2006:1463–1474.

Saad S, Duckett O. Urologic and gynecologic problems in children. In: Tintinalli JE, Kelen GD, Stapczynski JS, eds. *Emergency Medicine: A Comprehensive Study Guide*, 6th ed. New York: McGraw-Hill, 2004:900–905.

Schneider RE. Genitourinary system. In: Marx JA et al, eds. *Rosen's Emergency Medicine*, 6th ed. Philadelphia: Mosby, 2006:514–536.

Schneider RE. Male genital problems. In: Tintinalli JE, Kelen GD, Stapczynski JS, eds. *Emergency Medicine: A Comprehensive Study Guide*, 6th ed. New York: McGraw-Hill, 2004:613–620.

65 Scrotal Trauma

Anthony Ratanaproeksa

Definition

- Scrotal trauma encompasses injury to the scrotum and/or scrotal contents (testes, epididymis, spermatic cord; Fig. 65.1). The mechanism of injury can be used to classify scrotal trauma into three broad groups: blunt trauma, penetrating trauma, and avulsion injuries.
- Trauma to the testes can result in contusion, laceration, fracture/rupture, and dislocation.

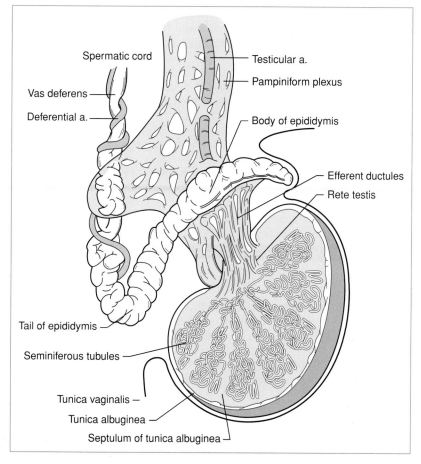

FIGURE 65.1: Normal testicular anatomy. (Reprinted with permission from Cosby KS, Kendall JL. *Practical Guide to Emergency Ultrasound*. Philadelphia: Lippincott Williams & Wilkins, 2005.)

Pathophysiology
- Blunt trauma accounts for 85% of scrotal trauma and generally includes sports-related injuries, kicks to the groin, motor vehicle accidents, falls, and straddle injuries. Penetrating trauma includes gunshot wounds, stab wounds, animal bites, and self-mutilation. Avulsion injuries most commonly occur as a result of farming/heavy machinery accidents where the scrotal skin is trapped or sheered off.
- Testicular dislocations are rare but may result following high-velocity blunt trauma, most commonly motorcycle accidents. Indirect inguinal hernias and atrophic testicles may be predisposing factors.
- A fibrous, bluish-white tissue called the tunica albuginea encapsulates the testis. A serous layer, the tunica vaginalis, envelops the tunica albuginea and also the epididymis. The tunica vaginalis comprises two layers, a visceral layer that is in direct contact with the tunica albuginea and a parietal layer. The space between the two layers of the tunica vaginalis is a potential space that normally contains a small amount of serous fluid.
- Violation of the tunica albuginea results in a rupture or fracture of the testicle. Rupture of the tunica albuginea can lead to extrusion of seminiferous tubules or blood (hematocele) into the tunica vaginalis layer.
- Disruption of the tunica vaginalis or epididymis can result in blood tracking through the facial planes into the scrotal wall resulting in a scrotal hematoma.

Diagnosis
- Suspicion for scrotal or testicular injury is usually straightforward given the mechanism of trauma and physical examination findings.
- Significant testicular injury via blunt trauma is highly suspected with complaints of severe scrotal pain, nausea, vomiting, or difficulty voiding. Physical findings include testicular swelling, tenderness, and visible scrotal or perineal hematoma/ecchymosis.
- The structural and vascular integrity of the testicle is best-evaluated utilizing color Doppler ultrasound and should be employed in any patient with a history of scrotal trauma and concerning examination findings. Ultrasound can identify disruption of the tunic layers, extrusion of testicular parenchyma, active bleeding, and vascular compromise. Identification of a hematocele (blood in the tunica vaginalis) is highly associated with testicular rupture (Fig. 65.2).

Evaluation
- Evaluation of scrotal trauma requires a thorough physical examination. The abdomen, pelvis, perineum, lower extremities, rectum, and each hemiscrotum should be examined to evaluate for coexisting injuries including vascular disruption.
- Particularly in penetrating scrotal trauma, detailed examination of all entrance and exit wounds is critical to determine the extent of potential vascular or structural injuries.
- Wound cultures are recommended for penetrating trauma and avulsion injuries.
- Following a thorough history and physical examination, color Doppler ultrasound should be performed to evaluate integrity of the testis in patients with scrotal trauma. Color Doppler will also be helpful to evaluate for trauma-associated torsion.
- Screening urinalysis should be obtained to assess for hematuria, which may indicate a concomitant urinary tract injury.

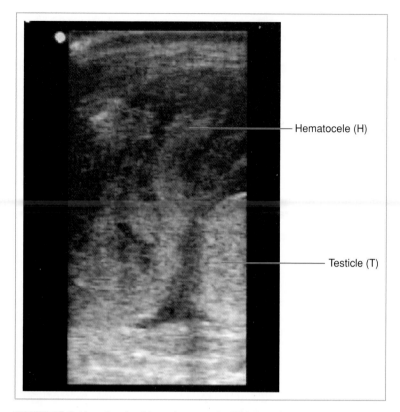

Hematocele (H)

Testicle (T)

FIGURE 65.2: Hematocele. A large hematocele (**H**) is noted superior to the testicle (**T**) in this patient who was involved in a motor vehicle crash. (Reprinted with permission from Cosby KS, Kendall JL. *Practical Guide to Emergency Ultrasound*. Philadelphia: Lippincott Williams & Wilkins, 2005.)

- Retrograde urethrography should be performed in patients with findings concerning for urethral injury (gross blood at the meatus, gross hematuria, perineal hematoma, or an absent or high-riding prostate).

Management
- Urologic consultation is required for all avulsion injuries, penetrating trauma, testicular fractures, hematoceles, hematomas, and dislocations. Surgical intervention is generally indicated.
- Antibiotic therapy and tetanus prophylaxis should be administered in all cases of penetrating trauma or avulsion injury. Clindamycin 900 mg IV q 8 hours and high-dose nafcillin 1–2 g IV q 4 hours are recommended in adults for coverage of *Clostridium perfringens*.
- Animal bites require coverage for *Pasteurella multocida* and *Streptococcus* with amoxicillin/clavulanate 500 mg PO TID or 875 mg PO BID for adults.
- Minor trauma in which there is no evidence of scrotal violation may be managed conservatively with nonsteroidal anti-inflammatory drugs, rest, elevation/support, and ice packs.

Special Considerations

- Scrotal/testicular injuries require immediate repair to preserve function. Delay in care increases the risk of infection, atrophy, necrosis, and loss of spermatogenesis and hormonal functions. Urology involvement should occur as early as possible.

Best Evidence/Clinical Decision Rules

What is the salvage/preservation rate of testicular function in scrotal trauma requiring operative intervention?

Depending on the mechanism of injury, the salvage rate ranges from 60% to 80%. There is better preservation of function in blunt trauma and worse in penetrating trauma, particularly in high-velocity penetrating trauma.

Do all hematoceles need evacuation?

All hematoceles bigger than 5 cm require surgical evacuation. There is some controversy surrounding the management of hematoceles smaller than 5 cm. Some urologists feel that exploration and evacuation of all hematoceles help achieve earlier pain resolution and shorter convalescence. Other urologists do not surgically explore hematoceles smaller than 5 cm and choose rather to follow up those patients with interval ultrasounds to ensure resolution.

Suggested Readings

Bandi G, Santucci RA. Controversies in the management of male external genitourinary trauma. *J Trauma*. 2004;56:1362–1370.

Jankowski JT, Spirnak JP. Current recommendations for imaging in the management of urologic traumas. *Urol Clin North Am*. 2006;33:365–376.

Morey AF, Metro MJ, Carney KJ, et al. Consensus on genitourinary trauma: external genitalia. *BJU Int*. 2004;94:507–515.

Section Editor: Sanjey Gupta

66

Soft Tissue Trauma: The First 15 Minutes, Algorithm, and Decision Making

Sanjey Gupta

 THE FIRST
15 MINUTES

ABCs
- Check vital signs and determine stability.
- Follow ATLS guidelines and Soft Tissue Trauma Algorithm.

History
- Crush injuries most commonly occur from "pedestrian struck" accidents, industrial accidents, and motor vehicle accidents and may lead to rhabdomyolysis.
- Compartment syndrome is a surgical emergency and is often associated with trauma and a fracture, especially tibia or forearm fractures.
- "Open fractures" is defined as a bone fracture underlying an open wound or laceration, most often occurring in the extremities.
- Peripheral amputations are often related to motor vehicle accidents, industrial accidents, or home power tool usage. Hemorrhage control is of extreme importance.
- Peripheral arterial injuries are most often related to penetrating trauma. Hemorrhage control and rapid diagnosis are of extreme importance.

Physical Examination
- Exposure of the limb and gross visual inspection is the first step
  - A full-length intact limb and intact skin rule out amputation and open fracture.
  - Look for signs of crush injury or fracture, including tissue maceration, contusion, skin laceration, pattern wounds, and limb deformity and consider further evaluation for rhabdomyolysis or compartment syndrome.
  - Brisk bleeding through a wound or an expanding hematoma within soft tissue may indicate an arterial bleed.
- Palpation
  - Any visible bone or wound/small laceration with underlying palpable bone is an open fracture.
  - A "firm" feeling compartment (e.g., gluteal, anterior tibial) with pain out of proportion to examination, especially upon passive stretching, may indicate compartment syndrome.
  - Palpable hematoma, arterial bruit or thrill, or reduced distal pulses indicate arterial injury.
  - Any peripheral appendage attached only by minor skin or tissue bridges is considered amputated.

TABLE 66.1: Compartment pressures and necessary intervention

Compartment pressure	Intervention
0 mm Hg	None, considered normal
<15 mm Hg	Observation, serial examinations
20–30 mm Hg	Observation, serial compartment pressures. May cause damage if persists for several hours
>30 mm Hg	Emergent fasciotomy

- Circulation
  - Classic "5 Ps" of arterial flow deficiency: **P**ain, **P**allor, **P**aresthesia, **P**aralysis, and **P**ulselessness.
  - "Hard signs" of arterial injury: pulsatile or rapidly enlarging hematoma, pulsatile visible arterial injury, bruit or thrill on palpating arterial pulse, or any of the 5 Ps.
  - "Soft signs" of arterial injury or flow deficiency: decreased distal pulses, decreased distal capillary refill, distal neurapraxia, and nonpulsatile hematoma.
- Neurologic
  - Pain on passive extension of extremity or pain out of proportion to examination is often the first sign of compartment syndrome.
  - Decreased sensation or strength to extremity may be present with ischemia or direct injury to nerve, even with an intact nerve sheath.
  - Loss of sensation or paralysis may indicate total/partial nerve lancination or extreme, long-standing pressure to the nerve.

Emergency Interventions
- **Suspected compartment syndrome (Table 66.1).**
  - Immediately measure compartment pressure with Stryker or similar device.
    - ▶ <15 mm Hg: considered safe.
    - ▶ 20–30 mm Hg: may cause injury if longstanding; must follow serially.
    - ▶ >30 mm Hg: consistent with compartment syndrome.
  - Immediate orthopedics or surgery consultation.
  - Do not elevate the affected limb; it does not improve venous return and impedes arterial flow, worsening tissue ischemia.
- **Open fractures** have a high risk of wound infection and osteomyelitis without acute intervention.
  - Remove gross contaminants, rinse with saline, wrap in sterile gauze.
  - Control hemorrhage with direct pressure.
  - Apply sterile pressure dressing to wound.
  - Intravenous (IV) antibiotics within 6 hours (Table 66.2).
  - Reduce fracture if weak or absent distal pulse and fashion rigid splint of extremity.
  - Update tetanus, if necessary.
  - Immediate orthopedics consultation.
- **Rhabdomyolysis**
  - Immediate treatment of early electrolyte abnormalities such as hyperkalemia, hyperphosphatemia, hypocalcemia, and metabolic acidosis as by-products of muscle breakdown.
  - Aggressive IV fluid hydration with normal saline (NS) to maintain urine output at 200–300 mL/hr.
  - Consider mannitol, urine alkalinization, and dialysis, especially in the presence of renal failure or life-threatening electrolyte abnormalities.

TABLE 66.2: Open fracture grading and antibiotic choice

Grade 1	Grade 2	Grade 3	Grade 3a	Grade 3b	Grade 3c
<1 cm laceration and minimal soft tissue damage	>1 cm laceration and minimal soft tissue damage	>1 cm laceration and extensive soft tissue damage	>1 cm laceration and extensive soft tissue damage with avulsion, flaps, muscle, neurovascular injury	>1 cm laceration and extensive soft tissue damage with periosteal stripping	>1 cm laceration and extensive soft tissue damage with vascular injury
Cefazolin 2 g (30 mg/kg) IV AND clindamycin 600 mg (10 mg/kg) IV		Same as Grades 1 and 2 or piperacillin/tazobactam 4.5 g (100 mg/kg) IV			

IV, intravenous.

- **Arterial injury:** time-sensitive treatment
  - Immediate vascular surgery consult because documented arterial injuries must be repaired within 6 hours to prevent irreversible tissue ischemia and damage.
  - Bleeding should be controlled with direct pressure or placement of a sterile pressure dressing.
  - If bleeding cannot be controlled with direct pressure, a tourniquet or blood pressure cuff inflated enough to control bleeding may be used as a temporizing measure.
  - Scalp lacerations should be immediately repaired with special attention to closure of the galea to prevent subgaleal hematoma development.
- **Amputation of extremity:** time-sensitive treatment
  - Amputated appendage should be replanted within 4–6 hours.
  - Bleeding should be controlled with direct pressure or proximal pressure with a tourniquet or blood pressure cuff.
  - IV antibiotics should given immediately.
  - Wound should be irrigated with sterile saline and wrapped with sterile dressing.
  - If the limb or appendage is still intact, irrigate the wound with saline, replace the skin to its original position, and wrap the wound with a sterile dressing.
  - If the limb or appendage is detached from the body, irrigate the wound with saline, wrap the appendage in saline-soaked sterile bandages, and then place in a resealable plastic bag and then place the appendage in an ice bath. Do NOT place the appendage directly on ice.
  - Immediate plastic/orthopedic/vascular surgery consults.
- **Memorable pearls**
  - Do not delay specialist consultation as early intervention may be life or limb sparing.
  - IV antibiotics given within 6 hours may reduce incidence of osteomyelitis.
  - Do not get distracted by an amputated, fractured, or bleeding limb—ATLS protocol must be followed for all trauma patients.

Essential Considerations
Consultations
- Trauma surgeon/team
- Orthopedic surgeon
- Vascular surgeon
- Plastic surgeon

DECISION
MAKING

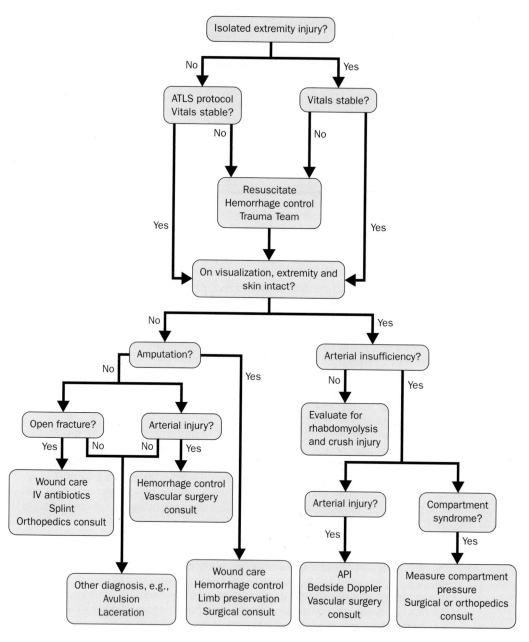

Soft tissue trauma: Decision making algorithm. ATLS, advanced trauma life support; API, arterial pressure index; IV, intravenous.

Suggested Readings

Amputation. http://www.nlm.nih.gov/medlineplus/ency/article/000006.htm. Published April 16, 2004. Accessed January 10, 2009.

Geiderman JM. General principles of orthopedic injuries. In: Marx JA, ed. *Rosen's Emergency Medicine: Concepts and Clinical Practice.* Vol 1. 6th ed. Philadelphia: Mosby, 2006:559–562.

Haller PR. Compartment syndromes. In: Tintinalli JE, ed. *Emergency Medicine: A Comprehensive Study Guide,* 6th ed. New York: McGraw-Hill Medical Publishing Division, 2004.

Levine B. 2009 *EMRA Antibiotic Guide.* Irving, Texas: Emergency Medicine Residents' Association, 2008.

Newton EJ. Acute complications of extremity trauma. *Emergency Medicine Clinics of North America.* Vol. 25, Issue 3. Philadelphia: Elsevier, 2007:751–761.

Newton EJ. Peripheral vascular injury. In: Marx JA, Hockberger RS, Walls RM, eds. *Rosen's Emergency Medicine: Concepts and Clinical Practice,* 6th ed. Philadelphia: Mosby, 2006:536–547.

Sauret J, Marinides G, Wang G. Rhabdomyolysis. *Am Fam Physician.* 2002;65(5): 907–913.

67

Amputation Trauma

Jose Dionisio Torres, Jr.

Definition
- Amputation is defined as the removal of any body protrusion by trauma or surgery.
- Most victims of traumatic amputation are males (80%) aged 15 to 30 years.
- Thirty thousand people in the United States lose a limb, digit, or other part of their body to accidental amputation annually.
- Motor vehicle crashes are a leading cause.
- Workplace accidents, especially in farm, factory, and construction environments, often result in traumatic amputation.
- Lawn mowers, saws, and other power tools contribute to limb severance.

Pathophysiology
- The longer the severed distal limb/extremity is starved of blood, the greater the amount of ischemia to muscle, nerve, bone, and other soft tissue.
- The amputation can become permanent regardless of reimplantation if the viable tissue of the amputated portion becomes necrotic.

Diagnosis
- Visual inspection often reveals the diagnosis of an amputated limb.
- Most amputated limbs bleed noticeably; examining the wound can help differentiate between arterial and venous bleeding (Fig. 67.1).

Evaluation
- Do not get distracted by the amputated limb!
- Follow ATLS guidelines and first consider all life-threatening emergencies, such as traumatic head injury, solid organ injury, pelvic fractures, spinal injuries, pneumothoraces, pericardial tamponade, etc.
- There is a risk for hemorrhage each time direct pressure is released from the amputated site. The wound should only be assessed by necessary parties.
- Radiologic studies are essential. X-rays can demonstrate whether the bones in the amputated limb are comminuted or cleanly transected, which has significant implications for management and success of reimplantation.

Management
General Guidelines
- Apply direct pressure to any hemorrhage with your hand and sterile cotton gauze.
- A tourniquet may be required to control hemorrhage of a limb if applying direct pressure is not enough. Options include:
  - A manual blood pressure cuff of appropriate size with pressure sufficient to occlude arterial blood flow.
  - A belt can be used as a temporizing measure in the nonclinical setting.

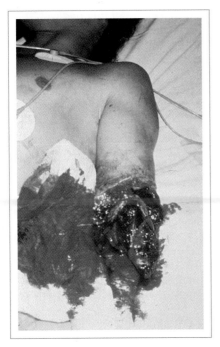

FIGURE 67.1: Avulsion injury to humerus. (Reprinted with permission from Bucholz RW, Heckman JD. *Rockwood & Green's Fractures in Adults*, 5th ed. Philadelphia: Lippincott Williams & Wilkins, 2001.)

- Obtain peripheral access in unaffected limb(s) with two large-bore intravenous lines (IVs) to administer a fluid bolus of 20 cc/kg.
- Transfuse packed red blood cells, platelets, and fresh frozen plasma as necessary.
- Be prepared to correct any acquired coagulopathy from medications such as aspirin, clopidogrel (Plavix), and warfarin.
- Consider giving tetanus toxoid with the addition of tetanus immunoglobulin if the tetanus status is unknown.
- Wound can be irrigated with saline or sterile water and then covered with wet sterile dressing.
- Wounds from amputation should be considered "dirty" wounds, necessitating broad-spectrum antibiotics.
    - Cefazolin and gentamicin IV.
    - If the patient is penicillin allergic, clindamycin can be used instead.
- Surgical consultation for definitive hemorrhage control by ligating arteries and veins that were lacerated or crushed during the amputation should be called early in the patient's clinical course.

Specific Amputated Limb Instructions
- If the finger or limb is still attached to the body, clean the wound surface with sterile water or saline solution. Then, if possible, gently place the damaged skin back to its normal position. Control bleeding and bandage the wound with bulky pressure dressings.
- If the limb is detached from the body, clean the wound surface with either sterile water or saline solution.
- Care of amputated limb:
    - Wrap the distal injured limb in sterile bandages soaked in sterile water.
    - Place the limb(s) into a resealable plastic bag.

- Place that bag in a solution of saline with ice. Label this bag with the name of the patient and time and date that the amputated part was obtained.
- Cold ischemia from direct contact with ice will lead to freezing and will harm the misplaced/amputated limb. Avoid dry ice.
- Because amputated digits have less muscle mass than extremities, they have a longer ischemic tolerance, or ischemia time, defined as the total time a body part can be without circulation but remain healthy enough for successful reimplantation.
  - The ischemic time for *digits* is up to *8 hours*.
  - The ischemic time for *extremities* is *4–6 hours*.
  - Cooling the amputated part may prolong this ischemic time.
- Reimplantation policies are institution dependent.
  - Obtain an immediate surgical consult.
  - Patient may be transferred to a reimplantation center if hemodynamically stable and an accepting surgeon is available.
- There are a number of considerations in determining whether reattachment of a severed body part is possible.
  - One of the key determinants is the mechanism of injury.
    - A crush injury typically results in extensive tissue damage, often irreversible. Severely crushed, mangled, or contaminated body parts are a contraindication to reimplantation.
    - A guillotine injury, also called a sharp amputation, refers to a body part that has been severed by a straight-edged laceration. A limb or digit cut off in a guillotine injury is more likely to be successfully replanted than one that is amputated by a crush or avulsion injury.
  - Patient's overall condition.
  - Time body part remains detached (ischemia time).
  - Method of preservation.

Special Considerations

- Many decision rules exist to indicate amputation or reimplantation.
  - Mangled Extremity Severity Score (MESS)
    - A score of seven points or higher *usually* indicates the need for amputation. This scoring system was originally devised to assess injuries to the lower limb.
    - Note that it is highly specific but has low sensitivity: low scores indicate to the surgeon that this patient likely has a viable limb for reimplantation, but low sensitivity of the indices has failed to support the validity of the scores as predictors of amputation.
  - Predictive Salvage Index (PSI)
  - Limb Salvage Index (LSI)
  - Nerve Injury Ischemia Soft tissue Skeletal injury, Shock, and Age (NISSSA) Score
- Although these indices are incapable of identifying patients who will eventually require an amputation, they might be useful as a screening test to support the entry of an extremity into the limb-salvage pathway.
- The decision for limb salvage is to be made by a collaboration of the emergency physician, vascular surgeon, orthopedic surgeon, trauma surgeon, and plastic surgeon involved in the care of the patient.

Best Evidence/Clinical Decision Rules

Do any perfect prediction rules exist to predict whether a mangled/amputated limb is salvageable?

None exists.

Suggested Readings

Clontz A, Annonio D, Walker L, et al. Trauma nursing: Amputation. rn.modernmedicine. com/rnweb/article/articleDetail.jsp?id=103342. Published 2004. Accessed July 1, 2004.

Haggerty M. Traumatic amputations. *Gale Encyclopedia of Medicine*. www.findarticles. com/cf_dls/g2601/0013/2601001392/p1/article.jhtml. Accessed April 16, 2004.

Microsurgeon.org. The decision for replantation. www.microsurgeon.org/decision_making.htm. Published 2004. Accessed April 16, 2004.

Pederson WC. Replantation. *Plast Reconstr Surgery*. 2001;107(3):823.

U.S. National Library of Medicine. Amputation-traumatic. www.nlm.nih.gov/medlineplus/ency/article/000006.htm. Published 2002. Accessed April 16, 2004.

Wilhelmi BJ, Lee A, et al. Hand, amputations and replantation. www.emedicine.com/plastic/topic536.htm. Published 2003. Accessed April 16, 2004.

68 Peripheral Arterial Trauma

Alison Suarez

Definition

- Arterial injury to the extremity involves both occlusive and nonocclusive mechanisms.
  - Occlusive causes include transection, thrombosis, and spasm.
  - Nonocclusive mechanisms involve intimal flap, pseudoaneurysm, formation of AV fistula, and compartment syndrome.
- Penetrating trauma accounts for approximately 70–90% of all vascular injuries to the extremities.
- Amputation rates have decreased from 50% to <5% over the past 50 years due to major technological advancements.

Pathophysiology

- The most common mechanisms of peripheral arterial injury involve both blunt and penetrating trauma. The majority of penetrating trauma is due to gunshot wounds and stab wounds.
- Blunt trauma is less common than penetrating trauma; however, its consequences can be more severe with associated significant collateral damage to the surrounding tissues including nerves, muscles, and bone.
- Peripheral arterial injury results in loss of cellular integrity and irreversible cell death to points distal to the injury, especially if collateral circulation is compromised.
- After 6 hours, 10% of patients will develop irreversible damage; therefore, time is crucial in both diagnosis and definitive management of arterial injury.
- It has been demonstrated that cooling of the affected extremity may prolong tissue tolerance of ischemia.

Diagnosis

- Physical findings on examination of peripheral arterial injury are categorized as "hard" and "soft" findings (Table 68.1).
- Hard findings account for <6% of patients with peripheral arterial injury and include pulsatile or rapidly enlarging hematoma, pulsatile arterial injury, bruit or thrill on palpating arterial pulse, or any of the 5 Ps classically seen in compartment syndrome (Pain, Pallor, Pulselessness, Paresthesias, paralysis).
- The incidence of arterial injury with any of the hard findings is 90%.
- "Soft" findings include decreased pulses, decreased capillary refill, peripheral nerve injury, and nonpulsatile hematoma.
- A "proximity wound" is defined as any wound 1 to 5 cm from a major vessel.
- If able to obtain a history from the patient, one should focus on the time and mechanism of injury, occupation, and hand dominance. Also inquire about comorbidities that might impede healing (diabetes mellitus, smoking, etc).

TABLE 68.1: Signs of peripheral arterial trauma

Hard signs	Soft signs
Pulsatile or rapidly expanding hematoma	Decreased pulses
Pulsatile arterial injury	Decreased capillary refill
Bruit or thrill present on palpating arterial pulse	Peripheral nerve injury

Any of the 5Ps of compartment syndrome
   Pain
   Pallor
   Pulselessness
   Paresthesias
   Paralysis
	Nonpulsatile hematoma

- On physical examination, note color, temperature, and capillary refill. Look for evidence of compartment syndrome. Document a thorough neurological examination as close proximity of structures often results in concomitant nerve injury.
- Distracting injuries or confounding coexistent trauma can mask crucial signs and symptoms associated with peripheral arterial injury.

Evaluation (Fig. 68.1)

- Peripheral arterial injury sustained during trauma requires prompt diagnosis and mobilization of the necessary resources with the initial and primary focus being stabilization of the patients according to ATLS protocol.
- Patients with hard findings should be taken immediately to surgery.
- Patents with "proximity wounds" have classically underwent exploratory surgery resulting in a high negative rate. Currently, non-invasive imaging is recommended prior to consideration of surgical exploration.
- Patients with soft findings also often require further investigation with noninvasive imaging.

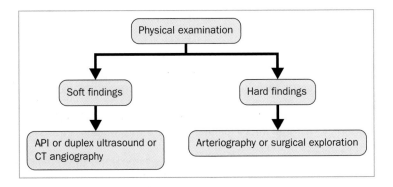

FIGURE 68.1: Arterial injury algorithm. API, arterial pressure index; CT, computed tomography.

- The following studies should be considered in patients with suspected peripheral arterial injury:
  - **Arteriography/angiography** is the gold standard. Its use is starting to lose popularity as it is time-consuming. It is often used in patients with high suspicion of peripheral arterial injury particularly after high-energy injury, and in those with proximity wounds.
  - **CT Angiography** is less invasive, readily available, and less time-consuming than arteriography. Its use in diagnosing peripheral arterial injury has yet to be directly compared with angiography; therefore, it is not considered the gold standard.
  - **Duplex ultrasound** is non-invasive and portable, and can readily detect the absence of blood flow; however, it is operator dependent.
  - **API/ABI (Arterial Pressure Index/Ankle Brachial Index)** can be easily obtained in the emergency setting and involves comparing the systolic pressures of both affected and uninjured limb. It is both sensitive and specific. A ratio of <0.9 is an indication for further evaluation.
  - **Handheld Doppler** can be used to detect a change in the triphasic quality of the pulse, which is indicative of arterial injury.
  - **X-ray** films are obtained to rule out a foreign body or associated fracture.

Management

- Arterial injury repair should be performed within 6 hours to avoid irreversible tissue damage.
- Patients with "hard" findings should undergo emergent surgical exploration (Fig. 68.2).
  - If the patient presents within the 6-hour window and is hemodynamically stable, one may opt to conduct further investigations; however, this should be performed in consultation with vascular surgeon.
- Proximity wounds can be observed for 12–24 hours while obtaining non-invasive imaging and monitoring hemoglobin or hematocrit levels, as overt signs of peripheral arterial injury may not be present.
- Profuse bleeding should be managed initially with direct pressure.
- Permissive hypotension involves avoiding aggressive fluid resuscitation with the thought that one may avoid dislodging a tenuous clot. This concept is controversial.
- The administration of antibiotics has not demonstrated a significant decrease in infection rates following peripheral arterial injury. The decision to administer antibiotics is up to the discretion of the provider.

Special Considerations

- Blind ligation of bleeding vessels is contraindicated in peripheral arterial injury.
- Vascular neuropathy occurs over hours, whereas primary neurological injury is immediate.
- Intravascular ultrasound holds promise for future investigative approaches.
- Late complications of arterial injury include delayed thrombosis, intermittent claudication, chronic pain, and aneurysm.
- Reperfusion of tissue after arterial repair can result in compartment syndrome. Patients should be frequently evaluated for the signs of compartment syndrome. Pain with passive range is the most sensitive sign.
- The presence of peripheral pulses can be misleading.
  - Thirty percent of patients with absent pulses have no arterial injury.
  - Forty percent of patients with pulses have arterial injury.

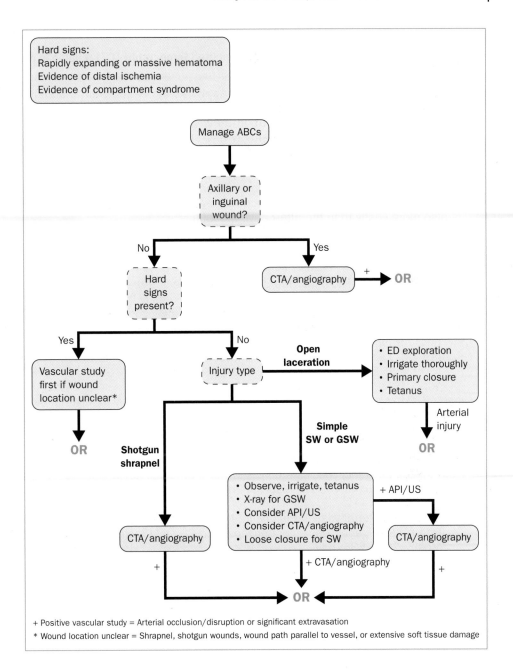

FIGURE 68.2: Penetrating extremity trauma algorithm. CTA, computed tomography angiography; ED, emergency department; SW, stab wound; GSW, gunshot wound; API, arterial pressure index; US, ultrasound. (Reprinted with permission from Bisanzo M, Bhatia K, Filbin MR. *Emergency Management of the Trauma Patient: Cases, Algorithms, Evidence.* Baltimore: Lippincott Williams & Wilkins, 2006.)

Best Evidence/Clinical Decision Rules

Is non-invasive imaging with multislice computed tomography (CT) reliable in diagnosing peripheral artery injuries?

The overall use of multislice CT angiography has increased tremendously over the last decade and is now showing promise for detection of arterial injury. Busquets et al. (2004) found no missed injuries in their study of 97 CT angiograms, and Inaba et al. (2006) reported 100% sensitivity and specificity in their retrospective review of CT angiography for penetrating arterial injury.

Contrast arteriography is still the gold standard imaging evaluation of potential arterial injury. It can detect the exact location and type of injury. However, it is not without risk. The procedure is invasive, requires contrast dye, and cannot be done at the bedside. It is also more costly than the alternative modalities.

Suggested Readings

Bizano M, Bhatia K, Filbin M. *Emergency Management of the Trauma Patient: Cases, Algorithms, Evidence.* Baltimore: Lippincott Williams & Wilkins, 2007.

Busquets AR, Acosta JA, Colon E, Alejandro KV, Rodriguez P. Helical computed tomographic angiography for the diagnosis of traumatic arterial injuries of the extremities. *J Trauma.* 2004;56(3):625–628.

Coates WC. Lacerations to the face and scalp. In: Tintinalli JE, Kelen GD, Stapczynski S. *Emergency Medicine: A Comprehensive Study Guide,* 6th ed. New York, USA: McGraw-Hill, 2004:1629–1630.

Inaba K, Potzman J, Munera F, et al. Multi-slice CT angiography for arterial evaluation in the injured lower extremity. *J Trauma.* 2006;60(3):502–506; discussion 6–7.

Kumar AK, Zane RD. Penetrating trauma to the extremities. In: Tintinalli JE, Kelen GD, Stapczynski S. *Emergency Medicine: A Comprehensive Study Guide,* 6th ed. New York, USA: McGraw-Hill, 2004:1629–1630.

Newton EJ. *Emergency Medicine Clinics of North America: Acute Complications of Extremity Trauma.* Vol. 25, Issue 3. Philadelphia: Elsevier Saunders, 2007: 751–761.

Newton EJ. Peripheral vascular injury. In: Marx JA, Hockberger RS, Walls RM, eds. *Rosen's Emergency Medicine: Concepts and Clinical Practice,* 6th ed. Philadelphia: Mosby, 2006:536–547.

69

Compartment Syndrome

Steven S. Wright and Daniel Irving

Definition

- Compartment syndrome occurs when tissue pressures in a confined space rise to the point of compromising tissue perfusion.
- Rising compartment pressures result in tissue hypoxia, damaging structures within the compartment (nerves and muscles are particularly susceptible). Prolonged hypoxia results in tissue necrosis, causing permanent muscle contracture (e.g., Volkmann's ischemic contracture).

Pathophysiology

- Elevated compartment pressures can result from three different processes.
  - **Increased compartment contents**: for example, trauma (most common), bleeding, excessive muscle use, burns, venous obstruction, venomous bites (especially rattlesnakes).
  - **Decreased compartment volume**: for example, excessive traction, closure of fascial defects.
  - **External pressure**: for example, tight circumferential casts/splints, pneumatic antishock garments, lying on limb.
- As tissue pressure increases, capillary perfusion pressure is exceeded and venous blood flow is impaired. Eventually, arterial capillary blood flow falls to the point that basic tissue metabolic needs are not met, causing ischemia and eventually necrosis.
- Tissues release histamine in an attempt to dilate capillaries, which leads to further increase of compartment pressure.
- Normal compartment pressure is near zero, up to 10 mm Hg. Capillary flow is compromised at pressures >20 mm Hg. Muscle and nerve tissues are at risk for ischemic necrosis at compartment pressures >30 mm Hg.

Diagnosis

- A history of trauma (especially crush injury) is common.
- Compartment syndrome can occur in any muscle compartment but is most frequently seen in the lower leg (anterior tibial compartment).
- Classically, the 5 Ps have been taught- **P**ain, **P**allor, **P**aresthesia, **P**aralysis, **P**ulselessness (poikilothermia). These are actually signs of arterial flow disruption, not necessarily compartment syndrome. Because arterial compromise is a later complication of compartment syndrome, these signs should not be used to exclude compartment syndrome. Pallor and Pulselessness are considered late, ominous findings.
- **The most reliable early sign is pain, especially on passive stretching of involved muscles, or pain out of proportion to examination.**
- Pain out of proportion to expectation and excessive use of analgesia should immediately raise the suspicion of compartment syndrome.

- Skin color, temperature, capillary refill, and distal pulses are unreliable indicators because the pressures required to produce compartment syndrome are well below arterial pressure.
- Compartment pressure can be measured with a device such as a STIC catheter (Stryker), which is a pressure monitor attached to a syringe. The catheter must be zeroed to atmospheric pressure and inserted at same level.
- Doppler ultrasound is not useful as good arterial flow may be observed in the presence of significant compartment syndrome.

Evaluation

- Compartment pressures <15 mm Hg are generally considered safe. Pressures between 20 and 30 mm Hg may cause damage if persisting for several hours and may be followed clinically with serial measurements. Pressures >30 mm Hg or neurovascular compromise is generally considered grounds for emergent fasciotomy.
- A secondary measurement allows for the compartment pressure (CP) to be >30 mm Hg difference from diastolic blood pressure (DBP). Normally the DBP > CP +30.
- Patient must also be monitored for possible complications of compartment syndrome including rhabdomyolysis, hyperkalemia, myoglobinuria, and lactic acidosis. These entities are a result of muscle cell breakdown from necrosis.

Management

- For cases of suspected compartment syndrome, follow the algorithm in Figure 69.1 and see Table 69.1.

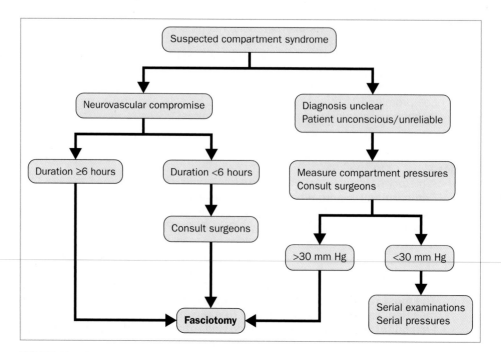

FIGURE 69.1: Emergency department management of suspected compartment syndrome.

TABLE 69.1: Emergency department interventions of compartment syndrome

Emergency department interventions

Rapid diagnosis of compartment syndrome
Remove casts and occlusive dressings
Place extremity in neutral position
Prophylactic antibiotics
Analgesia
Emergent fasciotomy or facilitating operating room fasciotomy

Inpatient postfasciotomy care

Debridement
Monitoring renal function
Continue antibiotics and analgesia
Consider skin flaps or grafts

- Complete fasciotomy is the only treatment that can reliably normalize elevated compartment pressures. This must be performed on emergent basis, as delays of more than 12 hours often result in irreversible muscle and nerve damage.
- Ensure adequate hydration to protect kidneys in case of rhabdomyolysis. Urinary alkalinization and/or dialysis may be necessary in cases of severe rhabdomyolysis with associated hyperkalemia, myoglobinuria, and lactic acidosis.
- DO NOT elevate the affected extremity. Elevation does not improve venous outflow and it reduces arterial inflow, worsening tissue ischemia.

Special Considerations
- Patients with risk factors for compartment syndrome or borderline measured compartment pressures require frequent monitoring of compartment pressures and for worsening clinical signs.
- Patients with compartment syndrome are also at risk for infection and tissue loss.
- Volkmann's ischemic contracture may be observed as sequelae of compartment syndrome.

Best Evidence/Clinical Decision Rules

Patients with critically elevated compartment pressures often have signs of good distal perfusion and palpable arterial pulses. Do these patients still require fasciotomy, or can they be managed more conservatively?

Compartment syndrome generally occurs at pressures of 30 mm Hg and above, well below arterial blood pressure. Therefore, arterial pulses and capillary refill may be detected distal to the compartment, even in the setting of compartment syndrome. Moderate elevations in compartment pressure can impede capillary blood flow, leading to tissue ischemia and necrosis, causing irreversible damage. Therefore, compartment pressures >30 mm Hg mandate emergent fasciotomy, even if pulses and capillary refill appear unaffected. Functional and cosmetic results of fasciotomy are acceptable when it is performed early. Permanent neuromuscular damage as a result of inadequate or delayed treatment is never acceptable.

Can compartment syndrome occur in a limb without a fracture?
Although it is more common in the setting of fractures, compartment syndrome can occur with isolated soft tissue trauma; in a study of 164 patients in the United

Kingdom, 69% involved a fracture (half involving the tibial shaft) but 31% had soft tissue injury without a fracture (McQueen et al., 2000).

Suggested Readings

Hallar P. Compartment syndrome. In: Tintinalli J, ed. *Emergency Medicine: A Comprehensive Study Guide*, 4th ed. Columbus, OH: McGraw-Hill, 1996:1746.

McQueen MM, Gaston P, Court-Brown CM. Acute compartment syndrome. Who is at risk? *J Bone Joint Surg Br*. 2000;82(2):200–203.

Siefert JA. Acute compartment syndrome. In: Wolfson AB, ed. *Clinical Practice of Emergency Medicine*. Philadelphia: Lippincott Williams & Wilkins, 2005:1109–1112.

70

Rhabdomyolysis

Amit Chandra and Steven S. Wright

Definition

- Rhabdomyolysis is a syndrome resulting from the breakdown of skeletal muscle.
- The by-products of this muscle degradation, including myoglobin, electrolytes, enzymes, and other cellular contents, enter peripheral circulation and may lead to deleterious end-organ consequences.
- Rhabdomyolysis is associated with acute renal failure, hyperkalemia, hypocalcemia, hyperuricemia, hyperphosphatemia, and other electrolyte abnormalities that can be potentially fatal.

Pathophysiology

- Skeletal muscle breakdown releases intracellular contents, including myoglobin, creatine phosphokinase (CPK), aldolase, lactate dehydrogenase (LDH), and potassium.
- Damage to the muscle sarcolemma disrupts the Na-K-ATPase pump and affects calcium transport, leading to increased intracellular calcium. The increased level of calcium in turn activates intracellular enzymes causing a cascade of cell necrosis.
- Myoglobin and other toxins accumulate in the renal tubules causing local damage and renal failure.
- Most common causes
  - Alcohol/drug abuse
    - Cocaine, amphetamines
    - Ethanol use or withdrawal
    - Ecstasy/MDMA
  - Trauma, near drowning, electrical injury, burns, and compartment syndrome
  - Strenuous activity (athletes, military recruits)
  - Seizures
  - Toxicity
    - Carbon monoxide
    - Medications: salicylates, propofol, statins
    - Malignant hyperthermia and neuroleptic malignant syndrome
    - Snake and spider bites
  - Hyperthermia or hypothermia
  - Hypothyroidism and hyperthyroidism
  - Diabetic ketoacidosis
  - Myopathies (e.g., dermatomyositis and polymyositis)
  - Infection (e.g., influenza, legionella, Epstein-Barr virus, human immunodeficiency virus, herpes simplex virus, West Nile, Coxsackie)

Diagnosis

- Signs and symptoms: Rhabdomyolysis is usually an acute process, characterized by myalgias, weakness, nausea, abdominal pain, dark urine, edema, and low-grade fever.

- Fifty percent of patients will present with symptoms that involve the thighs, calves, and lower back.
- Laboratory diagnosis
  - Myoglobin is a serum marker for rhabdomyolysis, though its short half-life makes it an unreliable diagnostic tool.
  - CPK is more sensitive than myoglobin in detecting rhabdomyolysis. CPK levels peak around 24 hours following an acute injury.
  - **Serum CPK analysis is 100% sensitive for rhabdomyolysis. Although there is no established cutoff, a level of 5–10 times normal values (>1,000) confirms the diagnosis.**
  - Urinalysis reveals brown urine as a result of myoglobinuria, with a large amount of blood and brown casts detected on dip but few red blood cells noted on urine microscopy.
  - Hyperkalemia, metabolic acidosis, hyperphosphatemia, hyperuricemia, and hypocalcemia or hypercalcemia are often present.

Evaluation

- Patients with traumatic rhabdomyolysis will likely have obvious signs of muscle damage, usually in an extremity that shows reddened overlying skin with local swelling, induration, or other signs of injury.
- In addition to following the CPK, it is essential to monitor renal function to screen for acute tubular injury, as this can be a complication of rhabdomyolysis in 5–30% of cases.
- Evaluate affected muscle areas for compartment syndrome.
- Hyperkalemia is by far the biggest initial life-threatening consequence of rhabdomyolysis and should be ruled out early in the clinical course. Hyperkalemia results from direct release of intracellular potassium into the extracellular fluid as a result of muscle cell necrosis.

Management

- The principle therapy for rhabdomyolysis is aggressive fluid resuscitation with normal saline to maintain a urine output of at least 2 mL/kg/hr. Fluid may be sequestered in extravascular spaces as a result of skeletal muscle damage, so large amounts of fluid may be necessary to achieve therapeutic urine output.
- Mannitol is an osmotic diuretic and free radical scavenger. It may be used as a therapeutic adjunct. Mannitol administration increases intravascular fluid and urine flow and therefore prevents tubular obstruction and necrosis.
- Urine alkalinization can be achieved with the administration of sodium bicarbonate to maintain urine pH >6.5. Alkalinization prevents the dissociation of myoglobin into more toxic by-products. Three amps of sodium bicarbonate is mixed with either 1 L of 0.45 normal saline or D5W and infused to maintain urine output at 100 mL/hr.
- Dialysis is indicated in patients with persistent hyperkalemia and metabolic acidosis. Fluid overload, pulmonary edema, and acute congestive heart failure seen in patients with acute oliguric renal failure should also be treated with hemodialysis. Only 4% of patients with acute renal failure due to rhabdomyolysis require hemodialysis.

Special Considerations

- The absence of symptoms does not exclude the diagnosis of rhabdomyolysis.
- Evaluate the patient for compartment syndrome, which can be both a predis-posing factor and consequence of rhabdomyolysis. Failure of CPK levels to fall may indicate an undiagnosed compartment syndrome or other ongoing process of muscle breakdown.

- Rhabdomyolysis causes 5–15% of all cases of acute renal failure in the United States.

Best Evidence/Clinical Decision Rules

If an area of muscle potentially undergoing rhabdomyolysis is not apparent from the history and physical examination, what is the best imaging test to identify the source?

Magnetic resonance imaging (MRI) with gadolinium enhancement has been found to be more sensitive than either computed tomography or ultrasound imaging in detecting muscle edema and inflammation. In one study consisting of 15 patients, the sensitivity for detecting muscle damage is 42% for ultrasonography, 62% for computed tomographic scan, and 100% for MRI (Lamminen et al., 1989). Although all three study modalities are nonspecific, in conjunction with history and physical examination, the MRI is the most sensitive.

Because of the cost and logistics of obtaining an MRI, ultrasonography may still play a role in diagnosing rhabdomyolysis, as demonstrated in one case report where the ultrasound showed classic findings of rhabdomyolysis: decreased echogenicity and "local disorganization of fascicular architecture."

Suggested Readings

Bontempo L. Rhabdomyolysis. In: Rosen P, Barkin RM, et al, eds. *Emergency Medicine: Concepts and Clinical Practice*, 6th ed. 2006.

Chawla S, et al. Rhabdomyolysis: a lesson on the perils of exercising and drinking. *Am J Emerg Med*. 2008;26(4): 521. e3-4.

Lamminen AE, Hekali PE, Tiula E, et al. Acute rhabdomyolysis: evaluation with magnetic resonance imaging compared with computed tomography and ultrasonography. *Br J Radiol*. 1989;62:326–330.

McGoldrick MD, Capan LM. Acute renal failure in the injured. In: Capan LM, Miller SM, Turndorf H, eds. *Trauma: Anesthesia and Intensive Care*. Philadelphia: JB Lippincott, 1991:755–785.

Newton EJ. Acute complications of extremity trauma. *Emerg Med Clin North Am*. 2007;25(3):751–761.

Steeds RP, Alexander PJ, Muthusamy R, Bradley M. Sonography in the diagnosis of rhabdomyolysis. *J Clin Ultrasound*. 1999;27:531–533.

71

Open Fractures

Joseph Walline

Definition

- Also known as "compound fractures," these injuries occur when a bone is broken and penetrates the overlying skin.
- Open fractures almost always occur with high-energy trauma, for example, motorcycle and motor vehicle accidents or auto versus pedestrian injuries.
- Associated injuries to the skull, chest, abdomen, or pelvis are present in 50% of open fracture cases and almost 10% are complicated by compartment syndrome when involving the lower extremity.

Pathophysiology

- Prior to modern antisepsis and antibiotic use, open fractures were historically ~80% fatal and the mainstay of treatment was amputation.
- Because of the broken skin, foreign particles and bacteria are able to enter the wound and infect the bones and surrounding soft tissues. These injuries are at very high risk for osteomyelitis.
- The tibia is the most frequent site of traumatic osteomyelitis because of the relatively sparse soft-tissue covering and reduced blood supply.
- The fractured bone(s) can lacerate arteries, veins, and nerves, causing neurovascular damage.

Diagnosis

- The diagnosis is obvious when bone is protruding from an open wound.
- The diagnosis is suggested when you see a fracture on plain radiograph underlying a surface wound or laceration (Fig. 71.1). Definitive diagnosis may require surgical exploration in an operating room.
- Usually involves extremities, but more proximal fractures (e.g., rib, clavicle, skull) may also occur.

Evaluation

- The risk of infection is stratified by the severity of injury. Although the severity of injury is a continuum, Gustilo and Anderson (1976) established a helpful classification system (Table 71.1).
- In an otherwise stable patient, computed tomographic (CT) scanning of the affected limb may provide more diagnostic detail and is often requested by the trauma/orthopedic team for operative planning purposes.
- An alternative diagnostic/evaluative method uses bedside ultrasound (linear array probe) to investigate the fracture site.

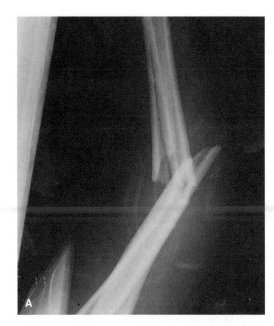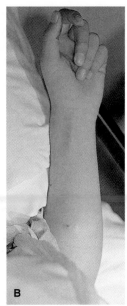

FIGURE 71.1: A: Radiograph showing a sharply angulated midshaft radius and ulnar fracture. **B:** A small laceration over the fracture suggests an open fracture that will require operative management. (Courtesy of Dr. Andrew Capraro.) (Reproduced with permission from Fleisher GR, Ludwig S, Baskin MN. *Atlas of Pediatric Emergency Medicine*. Philadelphia: Lippincott Williams & Wilkins, 2004.)

- Evaluation should focus on identifying associated injuries:
  - Palpate distal and proximal arteries to confirm arterial perfusion to the areas distal to the fracture site.
  - Test sensory and motor neurologic function proximally and distally to the fracture site.

TABLE 71.1: Open fracture grading system

Grade	Injury	Risk of infection
I	Puncture wound <1 cm with minimal contamination or crushing	0–2%
II	Laceration >1 cm with moderate soft tissue injury	2–10%
IIIA	Extensive soft tissue damage, severe crush component, massive contamination. Bone coverage adequate	10–50%
IIIB	Extensive soft tissue damage with periosteal stripping and exposure. Severe contamination and bone comminution. Flap coverage required	10–50%
IIIC	Arterial injury requiring repair	10–50%

Data from Gustilo RB, Anderson JT. Prevention of infection in the treatment of one thousand and twenty-five open fractures of long bones: retrospective and prospective analyses. *J Bone Joint Surg Am*. 1976;58(4):453–458.

TABLE 71.2: Emergency department open fracture treatment

Analgesia

Reduction of the fracture/dislocation

Antibiotics intravenously

Tetanus prophylaxis

Orthopedic consultation

Management (Tables 71.2 and 71.3)

- In the acute trauma scenario, an open fracture is an orthopedic emergency. However, it should not supersede traditional ATLS protocols.
- Do not allow the open fracture to distract from assessment of other life-threatening injuries.
- Given the significant risk for losing the extremity due to infection (~25% osteomyelitis risk in grade III open fractures), antibiotics should be started as soon as possible (standard of care is within 6 hours postinjury).
- Control pain with intramuscular/intravenous (IM/IV) morphine (0.1 mg/kg) or other narcotic analgesia.
- Remove gross contaminants and control bleeding with sterile pressure dressings.
- If time allows, rinse open fracture site with saline and wrap with sterile gauze.
  - Do not use povidone-iodine (Betadine)/chlorhexidine solutions as they can cause chemical damage to osteocytes and increase infection rates.
- Apply a rigid splint to affected extremity.
- Reduce the fracture if there is an absent or weak distal pulse, otherwise, do not attempt manipulation.
- Antibiotics:
  - Grades I and II:
    - Cefazolin 2 g (30 mg/kg) IV AND clindamycin 600 mg (10 mg/kg) IV
    - Alternative in penicillin-allergic patients: vancomycin 1 g (15 mg/kg) IV
    - If grossly contaminated with dirt or fecal matter: penicillin G 4 million units (100,000 units/kg) IV or gentamicin 5 mg/kg (2.5 mg/kg) IV
  - Grade III (adult)
    - As above, or piperacillin/tazobactam 4.5 g (100 mg/kg) IV
- Give tetanus vaccine (add tetanus immune globulin in non-immunized or for large crush wounds).

TABLE 71.3: Surgical open fracture treatment

Irrigation and debridement

Wound closure

Soft tissue reconstruction

Fracture stabilization

Secondary procedures: bone grafting to stimulate healing

- Suspect other serious injuries (particularly in patients with open fractures sustained after blunt trauma).

Special Considerations
- Open fractures often require significant trauma mechanisms. Have a low threshold for transferring the patient to a Level I trauma center. Apply splints and/or traction as feasible to maintain vascular function. Initiate antibiotics prior to transfer.
- Boxer's fractures (fourth or fifth metacarpal fracture from a direct blow) with an overlying laceration may be contaminated from the mouth of another person. It would be wise to treat this injury as a presumptive open fracture: apply a splint, give antibiotics and analgesia, and obtain an orthopedic consult.

Best Evidence/Clinical Decision Rules

What is the only grade 1A evidence-based recommendation for open fracture management?

Prophylactic antibiotic use to reduces risk of soft tissue infection and osteomyelitis.

Can compartment syndrome occur in the setting of open fractures?

Compartment syndrome can occur with open fractures as well as closed fractures; in one series, compartment syndrome was more common with open than closed fractures (DeLee and Stiehl, 1981). This reflects the fact that a great amount of energy/force is necessary to cause an open fracture leading to significant soft tissue trauma in addition to a fracture.

Suggested Readings
DeLee JC, Stiehl JB. Open tibia fracture with compartment syndrome. *Clin Orthop Relat Res*. 1981;(160):175–184.

Eastern Association for the Surgery of Trauma (EAST) working group. 1998. Practice management guidelines for prophylactic antibiotic use in open fractures. www.east.org/tpg.html. Accessed January 10, 2009.

Geiderman J. General principles of orthopedic injuries. In: Marx JA, ed. *Rosen's Emergency Medicine*. St. Louis, Missouri: Mosby, 2006:467–493.

Gustilo RB, Anderson JT. Prevention of infection in the treatment of one thousand and twenty-five open fractures of long bones: retrospective and prospective analyses. *J Bone Joint Surg Am*. 1976;58(4):453–458.

Levine B. *2009 EMRA Antibiotic Guide. Emergency Medicine Residents' Association*. Irving, Texas, 2008.

Zink B. Bone and joint infections. In: Marx JA, ed. *Rosen's Emergency Medicine*. St. Louis, Missouri: Mosby, 2006:1925–1943.

72

Scalp Laceration
Alison Suarez

Definition
- Lacerations to the scalp can result in massive blood loss if not addressed urgently and can lead to hemodynamic instability.

Pathophysiology
- The scalp receives its blood supply from branches of both the external and internal carotid arteries.
- The complex anatomy of the scalp lends to the development of significant pathology in the setting of trauma (Table 72.1).
- Bleeding can be substantial secondary to the limited retraction of vessels in the fibrous dermal tissues, especially when the galea is involved. This is commonly seen in blunt injuries with scalp avulsion.
- Infection and blood can collect in the potential space of the loose connective tissue of the scalp.

Diagnosis
- Close inspection of the scalp will reveal the diagnosis.
- It is not uncommon for scalp lacerations to bleed heavily (i.e., "arterial pumper"). Arterial scalp lacerations should be addressed immediately.

Evaluation
- Inspection of the scalp should focus on determining depth, presence of a galeal tear, and skull deformity/fracture.
- Injury to the scalp most often is a result of both sharp and blunt trauma.
  - Sharp trauma to the scalp creates wound edges that are often discrete and easily repaired.
  - Blunt injury to the scalp results in stellate wounds commonly associated with underlying skull fractures and significant soft tissue damage.
- When applicable, always maintain C-spine precautions when evaluating the scalp.

TABLE 72.1: Anatomy of the scalp layers arranged from most superficial to deepest layer

Skin
Connective tissue (superficial fascia)
Aponeurosis (galea)
Loose space (subaponeurotic space)—*potential space for infection/hematoma*
Pericranium

Management

- Bleeding vessels on scalp
    - A pressure dressing should be applied initially to avoid development of a hematoma.
    - Local infiltration of 1% or 2% lidocaine with epinephrine may provide enough vasoconstriction to stop small bleeding vessels.
    - Easily visualized bleeding vessels can be clamped followed by tying a suture around the vessel at the base of the clamp (termed "suture ligation") (Fig. 72.1).

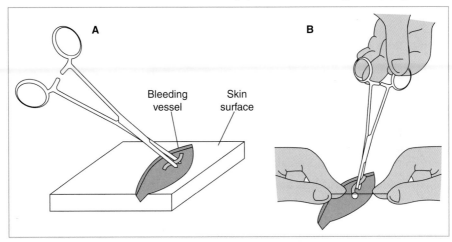

FIGURE 72.1: Control of a visualized bleeding vessel. **A:** Clamp the cut end of the vessel with a hemostat. **B:** Tie and secure a suture ligature around the base of the bleeding vessel.

- Vessels that are not easily visualized can be closed with a "figure-of-eight" stitch or a "purse-string" stitch (Fig. 72.2).

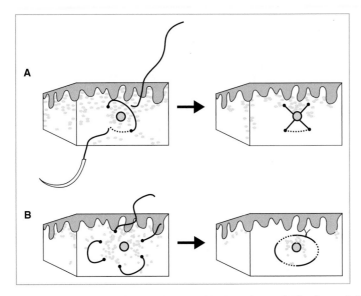

FIGURE 72.2: Control of a bleeding vessel in deep tissue. **A:** The figure-of-eight stitch. **B:** The purse-string stitch. Note that these stitches are not tied tightly for the sake of clarity here. In reality, these stitches must be tied tightly to seal the bleeding vessel.

- Definitive repair of scalp lacerations with staples/stitches will also stop bleeding by tamponading any lacerated vessels.
- Cutting or shaving of the surrounding hair should be avoided as this can increase the risk of infection.
- If the galea is involved, it should be repaired using 4-0 absorbable sutures. Repair of galea will minimize scalp depression and decrease the development of subgaleal hematoma.
- Staples can be used for simple lacerations of the scalp not involving the hairline or face.

Special Considerations

- The classic teaching is that hemorrhagic shock can occur from blood loss in the chest, abdomen, and pelvis but not inside the skull. While this is true, it is important to note that scalp lacerations can bleed heavily enough to cause hypotension and shock. Emergency medical services will often report a history of significant blood loss in the field.

Best Evidence/Clinical Decision Rules

Are staples or sutures preferred for repair of scalp laceration in adults?

Best best evidence topics (BETs) from the Manchester Royal Infirmary performed a shortcut review of the available literature and determined that there are no large prospective, randomized studies targeting adults with scalp lacerations and the only conclusion that can be drawn is that stapling is likely faster and cheaper than suturing for scalp wound closure. In children, stapling may be more effective (in addition to faster and cheaper), but further research is necessary.

Suggested Readings

Hogg K, Carley S. Towards evidence based emergency medicine: best BETs from the Manchester Royal Infirmary. Staples or sutures for repair of scalp laceration in adults. *Emerg Med J*. 2002;19(4):327–328.

Hogg K, Carley S. Towards evidence based emergency medicine: best BETs from the Manchester Royal Infirmary. Staples or sutures in children with scalp lacerations. *Emerg Med J*. 2002;19(4):328–329.

Section Editor: Joshua Quaas

73

Extremity Trauma: The First 15 Minutes, Algorithm, and Decision Making

Joshua Quaas

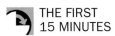 THE FIRST
15 MINUTES

ABCs and Vital Signs
- Follow advanced trauma life support (ATLS) guidelines. Resuscitation and management of life-threatening injuries supersedes extremity evaluation; only active hemorrhage should be initially addressed.
- Active extremity bleeding should be treated with direct pressure. Once the ABC's have been addressed and life-threatening pathology treated or stabilized, the extremity can be further examined and treated.

History
- Obtain as much history as possible regarding the mechanism of injury from the patient, witnesses, and emergency medical services personnel.
- High-energy mechanisms such as falls from significant height and high-speed motor vehicle crashes will raise your suspicions for significant injury and also for specific injuries (e.g., knee dislocation with spontaneous reduction is concerning for neurovascular injury at the popliteal level).
- Obtain history regarding patient's previous medical history and baseline of extremity function.
- Ask the patient about the function of their injured extremity. Pay close attention to complaints of motor/sensory deficit or weakness.

Physical Examination
- Carefully examine each extremity for injury. Examine bones, joints, and major nerves and arteries. A detailed examination can accurately predict specific injury and will guide imaging and treatment.
- Visually inspect each limb carefully. Compare the injured and uninjured limbs. Palpate the bones and soft tissues. Examine each joint for passive and active range of motion (especially if the patient is not able to identify the injured areas).
- Evaluate the motor function of extremity's major nerves (Table 73.1).
- Evaluation of sensation can be done by light touch as a screening examination; two-point discrimination is more definitive and is the standard of care for an injured extremity.

TABLE 73.1: Motor function of key nerves

Median: flexion of first and second digits into the "okay sign"

Radial: extension of wrist and fingers

Ulnar: abduction/adduction of the fingers

Femoral: knee flexion and extension

Peroneal: dorsiflexion and inversion of the foot

Tibial: plantar flexion of foot and toes

Emergency Interventions

- **Control active hemorrhage.** This is the only extremity intervention that should occur in the initial management of the multiple-injured trauma patient. Control should be achieved with direct pressure. Tourniquet or direct clamping of vessels is an alternative when direct pressure fails. Blind clamping may cause further injury to the vessel or nerves and is not recommended.
- **Identify associated injuries.** Do not let a severely mangled limb erroneously steer initial management away from immediate life-threatening injuries to the chest or abdomen.
- **Plain films** of the injury, including the joints above and below the site of injury, should be considered.
- **Reduction of fractures/dislocations** should occur as soon as possible. Radiography to characterize the injury and optimize treatment is recommended. Immediate attempts at reduction prior to imaging should occur only in the setting of obvious dislocation with obvious neurovascular compromise where delay to imaging risks harm to the patient. Neurovascular examination should be thoroughly performed and documented both before and after reduction.
- **Open fractures** should be irrigated with saline, covered with sterile gauze, and splinted without reduction unless neurovascular compromise is present. Intravenous antibiotics (usually first-generation cephalosporin) and tetanus prophylaxis should be administered. Definitive treatment should occur as soon as possible in conjunction with an orthopedic surgeon.
- **Splint stabilization** of the affected extremity should be performed after reduction, or to better immobilize the injury if the patient requires other evaluation (i.e., computed tomographic scan) prior to definitive treatment.
- Consider **fasciotomy** for the severely injured extremity with high compartment pressures. Evaluate often for compartment syndrome.

Memorable Pearls

- Fractures and/or dislocations should be reduced and splinted when definitive treatment will be delayed.
- Neurovascular injury is the most significant complication of extremity trauma and needs to be addressed promptly. Vascular injury should be treated within the first 6 hours to maximize salvage of distal tissues (Table 73.2).
- In general, injury to lower extremity vessels has a worse prognosis than upper extremity vessels; popliteal artery injury has the overall worst prognosis of any injured extremity vessel.
- Tourniquet use in the field is acceptable when hemorrhage control cannot be achieved. No patient should ever die from extremity exsanguination.

TABLE 73.2: Evaluate for hard signs of vascular injury

Active hemorrhage

Expanding or pulsatile hematoma

Bruit or thrill over wound

Absent pulses

Signs of distal ischemia: pallor, coolness, poor capillary refill

Essential Considerations

Consultations

- Trauma surgeon/team
- Orthopedic surgeon

DECISION MAKING

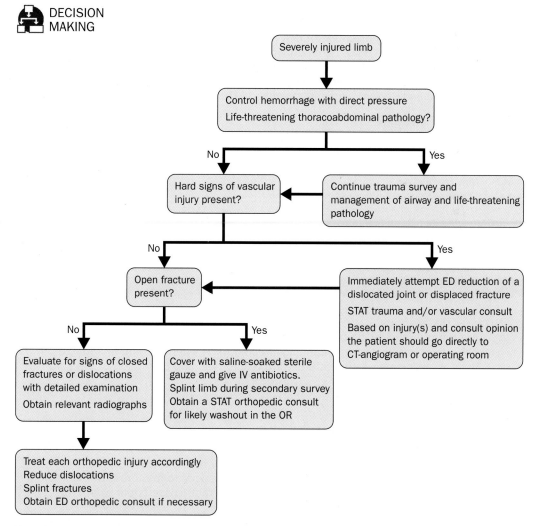

Extremity trauma: Decision making algorithm. ED, emergency department; STAT; CT, computed tomography; IV, intravenous; OR, operating room.

74 — Shoulder Dislocation

Jennifer Teng

Definition

- The most commonly dislocated large joint.
- Classified by location of the humeral head relative to the glenoid fossa: anterior, posterior, and less commonly inferior or superior.

Pathophysiology

Anterior Dislocations

- Represent >90% of shoulder dislocations.
- The most common mechanism is a fall or indirect blow on an externally rotated, abducted arm. The most common type of anterior dislocation is subcoracoid.
- Commonly associated injuries include rotator cuff tears, greater tuberosity fractures, Hill-Sachs deformity (posterior compression fracture of the humeral head following reduction) and Bankart's fracture (fracture of the anterior glenoid rim).

Posterior Dislocations

- The most commonly *missed* dislocation.
- This dislocation is often secondary to high-energy injuries (i.e., electrical injuries, tonic-clonic seizures, severe direct blow) when the arm is adducted and internally rotated.
- May be bilateral.
- The most common type is subacromial.

Inferior Dislocations (Luxatio Erecta)

- Represents <0.5% of all shoulder dislocations.
- This injury usually occurs secondary to a fall onto a hyperabducted shoulder or an axial load on an abducted arm, causing the humeral head to be displaced inferior to the glenoid.
- It is often associated with tears of the internal capsule.

Superior Dislocations

- Are the rarest of all dislocations.
- This injury is caused by a cephalad-directed force when the arm is adducted. It is often associated with fractures of the acromion and disruption of the acromio-clavicular (AC) joint.

Diagnosis

- Shoulder dislocations are clinically diagnosed by presentation, mechanism of injury, and radiography.
- Pre-reduction radiographs are recommended for multiple reasons, including definitive diagnosis and identification of any associated fractures. Some fracture patterns are inherently unstable and it is important to document whether a fracture existed prior to the reduction.
- The standard radiographic views are a scapular AP, lateral, and axillary. A Velpeau view may be obtained if the patient cannot tolerate an axillary view.

Anterior Dislocation

- The patient's arm is held in abduction, with loss of the normal round deltoid contour. The humeral head may be palpated anteriorly and a defect is seen just inferior to the acromion.
- Radiographs
  - On AP view, there is loss of the normal overlap of the humeral head with the glenoid.
  - On the lateral and axillary views, the humeral head is seen anterior to the glenoid fossa (Fig. 74.1).

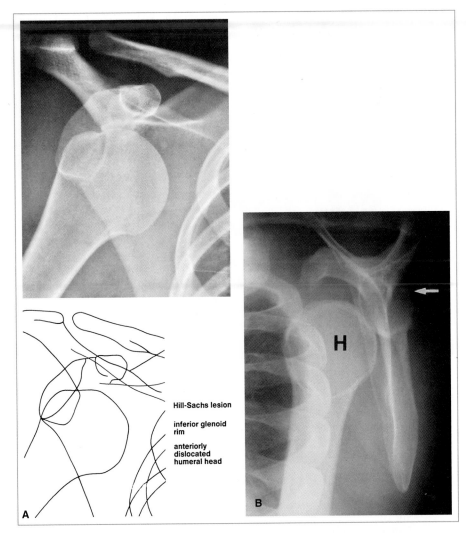

Hill-Sachs lesion

inferior glenoid rim

anteriorly dislocated humeral head

H

A

B

FIGURE 74.1: Anterior shoulder dislocation **A.** Anteroposterior film of the shoulder shows the typical appearance of anterior dislocation, with the humeral head beneath the inferior rim of the glenoid. **B.** A dislocation is well demonstrated on this trans-scapular (or Y) projection of the shoulder girdle. An arrow is pointing to the empty glenoid fossa. The humeral head (H) is medially and anteriorly displaced. (Reprinted with permission from Greenspan A. *Orthopedic Imaging: A Practical Approach*, 4th ed. Philadelphia: Lippincott Williams & Wilkins, 2004.)

Posterior Dislocation

- The arm is held in adduction with internal rotation, and patients are unable to abduct or externally rotate the arm. The humeral head may be palpable beneath the acromion.
- Look for radiographic signs of a posterior dislocation.
  - "Light bulb sign" shows the smooth contour of humeral head secondary to loss of greater tuberosity as the humerus is internally rotated.
  - "Rim sign" shows increased distance between the surface of the humeral head and the anterior glenoid rim (>6 mm) (Fig. 74.2).

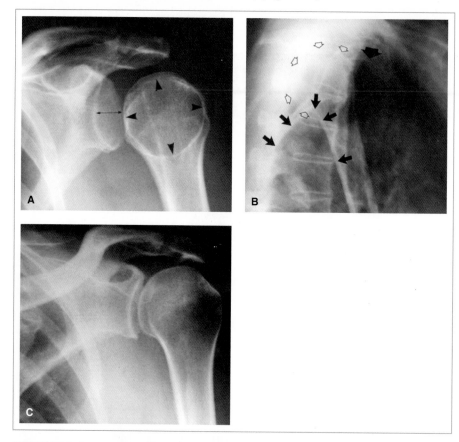

FIGURE 74.2: Pure posterior dislocation of the right humerus (**A**). On the lateral radiograph (**B**), although the relationship of the humeral head (open arrows) to the glenoid fossa cannot be evaluated, the humerus is clearly posterior to the acromion (large closed arrow), and the scapulohumeral angle (small closed arrows) is acute. Both of these observations confirm posterior dislocation of the humerus. The frontal projection of the normal right shoulder has been reversed for ease of comparison (**C**). (Reprinted with permission from Harris JH, Harris WH. *The Radiology of Emergency Medicine,* 4th ed. Philadelphia: Lippincott Williams & Wilkins, 2000.)

Inferior Dislocation

- Patient presents in severe pain with the affected arm held in 180 degrees of abduction with inability to adduct the arm. Radiographically, the humeral head is seen inferior to the glenoid fossa.

Superior Dislocation

- The arm is shortened and adducted with gross deformity over the A-C joint. On radiographs, the humeral head lies superior to the glenoid.

Evaluation

- In the acute trauma scenario, after the airway, breathing, and circulation have been addressed, it is important to fully expose the entire extremity, chest, scapula, clavicle, and C-spine. Conduct a full examination, noting any gross deformities, tenting of the skin, hematomas, lacerations, and abrasions. It is important, especially when abnormalities are noted, to examine the unaffected side for comparison.
- Evaluation should focus on identifying associated neurovascular injuries as a missed diagnosis may have serious ramifications for the patient.
- Assess the integrity of the radial pulse as well as integrity of the skin; if the skin is mottled or cool, or if pulses are weak or absent, procede with prompt reduction of the joint and bedside Doppler to assess vascular patency.
- Axillary neuropraxia is seen in up to 10% of anterior shoulder dislocations, which manifests as a lack of sensation over the lateral aspect of the deltoid with inability to abduct.
- In inferior/superior dislocations, there is a much higher percentage of associated injuries to the axillary artery and brachial plexus.

Management

- Prompt reduction is the priority of any dislocation after stabilization of life-threatening concomitant injury.
- Most reductions are performed with procedural sedation to achieve adequate analgesia and sedation. Agents often used are a combination of benzodiazepines and opiates, as well as newer agents such as propofol or etomidate (quicker onset and shorter half-lives). Intra-articular lidocaine (either alone or in conjunction with intravenous sedation) may also be considered.

Anterior Shoulder Reduction

- There are multiple techniques suitable for anterior shoulder reduction. The key to successful reduction is adequate muscle relaxation/sedation and gradual and constant application of force via manipulation and/or traction. Inability to reduce a dislocation (when there is adequate analgesia/sedation) may be secondary to fracture fragments or soft tissue entrapment.

Traction-Countertraction Technique

- Position the patient supine with the affected extremity near the edge of the bed.
- A sheet is looped around the patient's chest, under the affected axilla, to provide counter traction. The sheet can be grasped or tied around the assistant's waist to provide more stability.
- The practitioner provides gentle, continuous inferior traction on the affected limb. The reduction can be facilitated by both the practitioner and the assistant wrapping sheets (the practitioner's sheet will wrap around his/her waist and the patient's flexed elbow).
- Passive utilization of body weight to provide constant traction allows for a more stable and easier reduction (Fig. 74.3).

Stimson Technique

- This is the most passive technique and can be performed by the lone practitioner.
- The patient is placed in the prone position with the affected arm hanging off of stretcher. A 5 or 10 lb weight is applied at the wrist and allowed to hang until the joint reduces (Fig. 74.4).

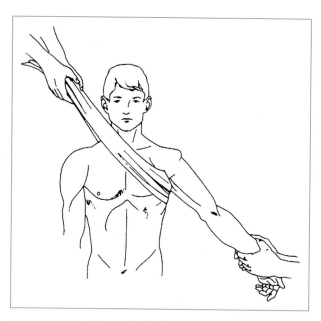

FIGURE 74.3: Traction-countertraction technique for reducing anterior shoulder dislocations. (From Simon RR, Sherman SC, Koenigsknecht SJ. *Emergency Orthopaedics: The Extremities.* McGraw-Hill, 2007:304.)

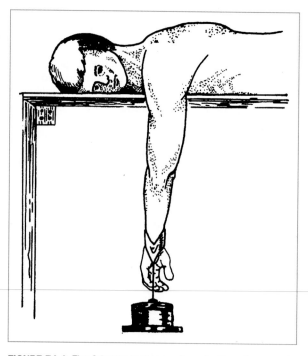

FIGURE 74.4: The Stimson technique for reduction of an anterior shoulder dislocation (Reprinted with permission from Simon RR, Brenner BE. *Emergency procedures and techniques,* 4th ed. Philadelphia: Lippincott Williams and Wilkins; 2002.)

Hennepin Maneuver
- Most often performed with the patient in an upright, seated position, but can be done with the patient lying supine.
- The practitioner gently grasps the affected arm and begins slow external rotation at the elbow to 90 degrees. If reduction has not yet occurred, the arm is then slowly abducted, while maintaining 90 degrees of external rotation (Fig. 74.5).

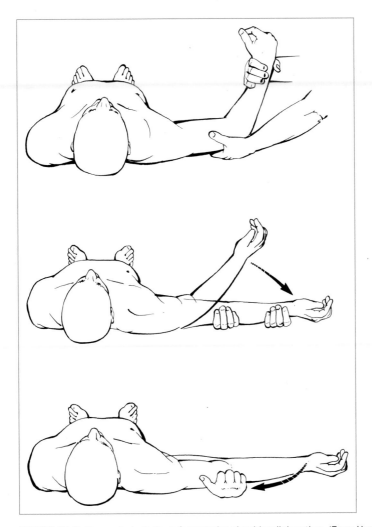

FIGURE 74.5: Hennepin technique for anterior shoulder dislocation. (From Harwood-Nuss, page 1037, Figure 189.5).

Scapular Manipulation
- This technique is performed with the patient in a seated position, and often can be done without parenteral medications.
- An assistant pushes medially on the inferior tip of the scapula and laterally on the superior aspect of the scapula, thus tipping the glenoid fossa downward.

- The practitioner takes the dislocated shoulder and performs one of two maneuvers:
  - Continued axial traction until the shoulder reduces.
  - Gently push the elbow medially across the patient's body. Slowly, passively raise (flex) the arm superiorly until the shoulder reduces. Do not continue if the patient has more than mild discomfort. (Can be done with or without scapular manipulation.)

Milch Technique
- The patient is placed supine in the bed.
- The practitioner externally rotates the shoulder. Then the shoulder is gently abducted into a position where the hand is behind the head.
- When the shoulder is fully abducted, apply axial traction and guide the humeral head over the glenoid.

Posterior Shoulder Reduction
- Place the patient in the supine position.
- Apply axial traction to the humerus.
- An assistant should apply gentle anterior pressure to the humeral head. Internally and externally rotating the humerus may assist in reduction.

Postreduction Care
- Place the shoulder in a sling. Mild abduction of the shoulder with a pillow in the axilla may aid in maintaining the reduction.
- Reassess and document post-reduction neurovascular status.
- Radiographs should be obtained after reduction to confirm anatomic placement and to evaluate and document any concomitant fractures occurring during reduction.
- Follow-up with an orthopedist should occur in 1–2 weeks.

Special Considerations
- Chronic dislocations (i.e., >1 week out) are often difficult to reduce and may require open reduction. They often are associated with a high incidence of neurovascular complications.
- The most common complication of shoulder dislocations is recurrent instability. The incidence of recurrent dislocations has been reported to be as high as 70–90%.
- Cases of neurovascular compromise or open fracture/dislocations warrant emergent orthopedic consultation.

Current Practices
Must one use parenteral procedural sedation ("conscious sedation") for shoulder reductions?
There are several advantages to procedural sedation, most notably patient comfort and relaxation of the shoulder musculature. Notable disadvantages include much more time and dedicated personnel (i.e., nursing support). The literature is littered with many small series of patients who have effective reductions with no analgesia, including the Milch technique or scapular manipulation technique. Many patients tolerate the procedure with minimal discomfort with oral analgesia alone. Patient discomfort and willingness to cooperate are the limiting factors; if the patient cannot tolerate the procedure or it fails after several attempts, another technique using standard procedural sedation is recommended.

Suggested Readings

O'Connor DR, Schwarze D, Fragomen AT, Perdomo M, et al. Painless reduction of acute anterior shoulder dislocations without analgesia. *Orthopedics*. 2006;29:528.

Roberts JQ, Hedges JR. *Clinical Procedures in Emergency Medicine,* 4th ed. Philadelphia: WB Saunders, 2004.

Shoulder DM. In: Marx JA, Hockberger RS, Walls RM, Adams JQ, eds. *Marx: Rosen's Emergency Medicine: Concepts and Clinical Practice,* 6th ed. St. Louis: Elsevier, 2006:670–701.

Ufberg JW, Vikle GM, et al. Anterior shoulder dislocations: beyond traction-countertraction. *J Emerg Med*. 2004;27(3): 301–306.

Zarkadas PC. Neurovascular injuries in shoulder trauma. *Orthop Clin North Am*. 2008; 39(4):483–490, vii

75

Clavicle Fractures

Jarone Lee

Definition

- The clavicle is an S-shaped bone that articulates with the sternum medially and the acromion (scapula) laterally.
- It acts as a strut between the shoulder and the axial skeleton and also protects vital structures such as the apex of the lung, brachial plexus, and the subclavian vessels.
- Clavicle fractures represent 2.6% of all fractures, with an incidence estimated at approximately 50 per 100,000 per year.
- Clavicle fracture has a bimodal distribution of age, with most patients either younger than 40 or older than 70 years.
- Classically, clavicle fractures are classified by dividing the clavicle into thirds. Furthermore, they are grouped from most to least common:
  - Group I—fracture of middle third (75%)
  - Group II—fracture of lateral third
  - Group III—fracture of medial third (<3%)
- Newer classification schemes also delineate each group into subgroups by fracture displacement and associated ligamentous tears.

Pathophysiology

- Clavicle fractures typically occur from direct high-energy trauma to the extremity.
- Eighty-five percent of fractures are caused by a fall or direct impact to the shoulder.
- The middle third of the clavicle is the most commonly fractured, as it is the only part that does not have any ligamentous and muscular attachments.
- Rarely, clavicle fractures result from penetrating injuries, direct blunt injuries, or from a scapulothoracic dissociation injury.

Diagnosis

- Most clavicle fractures are visualized on a chest or shoulder x-ray, and many clinicians do not order dedicated clavicular views for uncomplicated clavicle fractures (Fig. 75.1).
- Special x-ray film views:
  - A 45-degree cephalic tilt view can better evaluate for fracture displacement.
  - An axillary view can better highlight subtle injuries to the lateral third of the clavicle.
  - A serendipity view (40-degree cephalic tilt) allows comparison of both sterno-clavicular (SC) joints to look for dislocations and fractures of the SC.
- Computed tomographic (CT) scans add little to evaluate acute fractures. CT scans can be used to evaluate for chronic problems, such as nonunion or delayed union, or for vascular injury secondary to fracture.
- CT scan may help diagnose injury to the medial one-third of the clavicle, which can be difficult to see on plain films.

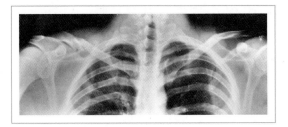

FIGURE 75.1: Fracture of both clavicles. Anteroposterior view of both shoulders demonstrates a comminuted fracture of the middle third of the right clavicle and a simple fracture of the midle third of the left. (Reprinted with permission from Greenspan A. *Orthopedic Imaging: A Practical Approach*, 4th ed. Philadelphia: Lippincott Williams & Wilkins, 2004

Evaluation

- Typically, clavicle fractures are easy to diagnose on physical examination:
    - Tenderness at fracture site
    - Obvious deformity
    - Skin tenting
    - Ecchymosis and swelling
- Since clavicle fractures may involve high-energy trauma, it is important to consider evaluation for other injuries depending on the clinical scenario and mechanism:
    - Rib and scapular fractures
    - Intrathoracic injuries such as pneumothorax or hemothorax
    - Neurovascular injury to the subclavian vessels and brachial plexus.

Management

- Non-operative treatment is recommended for most clavicle fractures, regardless of type:
    - Regular sling is preferred, though numerous others exist.
    - More restrictive braces, such as a figure-of-eight brace, do not improve outcomes.
    - Requires 2–6 weeks of immobilization and 4–6 months avoidance of heavy lifting and contact sports.
- Consider early operative treatment for:
    - Open fractures
    - Skin tenting that could convert to an open fracture
    - Neurovascular compromise
- Fractures of the medial third of the clavicle:
    - Frequently associated with other injuries including rib fractures, pneumothoraces, hemothoraces, and neurovascular injuries.
    - Treated nonoperatively with sling or brace immobilization.
- Fractures of the middle third of the clavicle:
    - A study from 1960 showed a 0.13% nonunion rate for these fractures treated with non-operative management as compared with 4.6% treated with operative management.
    - Nonunion and malunion rates increase with the degree of displacement. Newer studies have estimated that the rate of symptomatic malunion is between 18% and 35%.
        - Symptomatic malunion includes shoulder weakness, scapular winging, and/or thoracic outlet syndrome.
        - Patients at high risk for mal- or non-union should be considered for early, non-emergent surgical management (Table 75.1).
- Fractures of the lateral third are further subclassified (Table 75.2) (Fig. 75.2).

TABLE 75.1: Risk factors for clavicle mal- or non-union

100% displacement
Comminuted fractures
Advanced age
Shortening >2 cm
Female gender

TYPES OF CLAVICLE FRACTURES

A. Classification According to Involvement of the Anatomic Segment

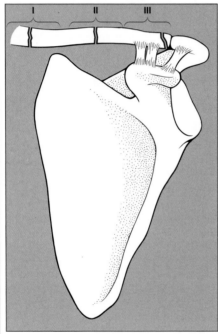

I. Proximal third

II. Middle third

III. Distal third

B. Neer Classification of Fractures of the Distal Clavicle

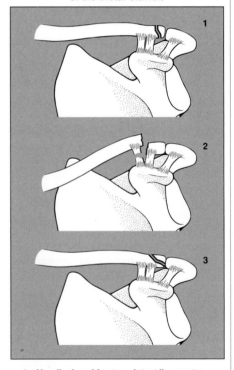

1. Nondisplaced fracture, intact ligaments

2. Displaced interligamentous fracture; conoid ligament torn, trapezoid ligament remains attached to the distal segment

3. Fracture extends to articular surface, ligaments intact

FIGURE 75.2: Classification of the fractures of the clavicle. (Reprinted with permission from Greenspan A. *Orthopedic Imaging: A Practical Approach*, 4th ed. Philadelphia: Lippincott Williams & Wilkins, 2004.)

TABLE 75.2: Neer Classification of clavicle fractures

Neer type	Injury pattern	Management
I	CC ligament intact	Non-operative
II	CC ligament torn off of medial fragment	Surgical correction because 22–37% nonunion rate
III	Intra-articular fracture involving the AC joint but with intact CC ligament.	Non-operative

CC, coracoclavicular; AC, acromioclavicular.

Special Considerations

- Most clavicle fractures can be treated non-operatively, solely with sling immobilization.
- Consider other injuries, especially if the mechanism is high-energy trauma.
- Consider early orthopedic consultation for:
  - Open fractures
  - Skin tenting or visible deformity
  - Shortening of the clavicle of more than 2 cm.
  - Lateral clavicle fractures with the coracoclavicular (CC) ligament torn (Neers type II)

Best Evidence/Clinical Decision Rules

Most patients with clavicle fractures require only non-operative immobilization. How do you decide which sling to use, regular sling versus figure-of-eight brace?

Currently, no single immobilization method has shown superiority. A study in 1987 by Anderson et al. compared a shoulder sling with a figure-of-eight brace. They found no functional or radiographic differences between the two groups. However, the authors did find that the figure-of-eight brace was more poorly tolerated than the sling.

Suggested Readings

Anderson K, Jensen PO, Lauritzen J. Treatment of clavicular fractures. Figure-of-eight bandage versus a simple sling. *Acta Orthop Scand.* 1987;58(1):71–74.

Harris JH, Harris WH. *Radiology of Emergency Medicine,* 4th ed. Lippincott, 2000.

Koval KJ, Zuckerman JD. *Handbook of Fractures,* 3rd ed. Lippincott, 2006.

Shoulder, DM. In: Marx JA, Hockberger RS, Walls RM, Adams JQ, eds. *Marx: Rosen's Emergency Medicine: Concepts and Clinical Practice,* 6th ed. St. Louis: Elsevier, 2006:670–701.

Simon RR, Sherman SC, Koenigsknecht SJ. *Emergency Orthopedics of the Extremities.* 5th ed. McGraw Hill Publishing Company, 2007.

76

Humeral Fractures

Christopher Cheng

Definition

- Proximal and midshaft humeral fractures account for up to 5% of all fractures.
- They are most common in the elderly.
- Supracondylar fractures occur mostly in children aged 4–9 years. They are rare in adults.

Pathophysiology

- Humeral fractures occur because of either direct trauma or via a fall on an outstretched arm (Fig. 76.1).
- The pectoralis major, deltoid, and rotator cuff muscles attach to the proximal humerus and influence displacement of fracture fragments.
- Neurovascular injury is uncommon with humeral fracture, though the radial nerve can be injured in midshaft fractures because of its close anatomic position.
- In the pediatric population, the anterior capsule ligaments about the distal humerus are stronger than the bone; therefore, fractures are more common than ligamentous injuries.

Diagnosis

- The patient with a humeral fracture is generally identified by physical examination. Sometimes a dislocated shoulder can present similarly: they both have proximal humeral swelling/deformity with painful and limited shoulder range of motion.
- Plain film radiography is sufficient for diagnosis in most cases.
- Four view radiographs of the shoulder can fully evaluate the proximal humerus:
  - Anteroposterior (AP) views with external rotation evaluate the greater tuberosity.
  - AP views with internal rotation evaluate the lesser tuberosity.
  - A scapular Y view identifies glenohumeral dislocation.
  - An axillary view evaluates the proximal humerus and articular surface. (This is often not tolerated because of pain).
- Three views of the elbow are recommended to evaluate for supracondylar fractures. Up to 25% of supracondylar fractures are nondisplaced and thus difficult to diagnose radiographically (Table 76.1; Fig. 76.2).

Evaluation

- Initial assessment should focus on the neurovascular status of the arm.
- Ulnar, median, and radial nerve function should be evaluated and documented.
- Radial and ulnar pulses should be assessed to evaluate for compromise of the brachial artery.
- Assess the shoulder and elbow for concomitant injuries.
- Look for any signs of open fractures around the joint. A search for associated fractures on x-ray film should be performed.

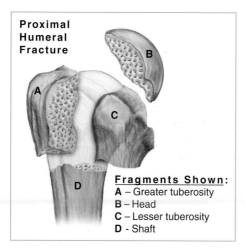

Proximal Humeral Fracture

Fragments Shown:
A – Greater tuberosity
B – Head
C – Lesser tuberosity
D - Shaft

FIGURE 76.1: Proximal humeral fracture. (Copyright © 2010. Anatomical Chart Company. Wolters Kluwer Health.)

TABLE 76.1: Methods to evaluate radiographs for supracondylar fractures

Anterior humeral line: A line drawn down its anterior surface on the lateral film should bisect the capitellum. Abnormality here suggests fracture.

Fat pads: Large anterior or any posterior fat pads raise suspicion for elbow fracture

Carrying angle: The angle between lines drawn through the midshafts of the humerus and ulna on an AP extension view should be <12 degrees. Fracture is associated when this carrying angle is >12 degrees.

AP, anterior-posterior.

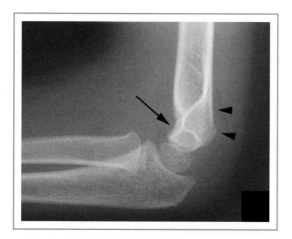

FIGURE 76.2: Nondisplaced supracondylar fracture. Close review of the radiograph shows the presence of a posterior fat pad (arrowheads) that is due to an effusion and suggests a high likelihood of a fracture. In addition, a subtle cortical defect is visible (arrow) on the anterior surface of the distal humeral metaphysis. (Reprinted with permission from Fleisher GR, Ludwig S, Baskin MN. *Atlas of Pediatric Emergency Medicine.* Philadelphia: Lippincott Williams & Wilkins, 2004.)

Management

Humeral Head Fracture

- The most common classification system for proximal humeral fractures is based on the Neer classification (Fig. 76.3).

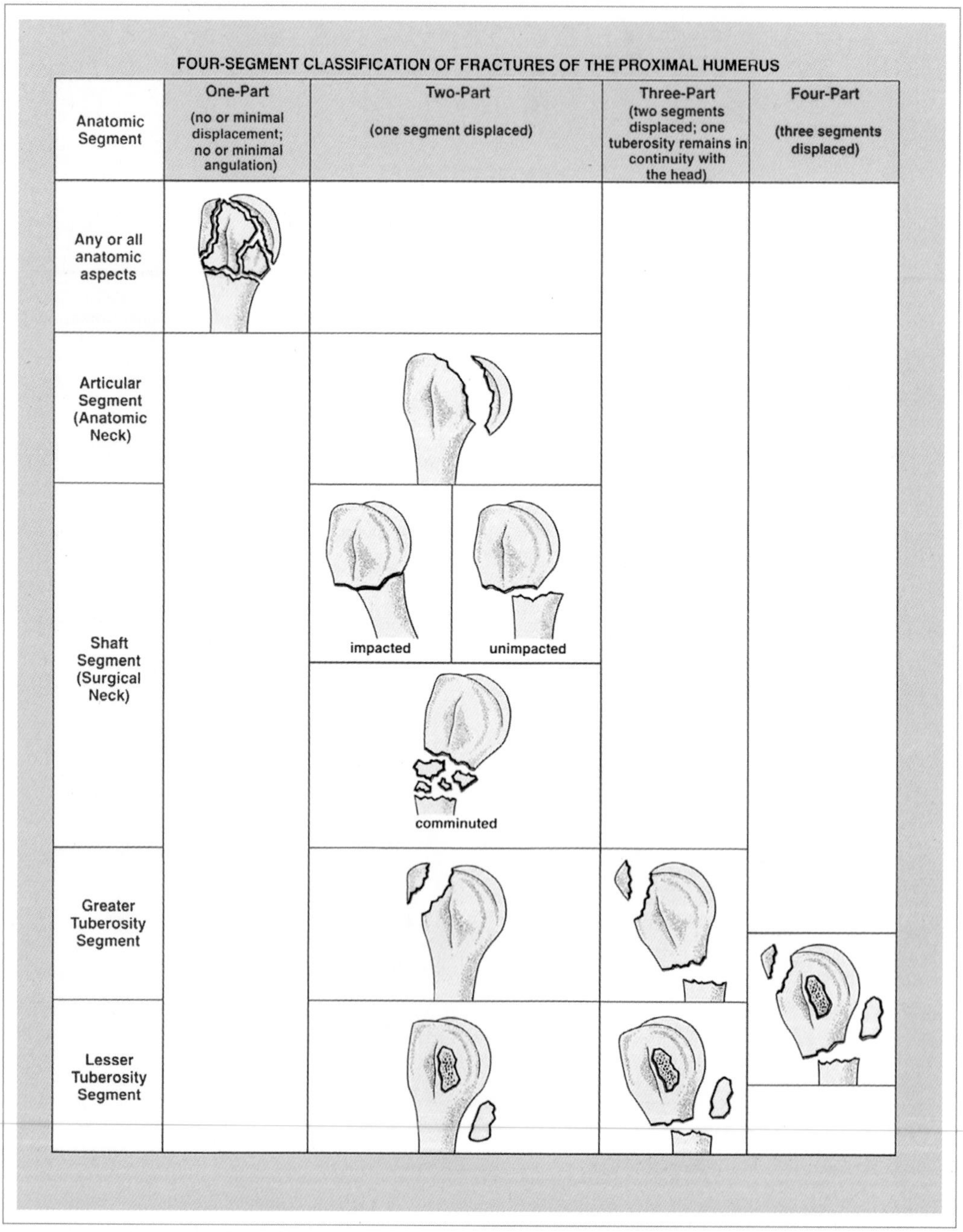

FOUR-SEGMENT CLASSIFICATION OF FRACTURES OF THE PROXIMAL HUMERUS
Anatomic Segment
One-Part
(no or minimal displacement; no or minimal angulation)
Two-Part
(one segment displaced)
Three-Part
(two segments displaced; one tuberosity remains in continuity with the head)
Four-Part
(three segments displaced)
Any or all anatomic aspects
Articular Segment (Anatomic Neck)
Shaft Segment (Surgical Neck)
impacted
unimpacted
comminuted
Greater Tuberosity Segment
Lesser Tuberosity Segment

FIGURE 76.3: Neer classification. Fractures of the proximal humerus based on the presence or absence of displacement of the four major fragments that may result from fracture. (Reprinted with permission from Greenspan A. *Orthopedic Imaging: A Practical Approach*, 4th ed. Philadelphia: Lippincott Williams & Wilkins, 2004. (*continued*)

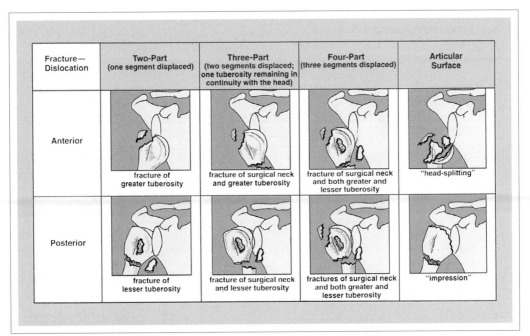

Fracture—Dislocation	Two-Part (one segment displaced)	Three-Part (two segments displaced; one tuberosity remaining in continuity with the head)	Four-Part (three segments displaced)	Articular Surface
Anterior	fracture of greater tuberosity	fracture of surgical neck and greater tuberosity	fracture of surgical neck and both greater and lesser tuberosity	"head-splitting"
Posterior	fracture of lesser tuberosity	fracture of surgical neck and lesser tuberosity	fractures of surgical neck and both greater and lesser tuberosity	"impression"

FIGURE 76.3: (*Continued*)

- More than eighty percent of proximal humerus fractures are nondisplaced with minimal angulation and are treated with a sling only. These simple fractures heal well without any surgical intervention. Patients generally require narcotic analgesia. These patients should still follow up with orthopedics for monitoring of the injury and to help with physical therapy (circumduction exercises to begin as soon as tolerated, with passive elbow and shoulder exercises at 2–3 weeks).
- Angulated fractures of >45 degrees generally require urgent referral for reduction under regional or general anesthesia. In elderly patients with low baseline physical demand, these fractures may not require intervention.
- Fractures with displacements of >1 cm require urgent referral for closed reduction under regional or general anesthesia. Percutaneous pinning may be required.

Humeral Shaft Fracture
- Diaphyseal fractures are classified as transverse, oblique, spiral, or comminuted.
- This fracture is usually treated with a coaptation splint.
- Reduction is generally not indicated because it is difficult to maintain and because minor angulation (<15 degrees) does not affect function. Operative repair is rare but is sometimes needed for significant angulation, interposed soft tissue that does not allow for alignment, pathologic fracture, or neurovascular injury.
- Diaphyseal fractures can be associated with radial nerve injury and occasionally brachial artery injury.
- The vast majority of fractures below the humeral head occur in middle third of the humerus. Patients with proximal fractures at the neck of the humerus should be evaluated for axillary nerve injury and avascular necrosis.

Greater Tuberosity Fracture
- Isolated greater tuberosity fractures are generally treated with a sling and referral to an orthopedist. Displaced greater tuberosity fractures are often complicated by rotator cuff injuries.

- Displaced fractures with significant rotator cuff injuries in young patients are generally repaired operatively.

Lesser Tuberosity Fracture

- Isolated lesser tuberosity fractures are uncommon. These fractures generally do not require more intervention than a sling as needed for comfort, though some orthopedists advocate surgical fixation.
- Lesser tuberosity fractures are associated with posterior shoulder dislocations. Do not miss it!

Supracondylar Fracture

- More than 95% of these fractures are of the extension type where the distal fragment is displaced posteriorly.
- Brachial artery injury, median nerve injury, and compartment syndrome are all associated with supracondylar fractures, so care to evaluate for these is paramount.
- Supracondylar fractures should be immobilized in a long arm posterior splint, from the axilla to the metacarpal heads, with the elbow in 90 degrees of flexion. The splinted arm should then be placed in a sling.
- Most patients with nondisplaced supracondylar fractures and all displaced supracondylar fractures should be admitted by an orthopedist for serial examinations, splinting or casting, and possible reduction or operation. Patients with very stable, nondisplaced supracondylar fractures that have been observed for 6–12 hours may be discharged with urgent orthopedic follow-up (Fig. 76.4).

Special Considerations

- Be aware of the neurovascular injuries associated with humeral fractures.
- Be extremely wary of discharging any patient with a supracondylar fracture that has not been evaluated by an orthopedist.

Current Concepts/Evidence

Why is the axillary view so important? Are there alternatives?

An axillary view is required to have a "complete view" of the shoulder to assess for humeral head and glenoid fracture, lesser tuberosity fractures, posterior dislocation, and anterior instability. It is difficult and sometimes impossible to achieve in patients presenting with dislocation and some humeral fractures. There are several modified views that can be useful where abduction of the arm is not required. The images obtained from these techniques are generally sufficient to assess for the concerned pathologies.

(1) *Trauma axillary view*: The patient lies supine, the x-ray plate is placed superiorly above the patient while the x-ray tube is positioned inferiorly.
(2) *Wheelchair axillary view*: The patient is positioned in a wheelchair at the edge of the radiograph table. The x-ray plate is placed on the arm of the wheelchair, and the patient leans forward into the cassette with slight abduction of the affected arm. The beam passes from above the patient's head with a 20-degree to 30-degree lateral angle of the beam (Routman, 2007).
(3) *Modified axillary view*: The patient stands upright and bends forward. There should be a craniocaudal tube inclination between 30 and 45 degrees (Geusens, 2006).

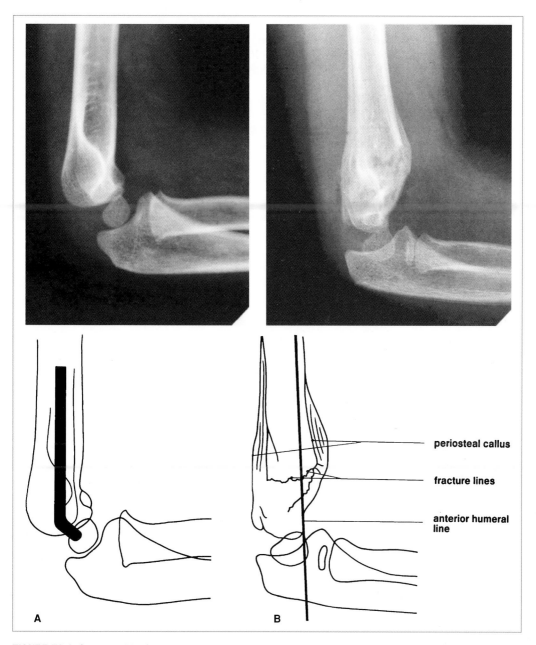

FIGURE 76.4: Supracondylar fracture. **(A)** Lateral view of the elbow joint in a 3-year-old child shows the normal hockey-stick appearance of the distal humerus. **(B)** Loss of this configuration, as seen in this film in a 3.5-year-old girl who sustained trauma to the elbow 4 weeks before this radiographic examination, serves as an important landmark in recognizing supracondylar fracture of the distal humerus. Note also that the anterior humeral line falls anterior to the capitellum, indicating extension injury. (Reprinted with permission from Greenspan A. *Orthopedic Imaging: A Practical Approach,* 4th ed. Philadelphia: Lippincott Williams & Wilkins, 2004.)

Suggested Readings

Geusens E, Pans S, Verhulst D, Brys P. The modified axillary view of the shoulder, a painless alternative. *Emerg Radiol*. 2006;(5):227–230.

Marx JA, Hockberger RS, Walls RM, et.al. *Rosen's Emergency Medicine*. Philadelphia: Mosby, 2006: 647–668.

Routmann H. The wheelchair axillary view of the shoulder. *Orthopedics*. 2007;(4): 265–266.

Simon R, Sherman S, Koenigsknecht S. *Emergency Orthopedics of the Extremities*, 5th ed. New York: McGraw-Hill, 2007:240–280.

77

Elbow Dislocation

Robert Favelukas

Definition

- An elbow dislocation is a complete separation of the articular surfaces of the proximal ulna and radius from the distal humerus.
- There are four types of dislocations: posterior, anterior, lateral, and medial. The dislocation is defined by the direction in which the forearm is displaced from the distal humerus.
- Pure lateral and medial dislocations without fracture are rare and are generally found as a component of a predominantly anterior or posterior dislocation (Fig. 77.1).

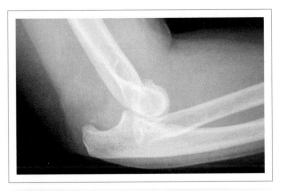

FIGURE 77.1: Posterior dislocation of the olecranon. This dislocation usually is evident clinically. (Courtesy of Robert Hendrickson, MD.) (Reprinted with permission from Greenberg MI, Hendrickson RG, Silverberg M, et al. *Greenberg's Text-Atlas of Emergency Medicine*. Philadelphia: Lippincott Williams & Wilkins, 2005.)

Pathophysiology

- Most elbow dislocations are posterior (90%).
- The mechanism of injury for posterior dislocation is usually a fall onto an outstretched hand with an extended elbow.
- The mechanism of anterior dislocation is usually a direct blow to the olecranon of a flexed elbow.
- All elbow dislocations result from rupture of the collateral ligaments and muscle attachments supporting the elbow joint.
- Elbow dislocations are complicated by fracture (60%), neurologic injury (20%), and vascular injury (8%).

Diagnosis

- The patient with a posterior dislocation generally presents with the arm in 45 degrees of flexion. Early in the course of injury the olecranon is prominent posteriorly. In addition, a defect may be palpable above the olecranon.

- Anterior dislocations present with the upper arm shortened and the forearm appearing elongated.
- Later in the course of any type of elbow dislocation, swelling may be so severe that nothing on palpation would suggest a dislocation. Anteroposterior (AP) and lateral views on x-ray film will diagnose the type of dislocation as well as any associated fractures.

Evaluation

- Initial assessment should focus on the neurovascular status of the arm.
- Ulnar, median, and radial nerve function should be evaluated and documented.
- Radial and ulnar pulses should be assessed to evaluate the integrity of the brachial artery.
- Assess the joints proximal and distal to the elbow for concomitant injuries.
- Look for any signs of open fractures around the joint. A search for associated fractures on x-ray film should be performed.

Management

- Prompt reduction is the priority of any dislocation, after stabilization of any life-threatening concomitant injury.
- Most reductions are performed with moderate sedation to achieve adequate analgesia and sedation. Agents often used are a combination of benzodiazepines and opiates, as well as newer agents such as propofol or etomidate (quicker onset and shorter half-lives).

Reduction of Posterior Dislocation

- Place patient in the supine position. An assistant stabilizes the humerus by wrapping both hands around the arm just distal to the axilla.
- Grasp the wrist with one hand and place the other hand just above the antecubital fossa with the thumb on the olecranon.
- Apply steady in-line traction while an assistant applies countertraction.
- Hold the elbow in slight flexion with the wrist supinated as traction is applied.
- Reduction is accompanied by a "clunk" that is heard or felt (Fig. 77.2).

Alternative Technique for Reduction of Posterior Dislocation

- Place the patient prone with the arm hanging flexed over the edge of the stretcher.
- The humerus lies on the bed with the forearm hanging down toward the floor.
- Downward traction is applied to the forearm, either by the physician or weights tied around the wrist (similar to the "Stimson technique" of shoulder reduction).
- Lateral and downward pressure can be applied to the olecranon with the physician's thumb (Fig. 77.3).

Reduction of Anterior Dislocation

- Place the patient in the supine position.
- An assistant encircles the humerus with both hands and applies countertraction.
- The physician grasps the wrist with one hand and applies in-line traction while the second hand is positioned at the proximal forearm applying downward pressure.
- Reduction is signaled by an audible or tactile "clunk."

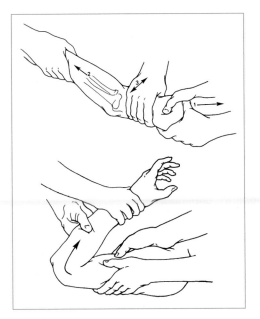

FIGURE 77.2: Technique for reduction of posterior dislocation of the elbow. (Reprinted with permission from Wolfson AB, Hendey GW, Ling LJ, et al. *Harwood-Nuss' Clinical Practice of Emergency Medicine,* 5th ed. Philadelphia: Lippincott Williams & Wilkins, 2009.)

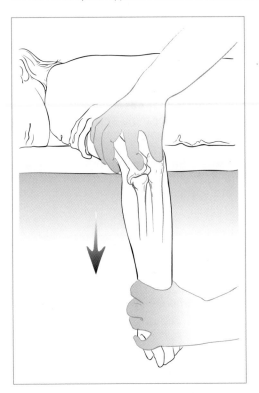

FIGURE 77.3: Technique for reduction of elbow joint dislocation. (Reprinted with permission from King C, Henretig FM et al. *Textbook of Pediatric Emergency Procedures* 2nd ed. Philadelphia: Lippincott Williams & Wilkins, 2008.)

Lateral and Medial Dislocation Considerations

- Lateral and medial dislocations are usually associated with predominantly anterior or posterior position and are treated as such. Scattered literature describing pure lateral and medial reductions generally recommends techniques similar to posterior reduction: longitudinal/posterior traction with force applied to relocate the olecranon into its correct position.

Postreduction Care

- Ensure stability of the joint by gentle range of motion.
- Repeat and document the neurovascular examination.
- Immobilize the elbow in 90 degrees of flexion with a long arm posterior splint.
- Obtain postreduction films to confirm reduction.

Special Considerations

- Observe for delayed vascular compromise, which may be a result of reduction techniques or soft tissue swelling.
- Anterior and open dislocations have a high rate of associated vascular injury. If you suspect any vascular injury, emergent orthopedic and/or surgical consult is warranted.
- Treat open dislocations like open fractures: administer intravenous antibiotics, update tetanus, and call for emergent orthopedic consult.
- Inability to properly range the elbow after reduction may be related to an entrapped medial epicondyle fracture fragment, which can require surgical intervention.

Current Practices

Patients with elbow dislocations may have delayed vascular compromise. Should patients with all simple dislocations be admitted for observation?

No. Most patients may be discharged in a posterior mold splint with a neurovascular check the following day and detailed instructions explaining the concerning symptoms that warrant immediate return to the emergency department. The patient should follow up with an orthopedic surgeon within a week. Early range of motion programs should be started 1–2 weeks postinjury. If there is question of neurovascular compromise, the patient should be seen by the appropriate specialty service.

Suggested Readings

Geiderman JM. Humerus and Elbow. In: Marx JA, Hockberger RS, Walls RM, Adams JQ, eds. *Marx: Rosen's Emergency Medicine: Concepts and Clinical Practice,* 6th ed. St. Louis: Elsevier, 2006:647–669.

Roberts JQ, Hedges JR. *Clinical Procedures in Emergency Medicine,* 4th ed. Philadelphia: WB Saunders, 2004.

78

Radial Head Fracture

Joseph Habboushe

Definition
- Radial head fractures are the most common elbow fracture in adults, accounting for 20% of elbow injuries.

Pathophysiology
- Radial head fracture usually occurs via a "FOOSH" mechanism (Fall On Out-Stretched Hand), which drives the radial head into the capitellum (distal end of humerus).
- The radial head provides 30% of the stability of the elbow, while the remaining 70% comes from the medial collateral ligament (MCL). Therefore, a concomitant MCL rupture can cause valgus instability.
- Ten percent of radial head fractures are accompanied by a radial head dislocation.

Diagnosis
- On physical examination, the radial head is tender to palpation and usually swollen. Pain is often elicited with both supination and pronation.
- Examine the wrist and forearm to evaluate for an **Essex-Lopresti lesion** (concomitant radial head fracture and disruption of the distal radioulnar ligaments from the interosseous membrane, which requires internal fixation), or **Monteggia fracture** (dislocation of the radial head and fracture of the proximal ulna).
- Always perform a full neurovascular examination of the upper extremity, in particular radial nerve function as assessed by wrist extension.
- Evaluate the MCL by valgus stressing while the elbow is flexed to 30 degrees.

Evaluation
- Plain film x-rays are nearly always adequate to evaluate for fracture. Often, the only positive finding is the presence of fat pads. The more common anterior fat pad sign, or "ship sail," has 85% sensitivity and 50% specificity. The posterior fat pad sign has 70% sensitivity and 80% specificity and is more diagnostically useful (Fig. 78.1).
- When the only positive finding is a fat pad sign, consider getting a "radial head—capitellum" view, which may increase the likelihood of identifying the fracture. However, in the presence of clinical findings suggestive of fracture and a fat pad (especially posterior) you should assume a diagnosis of radial head fracture (Fig. 78.2).

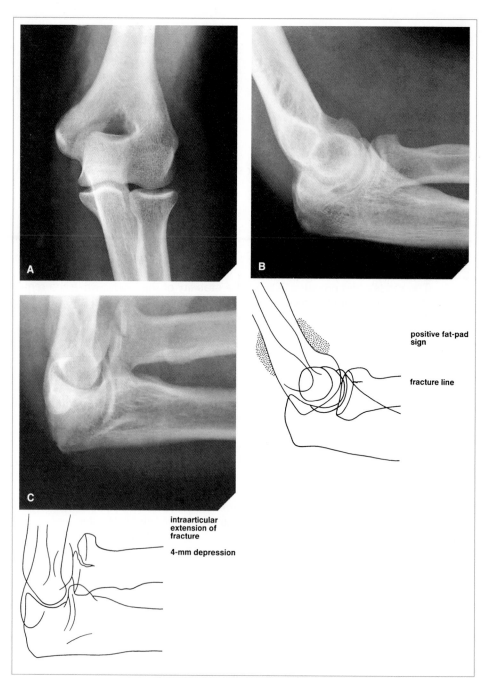

FIGURE 78.1: Fracture of the radial head. Anteroposterior **(A)** and lateral **(B)** films of the elbow show what appears to be a nondisplaced fracture of the radial head. On the radial head-capitellum view **(C)**, however, intraarticular extension of the fracture line and 4-mm depression of the subchondral fragment are clearly demonstrated (From Greenspan A, Norman A, Letter to the editor [Reply]. *AJR Am J Roentgenol* 1983;140:1273.) (Reprinted with permission from Greenspan A. *Orthopedic Radiology: A Practical Approach,* 3rd ed. Philadelphia: Lippincott Williams & Wilkins, 2000.)

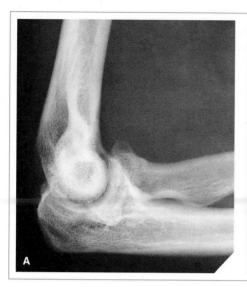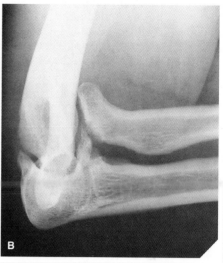

FIGURE 78.2: Fracture of the radial head. Standard lateral view of the eblow **(A)** demonstrates a fracture of the radial head, but bony overlap prevents exact evaluation of the extent of the fracture line and the degree of displacement. Radial head–capitellum view **(B)** reveals it to be a displaced articular fracture involving the posterior third of the radial head. (From Greenspan A, Norman A, Rosen H. Radial head-capitellum view in elbow trauma: clinical application and radiographic-anatomic correlation. *AJR Am J Roentgenol* 1984;143:355–359). (Reprinted with permission from Greenspan A. *Orthopedic Radiology: A Practical Approach,* 3rd ed. Philadelphia: Lippincott Williams & Wilkins, 2000.)

Management

- The Mason Classification System (Table 78.1) is a guide for treatment; individual treatment is determined by the patient's clinical scenario and the orthopedist. Most radial head fractures are treated in the emergency department with sling, analgesia, and outpatient orthopedic follow-up.
- While generally unnecessary, a patient with a large joint effusion may benefit from aspiration. Aspiration of the hemarthrosis is easily performed in the emergency department and can significantly decrease pain and lead to easier early range of motion (ROM).

TABLE 78.1: The Mason Classification system

Type I: Nondisplaced
Sling, elbow flexed at 90 degrees, and ROM within 3 days.

Type II: Displaced
<3 mm displaced: Treated conservatively with sling or splint, and early ROM.
>3 mm or >30 degrees displaced or involves >one-third of joint: Likely will require open reduction. Patient can be placed in a sling or posterior long arm splint with the elbow flexed at 90 degrees. Early orthopedic follow-up is important.

Type III: Comminuted
Usually requires open reduction and internal fixation. Patient should be placed in a long arm splint and follow up with an orthopedist as soon as possible.

- Start by visualizing a triangle made up by (a) the humeral lateral epicondyle, (b) the radial head, and (c) the olecranon.
- With an 18-gauge needle, enter the skin at the center of this triangle and aspirate 5 cc of blood.
- Injection of 1–2 cc of lidocaine or bupivacaine may be a welcome addition to oral analgesia (Fig. 78.3).

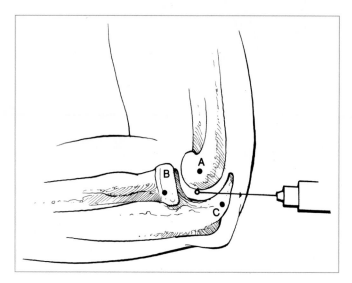

FIGURE 78.3: Elbow aspiration. The safest place to aspirate the elbow is in the center of a triangle produced by connecting **(A)** the lateral epicondyle of the humerus, **(B)** the radial head, and **(C)** the olecranon. (Reprinted with permission from Wolfson AB, Hendey GW, Ling LJ, et al. *Harwood-Nuss' Clinical Practice of Emergency Medicine,* 5th ed. Philadelphia: Lippincott Williams & Wilkins, 2009.)

Special Considerations

- Isolated radial head fractures are rarely associated with any significant complication. It is worth noting that the volar forearm compartment is one of the most frequent sites of compartment syndrome. Compartment syndrome is generally associated with a larger fracture, vascular injury, and significant soft tissue injury.

Suggested Readings

Hall-Craggs M, Shorvan P, Chapman M. Assessment of the radial head-capitellum view and the dorsal fat-pad sign in acute elbow trauma. *Am J Roentgenol.* 1985;145(3):607–609.

Irshad F, Shaw N, Gregory R. Reliability of fat-pad sign in radial head/neck fractures of the elbow. *Injury.* 1997;28(7):433–435.

O'Dwyer H, et al. The fat pad sign following elbow trauma in adults: its usefulness and reliability in suspecting occult fracture. *J Comput Assist Tomogr.* 2004;28(4):562–565.

79

Forearm Trauma

Zuleika Ladha

Definition

- The forearm, which consists of the radius and the ulna, is defined as the portion of the upper extremity located between the elbow and the wrist.
- Forearm injuries most commonly result from a fall on an outstretched hand. Less frequently, they are secondary to a direct blow or a crush injury.
- Forearm fractures are classified as involving the proximal, middle, or distal shaft of either the radius or ulna.

Pathophysiology

- The paired radius and ulna are bound together by joint capsules and ligaments proximally at the elbow and distally at the wrist. The intraosseous membrane connects the two bones along their lengths and also divides the forearm into volar and dorsal compartments.
- The ulna functions to stabilize the hand and wrist while the radius rotates upon it, allowing for pronation and supination.
- Fracture or displacement of one forearm bone is often associated with an injury to the other.
- Associated muscular, tendon, and nerve injuries can occur.

Diagnosis

- The forearm, elbow, and wrist should be evaluated for focal tenderness, swelling, ecchymosis, and range of motion with all suspected forearm injuries. Consider plain film x-rays for patients with focal tenderness.
- A thorough neurovascular examination should be performed. Sensory and motor evaluation of the radial, median, and ulnar nerves along with two-point discrimination should be documented.
- Definitive diagnosis requires imaging of the forearm. Obtain anteroposterior (AP) and lateral views of the forearm with additional elbow and wrist films as indicated.

Evaluation and Management of Radius Fractures

- Suspect radial head fracture in patients with tenderness over the radial head and pain with supination. Nondisplaced fractures are difficult to detect on plain films, but the presence of a posterior fat pad or a large anterior fat pad (sail sign) on a lateral x-ray film suggests the diagnosis (Fig. 79.1).
- Nondisplaced radial head fractures are treated with a sling and early mobilization within 48 hours. Immobilize displaced (over 10 degrees) or comminuted fractures with a posterior long arm splint and give early orthopedic referral.
- Radial shaft fractures occur most commonly at the border between the middle and the distal third of the bone. Displaced fractures at any point along the radial shaft require urgent orthopedic evaluation for reduction and likely operative open reduction and internal fixation (ORIF).

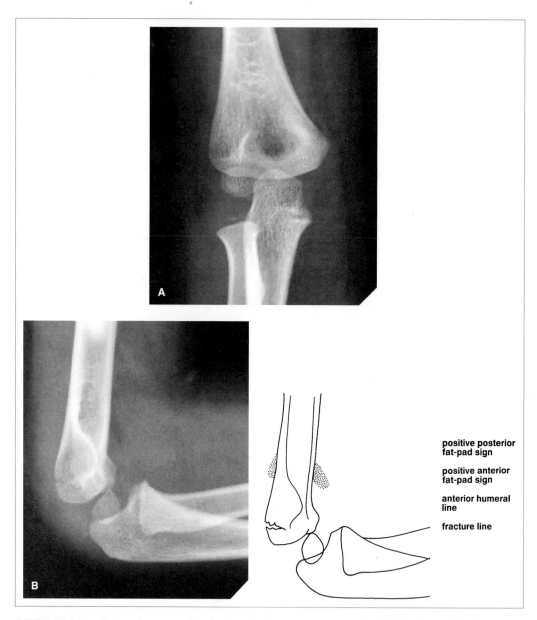

FIGURE 79.1: Nondisplaced supracondylar fracture. On the anteroposterior view **(A)**, the fracture line is practically invisible, whereas on the lateral view **(B)** it is more obvious. There is a positive posterior fat-pad sign, and the anterior fat pad is also clearly displaced. Note that the anterior humeral line intersects the posterior third of the capitellum, indicating slight anterior angulation of the distal fragment. (Reprinted with permission from Greenspan A. *Orthopedic Imaging: A Practical Approach*, 4th ed. Philadelphia: Lippincott Williams & Wilkins, 2004.)

TABLE 79.1: X-ray findings suggestive of distal radioulnar joint dislocation

Ulnar styloid fracture

Widening of the distal radioulnar joint space on AP view

Shortening of the radius by >5 mm

Dislocation of distal radius from ulna

- In patients with distal radius shaft fractures, look for an associated distal radioulnar joint dislocation or subluxation consistent with a Galeazzi fracture. These unstable fractures account for 7% of forearm fractures and require operative repair. Evaluate the distal radioulnar joint for tenderness and swelling (Table 79.1) (Fig. 79.2).

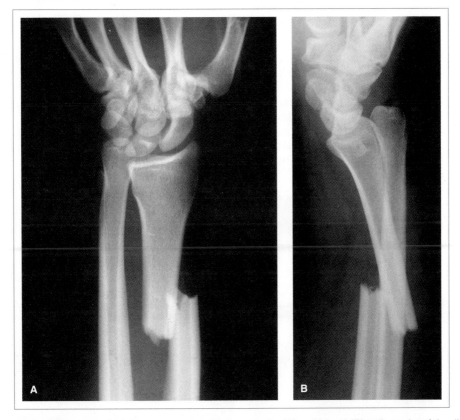

FIGURE 79.2: Galeazzi fracture-dislocation. Posteroanterior **(A)** and lateral **(B)** radiographs of the distal forearm show type I Galeazzi fracture-dislocation. The simple fracture of the radius affects the distal third of the bone, and the proximal end of the distal fragment is dorsally displaced and angulated. In addition, there is dislocation in the distal radioulnar joint. (Reprinted with permission from Greenspan A. *Orthopedic Imaging: A Practical Approach,* 4th ed. Philadelphia: Lippincott Williams & Wilkins, 2004.)

Evaluation and Management of Ulna Fractures

- Isolated ulnar shaft or "nightstick fractures" result from a direct blow to the ulnar border, classically while the arm is raised in self-defense. Nondisplaced fractures can be treated with a posterior long arm splint and orthopedic follow-up for casting in 7–10 days. Displaced fractures require reduction and likely ORIF (Fig. 79.3).

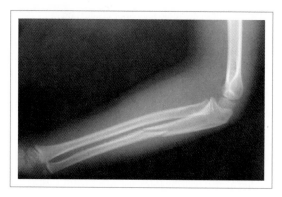

FIGURE 79.3: Nightstick fracture, showing an isolated ulna fracture. (Courtesy of Christy Salvaggio, MD.) (Reprinted with permission from Greenberg MI, Hendrickson RG, Silverberg M, et al. *Greenberg's Text-Atlas of Emergency Medicine*. Philadelphia: Lippincott Williams & Wilkins, 2005.)

▪ Monteggia fractures are located in the proximal third of the ulna with an associated dislocation of the radial head (Fig.79.4). Radial nerve injuries accompany 17% of these fractures.

▪ If a Monteggia fracture is suspected, obtain AP and lateral elbow films to assess for dislocation of the radial head. A line drawn along the radial shaft and head should intersect the capitellum in all views if dislocation is absent.

▪ Monteggia fractures should be immobilized in a long arm posterior splint. They require immediate orthopedic referral to arrange for ORIF as a delay in diagnosis and treatment increases risk of malunion and nonunion.

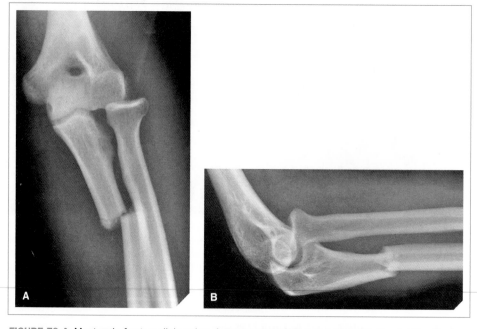

FIGURE 79.4: Monteggia fracture-dislocation. Anteroposterior **(A)** and lateral **(B)** views of the elbow that include the proximal third of the forearm demonstrate the typical appearance of type III Monteggia fracture-dislocation; fracture is at the proximal third of the ulna, associated with anterolateral dislocation of the radial head. (Reprinted with permission from Greenspan A. *Orthopedic Imaging: A Practical Approach,* 4th ed. Philadelphia: Lippincott Williams & Wilkins, 2004.)

Evaluation and Management of Combined Radius and Ulna Shaft Fractures
- Significant force is required to fracture both bones in adults.
- Nondisplaced fractures are rare and can be treated with a long arm anterior-posterior splint with subsequent casting.
- Displaced closed fractures require urgent orthopedic consult for likely ORIF. The time frame for operative repair is generally considered to be "as soon as practical," and most orthopedists recommend repair within 24–48 hours.
- Compartment syndrome can result from combined shaft fractures.

Special Considerations—Compartment Syndrome
- The forearm is the most common site for compartment syndrome in the upper extremity. It is most frequently seen in the volar compartment.
- The majority of compartment syndrome cases follow fractures, but soft tissue and vascular injuries have also resulted in this condition.
- Consider compartment syndrome in patients who require repeated or increasing doses of narcotic pain management for a forearm injury in excess to what would be expected. Maintain a high suspicion for this complication, particularly for those returning to the emergency department with complaints of worsening pain.

Suggested Readings
Roberts JQ, Hedges JR. *Clinical Procedures in Emergency Medicine,* 4th ed. Philadelphia: WB Saunders, 2004.

Woolfrey KGH, Eisenhauer MA. Wrist and Forearm. In: Marx JA, Hockberger RS, Walls RM, Adams JQ, eds. *Marx: Rosen's Emergency Medicine: Concepts and Clinical Practice,* 6th ed. St. Louis: Elsevier, 2006:622–646.

80

Wrist Fractures

Jamie Meade

Definition

- **Colles fracture:** Fracture of the distal radius in which there is dorsal displacement and dorsal angulation of the distal fragment.
- **Smiths fracture:** Fracture of the distal radius in which there is volar displacement and volar angulation of the distal fragment.
- **Barton fracture:** Intra-articular fracture of the distal radius with displacement of either the volar or dorsal rim.
- **Hutchinson fracture:** Avulsion fracture of the radial styloid.
- **Scaphoid fracture:** The most frequently fractured carpal bone. There are four types of fractures: waist (70%), proximal, distal, and tubercle.
- **Lunate fracture:** Most commonly a dorsal avulsion fracture or a fracture to the body of the lunate (Fig. 80.1).

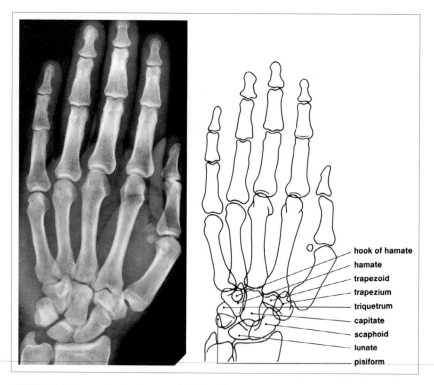

FIGURE 80.1: Dorsovolar (posteroanterior) view of the distal forearm, wrist, and hand. The distal radius and the ulna, as well as the carpal and metacarpal bones and phalanges, are well demonstrated. The thumb, however, is seen in an oblique projection; the bases of the second to fifth metacarpals partially overlap. In the wrist, there is also overlap of the pisiform and the triquentrum, as well as the trapezium and trapezoid bones. (Reprinted with permission from Greenspan A. *Orthopedic Imaging: A Practical Approach,* 4th ed. Philadelphia: Lippincott Williams & Wilkins, 2004.)

Pathophysiology

- The most common mechanism of a distal radius fracture is falling on an outstretched hand with the wrist in dorsiflexion.
- Scaphoid fractures result from forced hyperextension of the wrist and the specific type of fracture depends on the position of the forearm. For example, when the wrist is in radial deviation, the middle of the scaphoid gets compressed on the radial styloid, resulting in a waist fracture.
- Lunate fractures are produced by two different mechanisms. Dorsal avulsion fractures result from forced hyperextension of the wrist and body fractures are produced by axial compression.

Diagnosis

Distal Radius Fracture

- Distal radius fracture can be suspected on physical examination with obvious deformity such as the dinner fork deformity of the Colles fracture, or with tenderness over the distal radius.
- Typically the diagnosis of a distal radius fracture is determined on posteroanterior and lateral x-ray films of the wrist (Fig. 80.2).

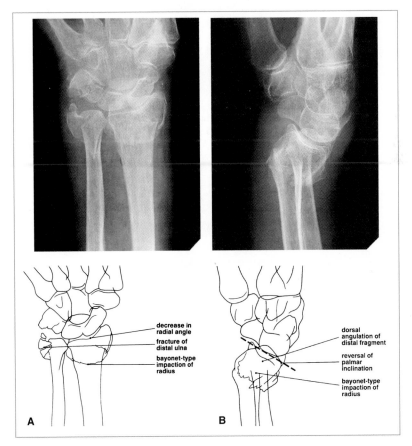

FIGURE 80.2: Colles fracture. Posterior (A) and lateral (B) views of the distal forearm demonstrate the features of Colles fracture. (Reprinted with permission from Greenspan A. Orthopedic Imaging: A Practical Approach, 4th ed. Philadelphia: Lippincott Williams & Wilkins, 2004)

- It is important to assess for normal wrist measurements when evaluating a wrist x-ray film. The maintenance of these measurements allows for the normal function of the wrist.
  - *Radial length*: The distal between the radial articular surface and the tip of the radial styloid ranges from 8 to 18 mm and averages 13 mm.
  - *Radial inclination*: The articular surface of the radius tilts between 12 and 30 degrees toward the ulna, with an average of 22 degrees.
  - *Volar tilt*: The radiocarpal angle on the lateral x-ray film is between 1 and 20 degrees in the volar direction with an average of 11 degrees (Figs. 80.3 and 80.4).

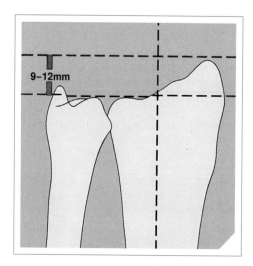

FIGURE 80.3: Neutral ulnar variance. As a rule, the radial styloid process rises 9 to 12 mm above the articular surface of the distal ulna. This distance is also known as the radial length. (Reprinted with permission from Greenspan A. *Orthopedic Imaging: A Practical Approach,* 4th ed. Philadelphia: Lippincott Williams & Wilkins, 2004.)

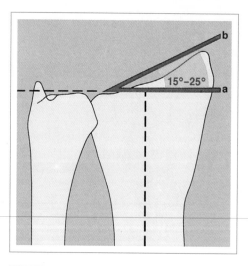

FIGURE 80.4: The ulnar slant of the articular surface of the radius is determined, with the wrist in the neutral position, by the angle formed by two lines: one perpendicular to the long axis of the radius at the level of the radioulnar articular surface (a) and a tangent connecting the radial styloid process and the ulnar aspect of the radius (b). (Reprinted with permission from Greenspan A. *Orthopedic Imaging: A Practical Approach,* 4th ed. Philadelphia: Lippincott Williams & Wilkins, 2004.)

Scaphoid Fracture
- Radiographic diagnosis of a scaphoid fracture is made on posterioanterior (PA), lateral, and oblique views of the wrist. A scaphoid view, in which the wrist is deviated to the ulnar side, can also be obtained to improve visualization of the scaphoid.
- In the acute setting, 30% of scaphoid fractures may not be seen on any radiographic view of the wrist. Provocation tests to diagnose clinical scaphoid fractures are useful:
  - *Anatomic snuffbox tenderness*: The anatomic snuffbox has a medial border formed by the extensor pollicis longus. The lateral border is formed by the parallel tendons of the extensor pollicis brevis and abductor pollicis longus. The base is the styloid process of the radius. Tenderness in this area has a sensitivity of 90% and specificity of 40% for a scaphoid fracture.
  - *Tenderness of the scaphoid tubercle.* The scaphoid tubercle can be palpated on the volar surface of the scaphoid, while the wrist is in radial deviation. A positive examination has an 87% sensitivity and a 57% specificity for fracture.
  - *Pain with axial loading of the thumb.*
  - *Pain in the snuffbox when the wrist is pronated and in an ulna deviated position.* In a small study, lack of this finding had a negative predictive value of 100% (Fig. 80.5).

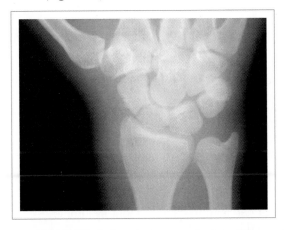

FIGURE 80.5: Nondisplaced, transverse fracture of the scaphoid. (Courtesy of Colleen Campbell, MD.) (Reprinted with permission from Greenberg MI, Hendrickson RG, Silverberg M, et al. *Greenberg's Text-Atlas of Emergency Medicine*. Philadelphia: Lippincott Williams & Wilkins, 2005.)

Lunate Fracture
- On examination, patients will have pain and tenderness over the lunate. The lunate can be palpated just distal to Lister tubercle, which is located on the dorsum of the distal radius. Patients will also have pain with axial compression of the third digit.
- It is difficult to diagnosis lunate fractures on x-ray film as overlying densities often obscure fracture lines. A definitive diagnosis is usually made with computed tomographic scan or magnetic resonance imaging (MRI). MRI can also evaluate for and stage lunate avascular necrosis (Kienbock's disease).

Evaluation
- Perform a thorough neurovascular examination of the affected hand:
  - **Median Nerve:**
    - *Motor*: Opposition of thumb and index finger.
    - *Sensory*: Volar surface of the first three and a half digits.

- *Radial Nerve:*
  - ▷ *Motor*: Dorsiflex the wrist or extension of the fingers at the metacarpal-phalangeal joint.
  - ▷ *Sensory*: Radial half of the dorsum of the hand.
- *Ulnar Nerve:*
  - ▷ *Motor*: Abduct and adduct the fingers. Flexion of the fifth finger.
  - ▷ *Sensory*: Dorsal and volar aspect of the ulnar half of the fourth digit and the entire fifth digit.
- It is also important to palpate for tenderness of the proximal ulna and radius, elbow, and shoulder for associated injuries.

Management

- Colles, Smiths, and Barton fractures should be reduced and splinted.
  - Use 1 or 2% lidocaine to perform a hematoma block.
  - Place the patient in traction with both the elbow and the shoulder at a 90-degree angle. Hang approximately 10 lb of weight from the forearm to provide traction.
  - Reduce the fracture.
    - ▷ *Colles*—First dorsiflex at the fracture site to disengage the volar edge of the distal fragment. Continue to reduce the fracture by moving the distal fragment into 20 degrees of volar flexion with an ulnar tilt (Fig. 80.6).
    - ▷ *Smiths*—Reverse deformity with longitudinal traction and attempt to realign distal fragments.
    - ▷ *Barton*—Apply pressure to move the fractured fragment distally, thereby reducing the intra-articular step-off.
  - Immobilize the fracture in a sugar tong splint.
  - Repeat and document the neurovascular examination.
  - Get a postreduction x-ray to reassess the wrist measurements. It is important to return the volar tilt to ≥0 degree.
  - Instruct the patient to keep the arm elevated for at least 48 hours to decrease swelling that can lead to compartment syndrome.
- Hutchinson fractures should be placed in a sugar tong splint.
- Scaphoid and lunate fractures, whether evident on x-ray film or solely clinically suspected, should be placed in a thumb spica splint. For a lunate fracture place the metacarpophalangeal joint in flexion to decrease compression of the lunate.

Special Considerations

- Smiths and Barton fractures are very unstable. In most cases, it is difficult to maintain a closed reduction; open reduction and fixation is often required.
- The majority of the blood supply to the scaphoid comes from a single blood vessel, which increases the rate of avascular necrosis. To decrease this risk it is important to immobilize any suspected fractures, even with negative x-ray films.
- Kienbock's disease is osteonecrosis, avascular necrosis, or osteomalacia of the lunate bone that results from disrupted blood flow to the lunate. It is more common in patients who have only one blood vessel supplying the lunate, compound fractures, repeated trauma, or in those of western European descent.

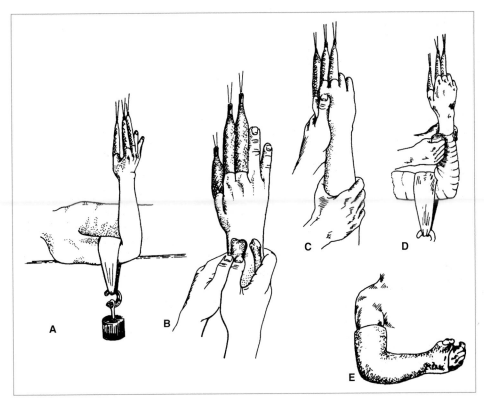

FIGURE 80.6: Colles fracture reduction. **A:** Fingers are placed in finger trap. **B:** After disimpaction of fragments with dorsal pressure, the fracture is reduced by applying a volar force to the distal segments. **C:** Adjust wrist into proper position for immobilization. **D:** Initial portion of splint is applied. **E:** Finished splint. (Reprinted with permission from Simon RR, Brenner BE. *Emergency Procedures and Techniques,* 4th ed. Philadelphia: Lippincott Williams & Wilkins, 2002.)

To reduce the risk of Kienbock's disease it is important to immobilize all suspected lunate fractures.

Current Concepts/Evidence

What is the incidence of fracture in patients suspected to have scaphoid injury with normal radiographs?

Several small case series are found in the literature. One recent (2008) sample of 100 consecutive patients in Britain found a fracture rate of 20%, diagnosed by MRI and/or bone scintigraphy. This is consistent with other reports citing up to a 25% incidence. It is interesting to note that when advanced imaging is done on the hand of a suspected scaphoid injury, fractures of the triquetrum and capitate are also found (though these are generally inconsequential in the long-term).

What is the best test to further evaluate a suspected scaphoid injury?

Making a definitive diagnosis is not critical in the emergency setting; however, the occasion may rise when it is necessary. Traditionally MRI and bone scintigraphy have been used; studies show roughly equal efficacy. Computed tomographic scanning has been shown to be superior to plain film in diagnosing occult fracture and can be done easily in the emergency department, though little evidence is available comparing it with MRI.

Suggested Readings

Beers FJ, Rhemrev SJ, den Hollander P, et al. Early magnetic resonance imaging compared with bone scintigraphy in suspected scaphoid fractures. *J Bone Joint Surg.* (British volume) 2008;90(9):1205.

Koval K, Zuckerman J. *Handbook of Fractures.* Philadelphia: Lippincott Williams & Wilkins, 2002:133–152.

Simon R, Sherman S, Koenigsknecht S. *Emergency Orthopedics: The Extremities.* New York: McGraw-Hill, 2001:184–209.

81 Metacarpal Fractures

Elan Levy

Definition and Anatomy

- Metacarpal fractures are generally divided into two groups: the first metacarpal and those involving metacarpals two through five. This distinction is made because the thumb is anatomically unique due to its high degree of mobility.

Pathophysiology

- Most first metacarpal fractures involve the base and are further subdivided into extra-articular or intra-articular fractures.
- Fractures of the second through fifth metacarpals are described based on the involved segment. These segments include the head, neck, shaft, and base.
- The fourth and fifth metacarpals have 15–25 degrees of anteroposterior motion. The fourth metacarpal can tolerate 20 degrees of angulation while the fifth can tolerate 30 degrees of angulation without functional impairment.
- In contrast, the second and third metacarpals have almost no mobility at their base and can tolerate only 15 degrees of angulation or less without functional impairment.
- Most thumb injuries are sprains, and thumb fractures can tolerate more angulation without loss of function than other metacarpal fractures.

Diagnosis

- Imaging for all of the fractures described can be accomplished with anteroposterior, lateral, and oblique views of the hand.
- A computed tomographic scan is sometimes performed to diagnose and delineate articular injury.

Evaluation

- Observe for swelling, deformity, and asymmetry compared to the uninjured side.
- Assess for rotation malalignment (Fig. 81.1).
- Palpate the hand carefully, including the wrist and fingers. Most fractures can be ascertained on the basis of examination.
- Evaluate and document motor and sensory testing of the ulnar, median, and radial nerves.
- Evaluate tendon function.
- Evaluate vascular function with, capillary refill and distal skin inspection.

Management

- Emergency management of all metacarpal fractures generally includes ice, elevation, and immobilization.

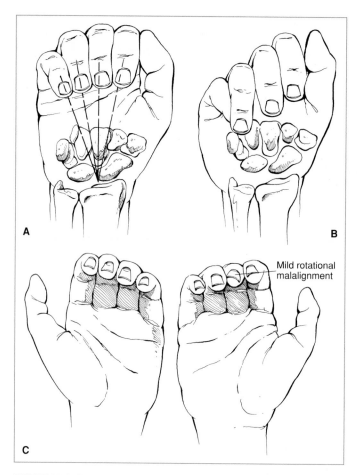

FIGURE 81.1: Clinical signs of rotational malalignment. **(A)** Normally, all fingers point to the same spot on the scaphoid when making a fist. **(B)** With rotational malalignment, the affected finger does not point to the scaphoid. **(C)** Loss of the usual parallel relationship of the finger nails with rotational malalignment. (Reprinted with permission from Wolfson AB, Hendey GW, Hendry PL, et al. *Harwood-Nuss' Clinical Practice of Emergency Medicine,* 4th ed. Philadelphia: Lippincott Williams & Wilkins, 2005.)

- Most closed injuries are treated nonoperatively and can be splinted in the emergency department and referred for outpatient orthopedic evaluation. It is important to know which injuries may require surgical intervention as these need a more urgent follow-up with an orthopedist or hand surgeon.
- Splint immobilization of the fracture should protect the injury and align the fracture as closely as possible, with the hand in the "position of function." The wrist is extended slightly (~20 degrees). The thumb is slightly abducted with the interphalangeal joint in slight flexion. The metacarpal-phalangeal, proximal interphalangeal, and distal interphalangeal joints are all slightly flexed, as if holding an imaginary can of soda.

First Metacarpal Fractures

Extra-articular

- Associated neurovascular injuries are uncommon.
- Mobility of the thumb metacarpal allows for 20–30 degrees of angulation without functional impairment. Fractures with a greater degree of angulation require closed reduction, postreduction films, and immobilization in a thumb spica cast for 4 weeks.

- Transverse fractures frequently angulate; these injuries require reduction and immobilization. Non-displaced transverse fractures can simply be immobilized.
- Oblique fractures and epiphyseal plate injuries require surgical referral for definitive management. Complications include rotational deformities with impairment of normal hand function.

Intra-articular

- The mechanism of injury is an axial force directed against a flexed metacarpal and is most often demonstrated by striking a fixed object with a clenched fist. The two types of intra-articular base fractures are the Bennett fracture and the Rolando fracture.
- A *Bennett fracture* is an intra-articular fracture at the base of the first metacarpal with subluxation or dislocation of the carpometacarpal joint. The ulnar portion of the metacarpal usually remains in place while the distal portion subluxes dorsally and radially. A thumb spica splint should be placed and urgent orthopedic consultation arranged. Because of the extensive pulling forces of the adductor pollicis muscles reduction should be done by the orthopedic or hand surgeon. Complications include joint stiffness, arthritis, and malunion (Fig. 81.2).

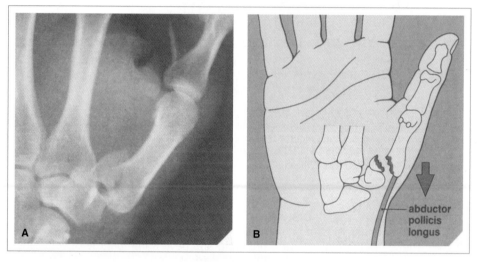

FIGURE 81.2: Dorsovolar radiograph of the hand **(A)** shows the typcial appearance of Bennett fracture. A small fragment at the base of the first metacarpal remains in articulation with the trapezium, while the rest of the bone is dorsally and radially dislocated. The accompanying schematic diagram **(B)** shows the pathomechanics of this injury. (Reprinted with permission from Greenspan A. Orthopedic *Radiology: A Practical Approach,* 3rd ed. Philadelphia: Lippincott Williams & Wilkins, 2000.)

- A *Rolando fracture* is a comminuted fracture of the base of the thumb, most commonly in a T- or Y-shaped pattern. This fracture is much less common than the Bennett fracture and has a worse prognosis. Emergency management and complications are similar to that of the Bennett fracture (Fig. 81.3).

Metacarpal Fractures of Digits II-V

Head Fractures

- The fracture is often distal to attachments of collateral ligaments. Examination reveals tenderness and swelling over the involved metacarpal-phalangeal joint. Complications include rotational malalignment, interosseous muscle fibrosis, extensor tendon injury, and chronic joint stiffness.
- The hand should be placed in a volar splint with the hand in position of function.

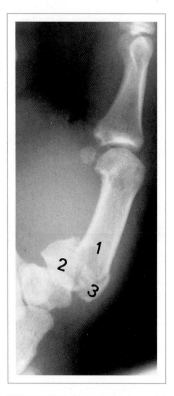

FIGURE 81.3: Rolando fracture of the base of the thumb metacarpal. This is the classic appearance of the Rolando fracture, with the large distal fragment (1) interposed between the proximal fragments (2, 3). (Reprinted with permission from Harris JH, Harris WH. *The Radiology of Emergency Medicine,* 4th ed. Philadelphia: Lippincott Williams & Wilkins, 2000.)

Neck Fractures
- The mechanism is most commonly a direct blow with a clenched fist.
- These fractures are usually unstable and have some degree of volar angulation. Fracture of the neck of the fifth metacarpal is quite common and frequently referred to as a *Boxer's fracture* (Fig. 81.4).
- Successful reduction depends on the anatomic mobility of the involved metacarpal.
- Nondisplaced or nonangulated fractures of the neck of the fourth or fifth metacarpal should be immobilized with volar and dorsal splints with 20 degrees of wrist extension and 90 degrees of flexion at the metacarpophalangeal joints. Fractures of the fourth and fifth digit with angulation >30% and >20%, respectively, should be reduced and, immobilized in a volar splint as described above with postreduction films. These fractures need close follow-up.
- Nondisplaced fractures of the neck of the second and third digits should be immobilized in a radial gutter splint. Close follow-up is recommended because displacement is difficult to correct beyond 1 week. Immediate referral is recommended for fractures with >10% displacement or angulation.
- Any neck fracture that exceeds allowable angulation after reduction and splinting generally requires surgical treatment to prevent loss of function. Complications of neck fractures include malalignment, extensor tendon injuries, collateral ligament damage, malpositioning, and pain with grasp.

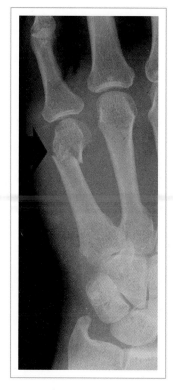

FIGURE 81.4: Boxer's fracture (arrow). (Reprinted with permission from Harris JH and Harris WH: *The Radiology of Emergency Medicine,* 4th ed. Philadelphia: Lippincott Williams & Wilkins, 2000.)

Shaft Fractures

- The most common mechanism for shaft fractures is a direct blow. There are three types: transverse, oblique or spiral, and comminuted.
- Shaft fractures are treated differently from other metacarpal fractures because rotational deformity and shortening are more likely and a lesser degree of angulation is acceptable.
- Any rotational deformity must be corrected. Immobilization should be done with a gutter splint with immediate referral to a hand surgeon. If manipulative reduction is necessary, operative fixation is usually indicated.
- Complications include malrotation, interosseous muscle damage, nonunion, and a chronic painful grip.

Base Fractures

- The mechanism is often from a direct blow, axial force along the digit, or torsion.
- Fractures at the base of the fourth or fifth digit may damage the motor branch of the ulnar nerve causing paralysis of the intrinsic muscles of the hand. There is also an association with carpal bone fractures.
- Immobilization is accomplished with a bulky compressive dressing or a volar splint. Complications include tendon damage, rotational malalignment, and chronic carpal joint stiffness.

Special Considerations

- Rotational and angular malalignment need to be corrected early.
- Be aware of the differences in acceptable malalignment for the specific metacarpals.

Current Concepts

Is there good evidence to validate current orthopedic trends for operative management of metacarpal fractures?

No. There is a paucity of literature, both in terms of large case series and in terms of anything resembling randomized trials. However, there are ample cases of healed fractures with malalignments that have resulted in long-term morbidity: poor grip strength, problems with fine motor tasks, and chronic pain. This anecdotal and experiential evidence has led orthopedists to have a low threshold to operate to decrease chances of impairment of this vital function.

Suggested Readings

Harris JH, Harris WH. *Radiology of Emergency Medicine,* 4th ed. Philadelphia: Lippincott Williams & Wilkins, 2000:419–427.

Simon S, Sherman S, Koenigsknecht S. *Emergency Orthopedics of the Extremities,* 5th ed. New York: McGraw Hill, 2007:143–152.

Tintinalli J. *Emergency Medicine: A Comprehensive Study Guide,* 6th ed. New York: McGraw-Hill Companies, 2004:1673–1674.

82

Phalanx Trauma

Erica Cavallo

Definition

Fracture

- Phalanx fracture usually occurs from a direct crush, twisting, or shearing force.
- Fractures are classified by anatomical segment as tuft, shaft, or intra-articular.
- Intra-articular fractures are classified by the joint involved: distal interphalangeal (DIP) joint and proximal interphalangeal (PIP) joint. The fractured segment can involve the dorsal or the volar surface.

Dislocation

- Injuries of the hand are very common. Dislocations can occur at the DIP, PIP, and metacarpal-phalangeal (MCP) joints.

Pathophysiology

Fracture

- Distal phalanx fractures account for approximately 25% of all hand fractures. Tuft fractures are frequently associated with nail bed injuries.
- Rotational deformity is common in phalangeal shaft fractures. This can lead to functional compromise, especially in the second and third digits.
- Angulation deformity can occur in any direction but is most common in the volar direction. Angulation is less impairing than rotational deformity.

Dislocation

- DIP joint dislocations are uncommon and are usually dorsal when they do occur.
- PIP joint dislocations are one of the most common ligamentous injuries of the hand, and are usually due to axial load and hyperextension.
- Volar dislocation is less common, but is associated with injury of the central slip (a ligament that inserts on the dorsal aspect of lip of the middle phalanx), leading to Boutonniere deformity.
- MCP joints are usually dislocated dorsally. Closed reduction may fail because of interposition of the volar plate between the base of the proximal phalanx and the head of the metacarpal.

Diagnosis

- Plain films of the injured digit are usually adequate to diagnose fractures and dislocations. Radiographs are generally advised to be done prior to reduction of an obvious dislocation to identify prereduction fractures.
- True lateral radiographs are required to determine the degree of angulation.
- Although not evidence-based, subungal hematoma >50% of the nail bed surface suggests an underlying nail bed injury.
- Dislocations are usually obvious from simple inspection. Remember to not let visually striking injuries delay the identification and treatment of other potentially life-threatening injuries (Fig. 82.1).

333

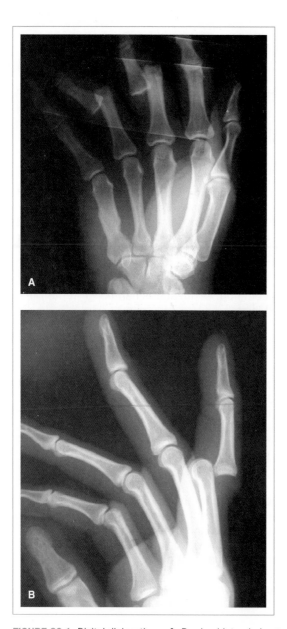

FIGURE 82.1: Digital dislocations. **A:** Proximal interphalangeal joint dislocation of the third and fourth digits. (Courtesy of Robert Hendrickson, MD.) **B:** Dorsal dislocation of the middle phalanx. (Courtesy of Colleen Roberts Campbell, MD.) (Reprinted with permission from Greenberg MI, Hendrickson RG, Silverberg M, et al. *Greenberg's Text-Atlas of Emergency Medicine*. Philadelphia: Lippincott Williams & Wilkins, 2005.)

Evaluation

- History—ascertain the time, cause, and position of hand at time of injury.
- Patient's occupation, avocations, prior hand injuries, and handedness should be noted.
- Physical examination should include detailed motor and sensory assessment including range of motion and strength against resistance of each joint in isolation.

- Rotational deformity can be assessed by having the patient flex the MCP and PIP joints while keeping the DIP joints in extension. The fingers should point to the same place on the wrist without overlapping (see Fig. 81.1).
- It is important that both hands are compared when assessing motor, sensory, and tendon function to better understand the baseline function.
- Range of motion should always be tested against resistance.

Management

Tuft Fracture

- Subungal hematomas are evacuated by heated cautery or boring a hole in the nail with a large bore needle.
- Lacerated nails are usually removed and nail bed lacerations repaired with absorbable sutures. The nail or an artificial stent is placed between the germinal nail matrix and the eponychial fold to prevent adhesions and allow for nail regrowth.
- Antibiotics are indicated for this open fracture that is managed as an outpatient (Fig. 82.2).

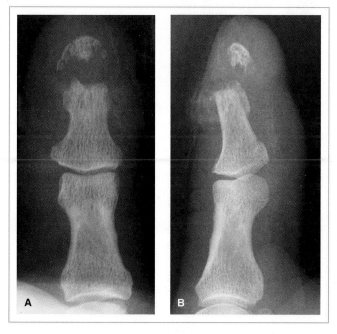

FIGURE 82.2: **A, B:** Comminuted displaced fracture of the subungual tuft. Note the associated soft tissue damage. (Reprinted with permission from Harris JH, Harris WH. *The Radiology of Emergency Medicine,* 4th ed. Philadelphia: Lippincott Williams & Wilkins, 2000.)

Mallet Finger

- Mallet finger is the loss of full extension at the DIP joint. This is caused by intra-articular avulsion fracture of the dorsal surface of the proximal distal phalanx.
- The DIP should be splinted in extension.
- When >30% of joint surface area is affected, a hand surgeon should be seen as these are sometimes repaired operatively (Fig. 82.3).

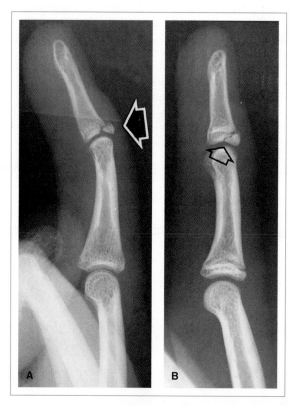

FIGURE 82.3: "Mallet" or "baseball" finger. **A, B:** The small triangular fragment (arrows) is proximally retracted by the common extensor tendon that inserts on this fragment. The flexion deformity results from the unopposed action of the flexor digitorum profundus tendon. **B:** Nondisplaced fracture of the dorsal aspect of the base of the distal phalanx. In this patient, the common extensor tendon inserts distal to the fracture fragment, and a mallet deformity did not result. (Reprinted with permission from Harris JH, Harris WH. *The Radiology of Emergency Medicine,* 4th ed. Philadelphia: Lippincott Williams & Wilkins, 2000.)

Shaft Fracture, Distal Phalanx
- Nondisplaced—protective hairpin splint for 2–4 weeks (Fig. 82.4).
- Displaced—longitudinal traction and dorsal splint for 4–6 weeks.

Middle/Proximal Phalanx
- Reduce and splint any displaced, angulated, or rotated fracture.
- Initially treat all with dorsal splint: MCP at 70 degrees, PIP at 15 degrees, and DIP at 10 degrees (position of function). Stable nondisplaced fractures may alternatively be placed in a dynamic splint (buddy tape).
- Surgical fixation is indicated for spiral, open, or comminuted fractures. Closed fractures with poor reduction, or fractures with >15 degrees of angulation may be considered for surgery as well.

Intra-articular Fracture, DIP
- Dorsal surface of the base of distal phalanx:
  - If <1/3 of the joint surface is involved, splint with DIP in slight hyperextension for 6 weeks.
  - If >1/3 joint surface is involved, splint as above and arrange close follow-up for consideration of surgical repair.

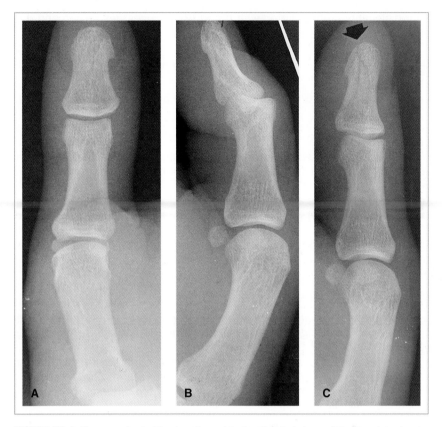

FIGURE 82.4: The comminuted fracture (arrow) in the distal phalanx of the thumb is clearly seen only in the slightly oblique projection **(C)**. (Reprinted with permission from Harris JH, Harris WH. *The Radiology of Emergency Medicine,* 4th ed. Philadelphia: Lippincott Williams & Wilkins, 2000.)

- Volar surface of base:
  - If <1/3 joint surface is involved, splint with DIP in 5–10 degrees of flexion for 6 weeks.
  - If >1/3 joint surface is involved, splint as above with close follow-up for consideration of surgical repair.

Phalanx Dislocations, General Guidelines
- A digital nerve block is recommended for pain control.
- Apply longitudinal traction with anterior/posterior manipulation to reduce into joint.
- Always test the collateral ligaments for stability after reduction.

Distal Interphalangeal
- If stable, put in full extension dorsal splint.
- If unstable, put in 30 degrees flexion dorsal splint.

Proximal Interphalangeal
- Dorsal dislocations are splinted in 15–30 degrees flexion. If there is evidence of complete ligamentous disruption, follow-up in 2–3 days should be arranged with a hand surgeon for possible operative repair.

- Volar dislocations are splinted with the MCP in 50 degrees flexion and the PIP and DIP in full extension.

Metacarpal-Phalangeal
- Splint in 50–70 degrees flexion.

All patients should have follow-up with a hand or orthopedic surgeon.

Special Considerations

- When there is an intra-articular fracture, it is important that the patient does not remove the splint and "test" the joint for 6 weeks or until appropriate orthopedic follow-up.
- Any unstable fractures amenable to closed reduction can be splinted from the forearm to the DIP with the wrist at 20 degrees extension and the MCP in 90 degrees flexion.
- Midshaft transverse fractures, spiral fractures, and intra-articular fractures involving >1/3 of the articular surface often require internal fixation.

Current Concepts/Evidence

Most phalanx fractures and dislocations need only orthopedic follow-up but many hand injuries can have significant morbidity. When is immediate hand surgery consultation recommended?

Consider immediate hand surgery consultation for vascular injuries with signs of ischemia or poorly controlled hemorrhage, severe crush injuries, high-pressure injection injuries, compartment syndrome, grossly contaminated wounds, irreducible dislocations, and finger amputation.

Do all nail injuries require nail removal and nail bed repair?

There is little evidence-based recommendation on this topic, and historically orthopedic practice has been to remove nearly all lacerated/injured nails for nail bed repair. The nail is removed to repair and align the nail bed, the theory being to allow for better nail regrowth. A mangled, avulsed nail should clearly be removed. However, some nail injuries have minimal nail bed injury, and the nail clearly adds support to the damaged phalanx. Leaving the nail in place when the eponychial fold is intact and the clinician suspects the healing nail will grow well is a practice that is performed as a judgment call by some emergency physicians.

Suggested Readings

Simon R, Sherman S, Koenigsknecht. *Emergency Orthopedics of the Extremities.* 5th ed. New York: McGraw-Hill, 2007:123–142.

Wolfson AB, Hendey GW, Hendry PL, et al. *Clinical Practice of Emergency Medicine.* Philadelphia: Lippincott Williams & Wilkins, 2005:1058–1068.

83

Hip Fracture
Mirtha Macri

Definition
- The hip joint is a multiaxial ball and socket joint enclosed within a fibrous capsule. A hip fracture occurs anywhere from the proximal femoral head to the first 4–5 cm of the femoral shaft (subtrochanteric region).
- Fractures of the hip are classified on the basis of relation to the capsule (intracapsular vs. extracapsular), anatomic location (femoral head, neck, trochanteric, intratrochanteric, and subtrochanteric), and the degree of displacement. Treatment and prognosis vary significantly with each fracture type.
- Most recent studies estimate that the incidence of hip fractures in the United States is approximately 80 per 100,000 population.
- Hip fractures carry significant morbidity and mortality. One-year mortality status after surgical repair is approximately 20% and is much higher without surgical repair.
- Morbidity is often a result of immobilization and includes subsequent development of deep venous thrombosis, pulmonary embolism, pneumonia, and urosepsis from indwelling catheters. Approximately one-third of survivors will not regain the ability to ambulate.

Pathophysiology
- Femoral head fractures (intracapsular) are rare and are associated with hip dislocation. These fractures are often diagnosed with postreduction radiographs for hip dislocation. Intracapsular fractures can compromise femoral vasculature which courses along the femoral neck secondary to intracapsular hemarthrosis (Fig. 83.1).
- Femoral neck fractures (intracapsular) generally occur in the elderly osteoporotic patient and are usually the result of minor trauma or fall (90%). Fractures of the femoral neck are classified as displaced or nondisplaced, and these fractures are more concerning for intracapsular hemarthrosis.
- Trochanteric fractures (extracapsular) are secondary to avulsion fractures at the greater and lesser trochanters and usually occur in children and young athletes.
- Intertrochanteric fractures occur anywhere between the lesser and greater trochanters and are often the result of high-speed accidents in young adults and falls in the elderly.
- Subtrochanteric fractures occur between the lesser trochanter and the first 5 cm of the femoral shaft. Approximately 40% of all subtrochanteric fractures have an associated fracture of the pelvis, spine, or other long bones.

Diagnosis
- Most radiological anteroposterior (AP) and lateral views of the hip will demonstrate a hip fracture.
- Fractures of the femoral neck, specifically stress fractures may not be visible on plain film. An AP view with maximal internal rotation of the limb provides a better view of the femoral neck. Look for asymmetry of Shenton's line (curvilinear

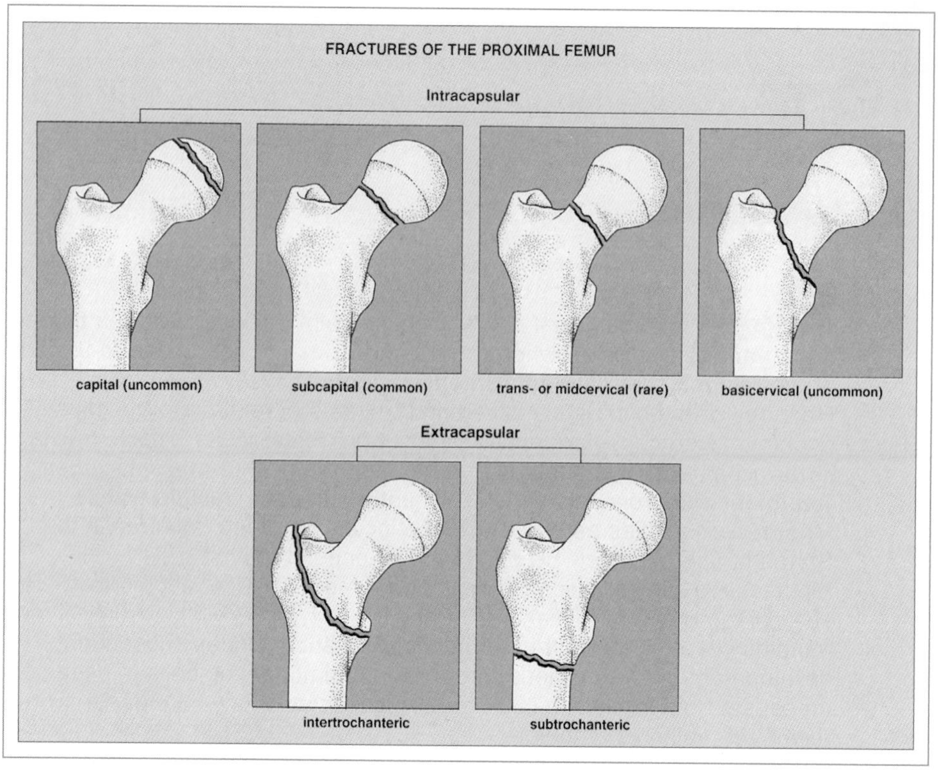

FRACTURES OF THE PROXIMAL FEMUR

Intracapsular

capital (uncommon)   subcapital (common)   trans- or midcervical (rare)   basicervical (uncommon)

Extracapsular

intertrochanteric   subtrochanteric

FIGURE 83.1: Fractures of the proximal femur. (Reprinted with permission from Greenspan A. *Orthopedic Imaging: A Practical Approach,* 4th ed. Philadelphia: Lippincott Williams & Wilkins, 2004.)

line along superior border of obturator foramen and medial aspect of femoral metaphysis).
- In addition, the neck-shaft angle, which is measured by drawing a line through the center of the femoral shaft and neck, can be measured. The normal angle is between 120 and 130 degrees.
- Suspect an occult hip fracture in a patient with significant hip pain upon weight bearing and normal radiographs. Computed tomography or magnetic resonance imaging (MRI) should be considered for further evaluation in the patient who has trauma, hip pain, and inability to ambulate.
- Physical examination holds clues to the type of hip fracture that may be present (Table 83.1).

TABLE 83.1: Type of fracture indicated by specific physical examination findings

Fracture	Physical examination findings
Femoral neck	Leg appears externally rotated, abducted, and shortened
Greater trochanter	Pain with abduction and extension of hip
Lesser trochanter	Pain with flexion and internal rotation
Intertrochanter	Leg is significantly shortened, often with hip edema and ecchymosis
Subtrochanter	The limb is internally rotated and held in flexion

Evaluation and Management

- In the trauma setting, a primary survey and a detailed secondary survey are performed upon arrival. Life-threatening injuries are addressed first. Up to 70% of patients with femoral head fracture and dislocation experience major associated injuries such as intra-abdominal, intra-pelvic, head, and neck injuries.
- Vital signs and secondary signs of hypovolemic shock should be addressed as hip fractures can have a blood volume loss of up to 3 L, though this is uncommon without a significant mechanism of injury.
- Always perform a detailed neurovascular examination of the affected extremity.
- Inspect the lower extremity for deformity, shortening, rotation, and ecchymosis. Palpate the pelvis for stability and the greater trochanters laterally for pain. Range of motion of the hips should be assessed only if no abnormalities are found. If pain is elicited during rotation of the hip with the leg extended, all other maneuvers should be exercised cautiously.

Management

- Management of the patient with the hip fracture should focus on diagnosis of concomitant injury, pain management, and consultation with orthopedic services. Nearly all patients with hip fracture require operative repair (the notable exception being isolated greater or lesser trochanter injury).
- Following the primary and secondary survey, the injured hip should either be immobilized or efforts instituted to severely limit any movement of the injury to prevent additional hemorrhage and pain.
- Intertrochanteric hip fractures may be immobilized with traction splints or application of traction to help with hemorrhage or intractable pain. Skeletal traction is contraindicated in femoral neck fractures because it may further compromise blood flow. Most patients with hip fracture do not require traction.
- Large-bore intravenous access should be obtained if there is a significant mechanism of injury (i.e., high-speed motor vehicle collision, fall from height).
- Preoperative laboratory work should be collected, and the patient should be made NPO. Begin intravenous analgesics promptly.

Special Considerations

Common medicolegal pitfalls:

- Failure to consider fracture of the femoral neck in elderly patients with hip pain and normal radiographs.
- Failure to make a patient non–weight bearing with a stress fracture of the femoral neck, as it may progress to complete fracture.
- Failure to diagnose other injuries, that is, 10% incidence of ipsilateral femoral shaft fractures occurring with femoral neck fracture.

Best Evidence

How often do patients with negative radiographs but persistent pain have occult fracture identified on advanced imaging?

Plain radiography is known to have limited sensitivity for femoral neck fractures, but little data are published regarding sensitivities. A recent small Norwegian study prospectively followed 52 patients admitted to a hospital with hip pain and negative radiographs. Those 52 patients underwent MRI which revealed: femoral neck fracture in 12 (23%), intertrochanteric fracture in 15 (29%), pubic rami fracture in 4 (8%), greater trochanter fracture in 3 (6%), acetabular fracture in 2 (4%), and normal imaging in 6 (12%). The remaining patients mostly had soft tissue injury and two had malignant disease diagnosed.

The take home point: the patient with persistent hip pain (especially the inability to bear weight) after hip trauma with negative radiographs needs advanced imaging (MRI, CT, bone scintigraphy are all considered reasonable tests).

Suggested Readings

Davenport M. Fracture: Hip. eMedicine. http://emedicine.medscape.com/article/825363.

Frihagen F, Nordsletten L, Tariq R, Madsen JE. MRI diagnosis of occult hip fractures. *Acta Orthop.* 2005;76(4):524–530.

Gibbs MA, Newton EJ, Fiectl JF. Hip and Femur. In *Marx: Rosen's Emergency Medicine: Concepts and Clinical Practice,* 6th ed. St. Louis: Elsevier, 2006:735–769.

Steele MT, Ellison SR. Trauma to the pelvis, hip and femur. In: Tintinalli JE, et al, eds. *Emergency Medicine: A Comprehensive Study Guide.* Tintinalli, New York: The McGraw-Hill Companies Inc, 2004:1717–1726.

84

Hip Dislocation

Aparajita Sohoni

Definition

- A hip dislocation is defined as the displacement of the femoral head from the acetabulum.
- Hip dislocations are classified by the direction in which the femoral head is displaced.
  - Posterior dislocations account for almost 85% of hip dislocations.
  - Anterior and central dislocations occur in less than 10% of cases.

Pathophysiology

- The hip joint is a ball-and-socket joint consisting of the femoral head (ball) and the acetabulum (socket). The cartilaginous labrum provides additional structural support to the acetabulum. The entire joint is contained within a thick fibrous capsule and bolstered by the ischiofemoral ligaments, gluteal, and upper thigh muscles.
- The pathophysiology of hip dislocation:
  - Posterior dislocation: A direct force applied to the flexed hip results in posterior dislocation of the femoral head. This "dashboard injury" is so named because it occurs most often after a motor vehicle accident in which the impact of the knee on the car dashboard results in the posterior hip dislocation (Fig. 84.1).

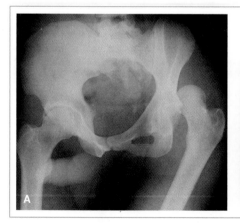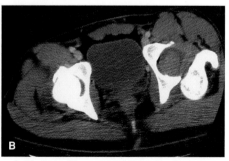

FIGURE 84.1: **Posterior hip dislocation as seen on plain film (A) and computed tomographic scan (B).** Note the left femoral head displaced posteriorly and superiorly. (Courtesy of Alameda County Medical Center—Highland Hospital, Oakland, CA.)

  - Anterior dislocation: This type of dislocation usually results from forced external rotation of an abducted hip, or from forced extension of the entire limb in a high-energy setting, such as during ejection from a vehicle (Fig. 84.2).

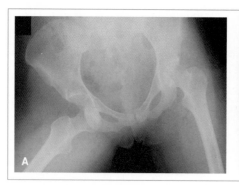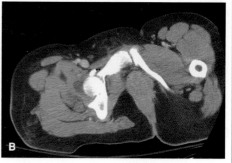

FIGURE 84.2: Anterior hip dislocation as seen on plain film (A) and computed tomographic scan (B). Note the right femoral head displaced anteriorly and inferiorly on plain film, while the computed tomographic scan shows the compression of the femoral head against the pelvis with associated fractures (Courtesy of Alameda County Medical Center—Highland Hospital, Oakland, CA.).

- Central dislocation: Multiple fractures in the floor of the acetabulum can allow the femoral head to dislocate medially (Fig. 84.3).

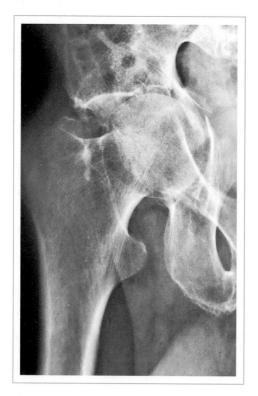

FIGURE 84.3: Central hip dislocation. Anteroposterior view of the right hip shows a typical central dislocation in the hip associated with a comminuted fracture of the medial acetabular wall. Note the protrusion of the femoral head into the pelvic cavity. (Reprinted with permission from Greenspan A. *Orthopedic Imaging: A Practical Approach,* 4th ed. Philadelphia: Lippincott Williams & Wilkins, 2004.)

- Note that each type of hip dislocation is frequently associated with acetabular fracture(s).

▪ Sheering forces applied to the joint capsule can result in vascular compromise of the femoral head.

Evaluation

▪ Clinical suspicion for the presence of a hip dislocation begins by assessing the history and mechanism of injury. A hip dislocation should be considered in all high-speed or high-energy collisions or falls.

▪ On review of systems, patients with a hip dislocation will generally complain of pain in the hip joint. However, patients may not be able to provide this history or may be distracted by another injury.

▪ On physical examination, the following features may be observed:
  • The affected leg is generally shortened.
  • Posterior dislocation—leg held in internal rotation, flexion, and adduction.
  • Anterior dislocation—leg held in external rotation, flexion, and abduction.

▪ Atypical presentations, such as hip dislocations presenting with the lower limb in full extension or with lengthening of the affected limb instead of shortening, have been reported rarely.

▪ Clinical evaluation includes assessing for preservation of vascular flow to the lower extremity and intact function of the sciatic nerve.

Diagnosis

▪ Start with a plain anteroposterior radiograph of the pelvis. Lateral or oblique Judet views can also be obtained to better assess the femoral head/neck and acetabulum. Computed tomographic scans of the pelvis can also be obtained to better assess the hip dislocation or if plain films are inadequate (Figs. 84.1 and 84.2).

▪ It is important to specifically evaluate for a hip dislocation even if another injury to the femur or acetabulum is identified, as these injuries will often coexist.

Management

▪ The force required to disrupt the hip joint space is significant and should prompt immediate search for other serious injuries. Approximately 30–40% of patients with a hip dislocation have additional musculoskeletal injuries. The hip dislocation should be addressed following the trauma initial survey and management of immediate life-threatening injury.

▪ Reduction of a hip dislocation is an emergency. The compromised vascular supply to the femoral head can result in chondrolysis and degenerative changes with lifelong morbidity. Avascular necrosis of the femoral head occurs in approximately 50% of hip dislocations reduced after 6 hours versus only 5% of cases if reduction occurs within 6 hours from the time of injury.

▪ Hip dislocations should be reduced with moderate sedation or in the operating room under general anesthesia.

▪ Posterior and anterior hip dislocations are reduced in a similar fashion (Fig. 84.4).

▪ Following reduction, the hip should be easily ranged through a full range of motion to ensure stability of the joint and that there is no recurrence of the dislocation. If stable, the affected extremity should be secured in a knee immobilizer. Repeat radiographs should be obtained to confirm reduction. If unstable, a femoral pin should be placed for longitudinal traction.

▪ A hip dislocation that fails initial attempts at closed reduction warrants immediate orthopedic consultation for further evaluation. Multiple closed-reduction attempts are associated with poor long-term outcomes.

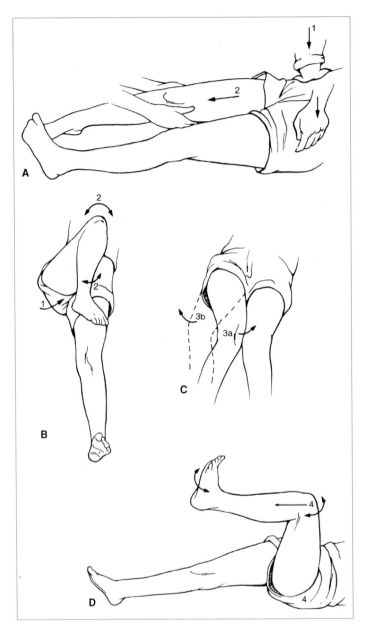

FIGURE 84.4: Posterior dislocation of the hip: method of manipulative reduction. **(A)** The assistant holds downward pressure (*1*) on the anterior–superior iliac spine. With the knee flexed (*2*), the operator pulls on the limb in the line of deformity. **(B)** The assistant slowly brings the thigh (*1*) to 90 degrees of flexion. The assistant gently rotates the thigh internally and externally and rocks the thigh (*2*) backward and forward to disengage the head from the external rotator muscles and the posterior capsule. **(C)** The assistant relocates the femoral head by further internal rotation and extension of the thigh (*3a*), or external rotation and extension of the thigh (*3b*). **(D)** The assistant pushes firmly on the trochanter to direct the femoral head into the acetabulum while the limb is rotated and extended (*4*). Forceful rotation should be avoided, because it can fracture the femoral neck. If the reduction is not accomplished with two adequate attempts, open reduction is indicated. (Reprinted with permission from Wolfson AB, Hendey GW, Hendry PL, et al. *Harwood-Nuss' Clinical Practice of Emergency Medicine*, 4th ed. Philadelphia: Lippincott Williams & Wilkins, 2005.)

Special Considerations

- Hip dislocations have a high incidence of long-term morbidity, either due to necrosis of the femoral head or from injury to the joint and joint capsule, resulting in degenerative arthritis. **Early reduction of the hip is paramount!**
- Orthopedic consultation should be obtained if recurrence of the dislocation occurs to evaluate for placement of a femoral pin for traction versus operative repair.
- Orthopedic consultation should also be obtained prior to reducing the hip in cases of significant acetabular or femur fractures.

Current Concepts

It is recommended that dislocated prosthetic hips be left for orthopedists to reduce due to concern for damage to hardware. What if there is no orthopedist available?

A retrospective chart review at an academic emergency department (ED) sheds some light on this question. Orthopedics was not formally consulted on many of the hips primarily. Of those done in the ED by EM physicians, reduction was successful in 74/81 (91%). Interestingly, in those cases in which the orthopedic service was consulted to perform the reduction in the ED in concert with EM physicians, the results were similar: 28/31 (90%). All failed ED reductions were reduced subsequently in the operating room. There were no significant neurovascular complications documented in any of the patients who were reduced in the ED.

Suggested Readings

Brooks RA, Ribbans WJ. Diagnosis and imaging studies of traumatic hip dislocations in the adult. *Clin Orthop Relat Res.* 2000;(377):15–23.

Germann CA, Geyer DA, Perron AD. Closed reduction of prosthetic hip dislocation by emergency physicians. *Am J Emerg Med.* 2005;23(6):800–805.

Goddard NJ. Classification of traumatic hip dislocation. *Clin Orthop Relat Res.* 2000;(377):11–14.

Phillips AM, Konchwalla A. The pathologic features and mechanism of traumatic dislocation of the hip. *Clin Orthop Relat Res.* 2000;(377):7–10.

Yang EC, Cornwall R. Initial treatment of traumatic hip dislocations in the adult. *Clin Orthop Relat Res.* 2000:24–31.

85

Femur Fracture

Patricia Van Leer

Definition

- Any fracture of the femur that occurs distal to the subtrochanteric region of the hip and proximal to the supracondylar region of the knee.
- Most common type of facture is transverse; however, spiral, comminuted, and open fractures can also occur.

Pathophysiology

- Fracture requires a large amount of force applied directly to the femur (falls, motor vehicle collisions, industrial accidents, etc.).
- Because the femur is the largest long bone and has significant musculature attached, fracture is usually associated with an impressive mechanism of injury.
- In special cases such as osteoporosis or lytic lesions of the bone, fractures can occur with far smaller amounts of force.

Diagnosis

- Femur fracture is often diagnosed on the basis of physical examination. Findings of fracture include obvious deformity, shortening, and/or swelling.
- Anteroposterior (AP) and lateral films will provide details of the fracture but are not a high priority in an unstable trauma patient (Fig. 85.1).

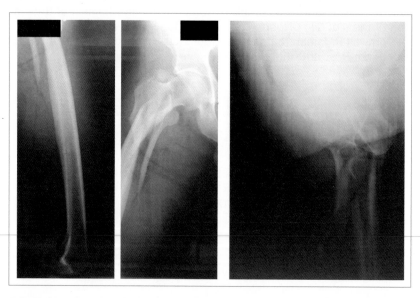

FIGURE 85.1: The injury films show a subtrochanteric femur fracture with proximal extension and severe comminution. (Reprinted with permission from Bucholz RW, Heckman JD. *Rockwood & Green's Fractures in Adults,* 5th ed. Lippincott Williams & Wilkins, 2001.)

Evaluation
- Physical examination should focus on the neurovascular status.
- The adductor hiatus is the point at which the femoral artery becomes the popliteal artery and it also represents the area in which arterial tears often occur. This is approximately at the juncture of the middle and distal thirds of the femur. Absent or diminished distal pulses are signs of possible vascular compromise and should prompt vascular surgery consultation and arteriography.
- Sciatic nerve damage is not common but can occur. Sciatic nerve damage is a contraindication to traction splinting since traction can cause further damage. A neurological deficit can also signify vascular injury and may also require vascular surgical consult.
- As mentioned above, x-ray films of the femur are diagnostic but not emergent.

Management
- Traction splints are the hallmark of prehospital care for femoral shaft fractures.
  - Several splints exist; some examples are the Hare and Thomas splints.
  - Each splint works on the principle of applying traction to the ankle and providing realignment of the affected femur.
  - Splinting usually helps significantly with pain relief.
  - Pneumatic splints are doubly beneficial as they also provide direct pressure.
  - Contraindications to traction splinting are suspected sciatic nerve injury and open fracture.
- Initial emergency department care focuses on patient resuscitation and identifying concomitant injury. Blood loss can be significant and patients may require fluid resuscitation and blood products.
- If realignment was not achieved in the prehospital setting, splinting should be adjusted.
- Pain control is essential and usually requires parenteral opioids.
- **Definitive management is surgical and will require orthopedic consultation.**
- Open fractures, as mentioned above, are a contraindication to traction splints. Patients require intravenous prophylactic antibiotics, usually a first generation cephalosporin. The wound should be covered with saline-soaked gauze. Emergent orthopedic consultation is important for operative irrigation and surgical repair (Fig. 85.2).

Special Considerations
- Because of the significant force required for femoral shaft fractures, many patients will present with multiple injuries. Do not assume that the femoral fracture is an isolated injury.
- Respiratory sequelae can occur. Early complications include fat embolism and acute respiratory distress syndrome (ARDS). Late complications due to prolonged immobilization include deep vein thrombosis (DVT) and pulmonary embolus (PE).

Current Concepts/Evidence
Are femoral fractures in children usually the result of child abuse?
Reports in the literature vary. One recent study from 2000 says "no." One hundred thirty-nine charts were retrospectively reviewed. Charts were examined for physician and social work notes, the use of child protective services, and for whether accidents had witnesses (i.e., clearly a motor vehicle accident). Reviewers then categorized each

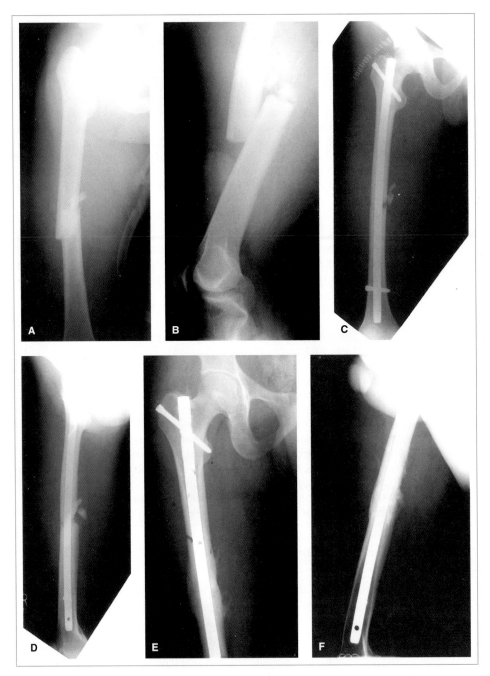

FIGURE 85.2: Radiographs showing a grade IIIA open femur fracture **(A, B)**. Patient underwent immediate irrigation and debridement of open wounds. All devitalized bone fragments were removed. Then, reamed nailing of the femur was performed **(C, D)**. One year after surgery, radiographs reveal a solid union of the femur fracture **(E, F)**. (Reprinted with permission from Bucholz RW, Heckman JD. *Rockwood & Green's Fractures in Adults,* 5th ed. Lippincott Williams & Wilkins, 2001.)

case into several categories of likelihood. 13/139 (9%) were identified as "likely due to abuse" while the remainder were classified as "unlikely to be due to abuse." Of note, 10/13 cases of likely abuse occurred in patients who were not ambulatory (due to age or chronic illness). The authors conclude that most femoral fractures in children are not due to abuse; however, **a femoral fracture in a nonwalking child is a red flag and should raise serious suspicion for abuse** (Fig. 85.3).

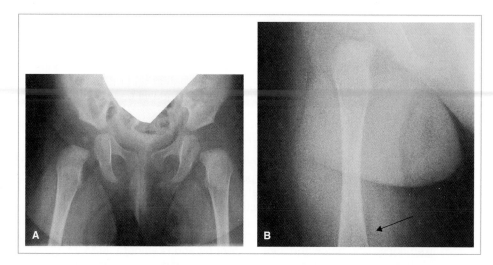

FIGURE 85.3: Femur fracture secondary to child abuse. **A:** Initially hip films were obtained and are normal, but a full femur radiograph **(B)** shows a spiral femur fracture (arrow) consistent with child abuse. (Reprinted with permission from Fleisher GR, Ludwig S, Baskin MN. *Atlas of Pediatric Emergency Medicine*. Philadelphia: Lippincott Williams & Wilkins, 2004.)

Suggested Readings

Marx JA. *Rosen's Emergency Medicine: Concepts and Clinical Practice*. Philadelphia: Mosby Elsevier Publishing, 2009:735–768.

Schwend RM, Werth C, Johnston A, et al. Femur shaft fractures in toddlers and young children: rarely from child abuse. *J Pediatr Orthop*. 2000;20(4):475–481.

Simon R, Sherman S, Koenigsknecht S. *Emergency Orthopedics of the Extremities*, 5th ed. New York: McGraw-Hill, 2007:380–388.

86

Knee Dislocation

Liz Kwan

Definition

- Knee dislocation refers to displacement of the tibia from the femur, a rare but limb threatening emergency due to high rates of vascular complications.
- Multiple classification systems exist. The simplest and most common refers to the position of the tibia relative to the femur, and will be used in this chapter.

Pathophysiology

- Knee dislocation results from the disruption of two or more major knee ligaments.
- Anterior (50–60% of cases) and posterior dislocations are most common and have the highest risk for popliteal artery injury (Fig. 86.1).
  - Anterior dislocations occur with hyperextension.
  - Posterior dislocations classically occur when a flexed knee hits a dashboard.
- The neurovascular bundle (popliteal artery, popliteal vein, and peroneal nerve) is fixed above and below the joint posteriorly and is vulnerable to injury.
  - Peroneal nerve injury occurs in about a quarter of dislocations, and half of these will result in permanent neurological deficits.
  - Reported rates of popliteal artery injury with knee dislocation, vary from 7% to as high as 80%.
- A normal pulse and ankle-brachial index (ABI) does not reliably rule out significant popliteal artery injury.
  - Intimal tears are associated with traction and hyperextension.
  - Occult vascular injuries may cause thrombosis and delayed occlusion, especially during tourniquet use in operative repair of ligaments.
  - The clinical significance and management of these tears remains controversial.

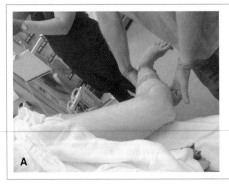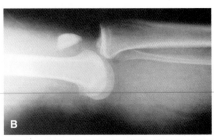

FIGURE 86.1: A: Posterior knee dislocation. **B:** Anterior knee dislocation. (Reprinted with permission from Greenberg MI, Hendrickson RG, Silverberg M, et al. *Greenberg's Text-Atlas of Emergency Medicine*. Philadelphia: Lippincott Williams & Wilkins, 2005.)

Diagnosis

- Clinical presentation of knee dislocation may be subtle, especially in obese patients.
- Plain film x-rays will identify knee dislocations but physical examination and history are essential to identifying those patients with dislocation followed by prehospital spontaneous reduction.
  - Over half of dislocations have spontaneously reduced by the time of evaluation in the emergency department.
- Suspect knee dislocation and vascular injury in any patient with a significant mechanism or unstable knee.
  - The frequency of major and minor vascular abnormalities in patients with severe ligamentous injury is the same as in those with documented knee dislocation.
  - Trauma patients may have altered mental status or other injuries that delay a complete secondary survey.
  - The incidence of low-energy knee dislocation has increased with the prevalence of obesity.

Evaluation

- Suspect other injuries and use Advanced Trauma Life Support protocols as appropriate.
  - More than a quarter of high-velocity knee dislocations are associated with other life-threatening injuries. Greater than half may have an associated fracture.
- The timely diagnosis of arterial injury is critical.
  - The amputation rate is 85% when repair delayed is more than 8 hours, compared to 11% when repair is done within 6 hours.
  - Prolonged ischemia also increases the risk of compartment syndrome postrevascularization.
- Document a neurovascular examination pre- and postreduction.
  - Check both dorsalis pedis and posterior tibial pulses.
  - Check peroneal nerve function: sensation at the dorsal web space between the first two toes and strength of toe and foot dorsiflexion.

Management

- Reduce with longitudinal traction, avoiding pressure and further injury to the popliteal area. Sedation and pain analgesia will likely be necessary.
- Get postreduction x-ray films (Figs. 86.2 and 86.3).

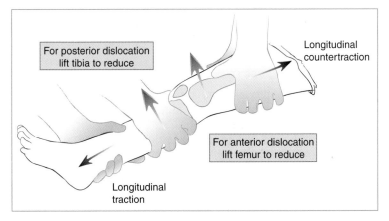

FIGURE 86.2: Technique for reduction of knee joint dislocation. (Reprinted with permission from Young GM. Reduction of common joint dislocations and subluxations. In: Henretig FM, King C, Joffe MD, et al, eds. *Textbook of Pediatric Emergency Procedures.* Philadelphia: Lippincott Williams & Wilkins, 1997.)

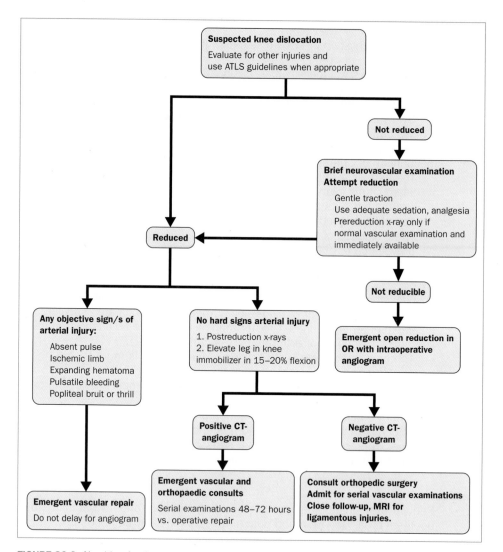

FIGURE 86.3: Algorithm for the management of suspected knee dislocation. ATLS, advanced trauma life support; OR, operating room; CT, computed tomography; MRI, magnetic resonance imaging.

Best Evidence
Is it safe to do selective angiography?

- Because the incidence of popliteal injury in patients with normal pulses has been found to be as high as 23%, angiography or surgical exploration has traditionally been recommended for all knee dislocations.
- A growing surgical literature is now proposing selective angiography. It argues that most of these occult cases involve intimal flaps, which are commonly observed with 48–72 hours of serial examinations. An animal model showed that only 3% of intimal injuries with <50% luminal narrowing formed thrombus. There is also concern for the costs, complications, and false-positive angiograms that would be associated with routine angiograms.
- A meta-analysis reports that the finding of abnormal pulses has a sensitivity of only 79% for a surgical popliteal artery injury. The evidence to support ABI and/or duplex Doppler examinations in place of angiogram is as yet insufficient.

Can ABI predict popliteal injury in knee dislocation?

- ABI is commonly used for peripheral vascular disease or penetrating trauma.
- A single study of only 38 patients looked at ABI and vascular injury associated with knee dislocation. Abnormal ABI appears to be more sensitive for vascular injury than pulse examination, but normal ABI was not compared with angiogram.

How well does angiogram predict popliteal artery injury?

- Significant popliteal artery injury can be missed by both examination and angiography.
  - In a series of 72 knee dislocations, 3 of 12 popliteal artery injuries were missed on both examination and angiography. All three were discovered during the ligament reconstruction weeks later. Two had absent pulses when the tourniquet was released, and one had postoperative bleeding from a popliteal aneurysm.
  - Patients and their orthopedic surgeons should know the limitations of angiography and be given explicit precautions for return.

Suggested Readings

Abate J. Dislocations and soft tissue injuries of the knee. In: Browner BD, Jupiter JB, Levine AM, Trafton PG, Kretteck C, eds. *Browner: Skeletal Trauma,* 4th ed. Philadelphia: W.B. Saunders, 2008:2167–2200.

Barnes CJ, Pietrobon R, Higgins LD. Does the pulse examination in patients with traumatic knee dislocation predict a surgical arterial injury? A meta-analysis. *J Trauma*. 2002;53(6):1109–1114.

Everett L, Pallin D, Antosia, Robert E. Knee and lower leg. In: Marx JA, Hockberger RS, Walls RM, Adams JQ, eds. *Marx: Rosen's Emergency Medicine: Concepts and Clinical Practice,* 6th ed. St. Louis: Elsevier, 2006:770–807.

McDonough EB Jr, Wojtys EM. Multiligamentous injuries of the knee and associated vascular injuries. *Am J Sports Med*. 2009;37(1):156–159.

Mills WJ. The value of the ankle-brachial index for diagnosing arterial injury after knee dislocation: a prospective study. *J Trauma*. 2004;56(6):1261–1265.

Newton EJ, Love J. Emergency department management of selected orthopedic injuries. *Emerg Med Clin North Am*. 2007;25(3):763–793.

Seroyer ST, Musahl V, Harner CD. Management of the acute knee dislocation: the Pittsburgh experience. *Injury*. 2008;39(7):710–718.

87

Patellar Fracture and Dislocation

Jean Yang

Definition

- Patellar fractures account for approximately 1% of all skeletal injuries in children and adults. Major types of patellar fractures include:
  - *Transverse*: **most common**; course in medial-lateral direction, often in the central aspect or distal one-third of patella.
  - *Vertical*: rare, extend superiorly to inferiorly in sagittal plane.
  - *Marginal*: involve edge of patella with no disruption of extensor mechanism.
  - *Osteochondral*: occur more often in children, along with acute patellar dislocation in 5% of patients. Defined by a separate fracture fragment that contains articular cartilage, subchondral bone, and supporting trabecular bone. A subtype of this class, a sleeve fracture, uncommonly occurs when there is avulsion of part of the articular surface (often at the inferior pole).
- Any type of fracture may be displaced, stellate, or comminuted.
- Patellar dislocation accounts for ~2–3% of all knee injuries and are much more common in females.
- Lateral dislocations are seen more often than medial and intra-articular.

Pathophysiology

- Patellar fractures occur as a result of two types of force/injury:
  - Direct (onto flexed knee; i.e., after fall or striking dashboard during motor vehicle accident).
  - Indirect (with sudden contraction of quadriceps; i.e., landing after jumping or abrupt stop after full sprint).
- Patellar dislocations arise frequently as a result of twisting movement about the knee, especially with valgus position. Like fractures, they may also be a consequence of direct or indirect trauma.

Evaluation

- **Emphasis should be placed on assessing knee extension** since this is the primary functional role of the patella. Stress testing is important as well as comparison to the normal knee for all aspects of examination.
- Adequate analgesia may be required before proper evaluation of the knee can be performed.

Diagnosis

- Suspicion of patellar fracture should be high based upon history of direct or indirect trauma. Clinically, patients often present with persistent patellar tenderness and pain or an acutely swollen knee, indicating joint effusion.
- Clinical presentation of patellar dislocation is similar to that of fracture. Patients often state that they heard a pop or a tear at the time of injury. The knee is typically held in 20–30 degrees flexion.

- Diagnostic imaging includes:
  - *Radiography*: Preferred modality of imaging. Anteroposterior (AP), lateral, and oblique views of the knee should be obtained. For better imaging of the patella, consider a sunrise, tunnel, or Merchant view; **sunrise view is best for suspected patellar fracture or dislocation** (Figs. 87.1 and 87.2).
  - *Computed tomography*: Best for occult or osteochondral injuries. Limited for soft tissue evaluation, however, detects loose bone fragments well.
  - *Magnetic resonance imaging*: Useful when clinical diagnosis is difficult, such as with osteochondral sleeve fractures or stress fractures in athletes. Identifies bone bruises and soft tissue injury.
  - *Bone scan*: If normal, fracture may be excluded. Results may be positive for up to 24 hours after time of injury.
  - *Ultrasound*: Rarely used. Ultrasound has limited utility due to the close proximity of posterior articular patellar cartilage to the femur.

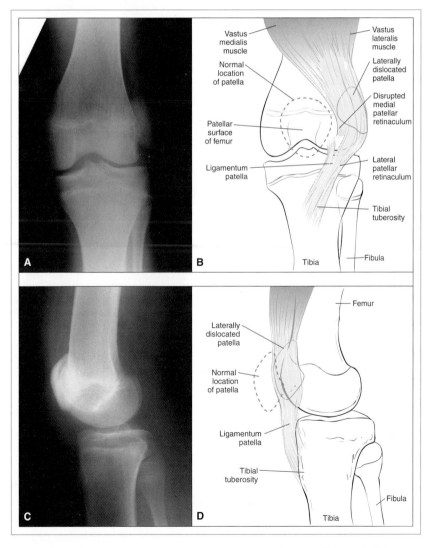

FIGURE 87.1: Patellar dislocation. (Reprinted with permission from King C, Henretig FM et al. *Textbook of Pediatric Emergency Procedures* 2nd ed. Philadelphia: Lippincott Williams & Wilkins, 2008.)

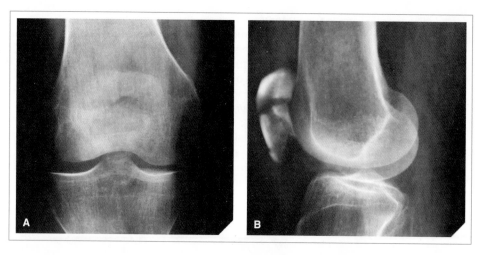

FIGURE 87.2: Fracture of the patella. After a fall on the stairs, a 63-year-old man presented with severe pain in the anterior aspect of the right knee. Anteroposterior (A) and lateral (B) radiographs show the typical appearance of fracture of the patella. Note the significant suprapatellar effusion. (Reprinted with permission from Greenspan A. *Orthopedic Imaging: A Practical Approach,* 4th ed. Philadelphia: Lippincott Williams & Wilkins, 2004, p. 265, image 9.38.)

Management
Reduction of Patellar Dislocation
- Patient is placed in supine position with hips flexed.
- Affected knee should be held in mild flexion with distal thigh fixed in place.
- While slowly extending the knee, apply slight pressure to the lateral aspect of the patella to successfully reposition it medially (Fig. 87.3).

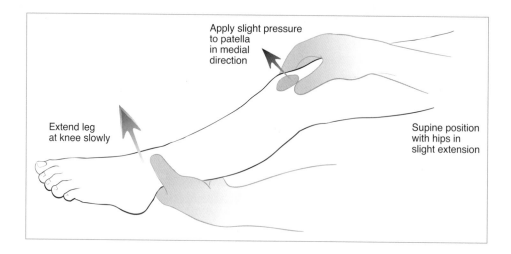

FIGURE 87.3: Technique for reduction of patellar dislocation. (Reprinted with permission from King C, Henretig FM et al. *Textbook of Pediatric Emergency Procedures* 2nd ed. Philadelphia: Lippincott Williams & Wilkins, 2008.)

- Postreduction, patients should be placed in a knee immobilizer or extension splint.
- Fractures or fracture-dislocations of the patella may require a cylinder/long-leg cast from groin to ankle placed 5–7 days following injury and maintained for 4–6 weeks.

TABLE 87.1: Indications for operative management of **patellar fractures**

Disruption of the extensor mechanism

Articular step-off of more than 2 mm

Separation of more than 3 mm between fractured patellar fragments

Severely comminuted fractures

TABLE 87.2: Indications for operative management of **patellar dislocations**

Presence of osteochondral fracture

Substantial disruption of the medial patellar stabilizers

Magnetic resonance imaging findings of chondral injury

- Nonsurgical management mainstay is **RICE**: Rest, Ice, Compression, Elevation. As with other orthopedic injuries, this combination is key in controlling pain and swelling.
- Indications for operative management of patellar fractures and dislocations are listed in Tables 87.1 and 87.2, respectively.

Special Considerations

A bipartite patella develops when two or more ossification centers exist during bone development. Two separate pieces are formed when one of these centers fails to fuse with the main patella. In many cases, it is difficult to differentiate a bipartite patella from an acute patellar fracture and further diagnostic tests may have to be performed. Bipartite patellas have smooth, well-corticated borders and minimal separation between the two parts. Tangential views on radiograph or magnetic resonance imaging are most helpful in these cases. In addition, bipartite patellas are often bilateral, so films of the contralateral knee are quite useful.

Suggested Readings

Lamoureux C. Patella, fractures. *emedicine*. http://emedicine.medscape.com/article/394270-overview. Published January 23, 2009. Accessed February 3, 2009.

Stefancin JJ, Parker RD. First-time traumatic patellar dislocation. *Clin Orthop Relat Res.* 2007;455:93–101.

88

Tibial Plateau Fracture

Prakash Ramsinghani

Definition

- The tibial plateau is one of the most critical load-bearing structures in the human body. Tibial plateau injury can cause serious disability and ambulation limitation.
- This injury comprises 1% of all fractures.

Pathophysiology

- The normal force placed on the tibial condyles is axial compression and rotation. The most common mechanism of injury is a strong valgus force with an axial load.
- Tibial fractures often occur with high energy, such as motor vehicle crashes (used to be referred to as a "fender fracture") and falls from height; however, the elderly with osteoporosis can sustain stress fractures from low-energy compressive forces (Fig. 88.1).

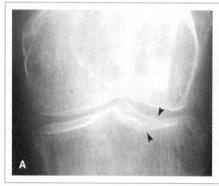 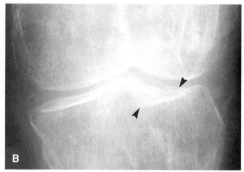

FIGURE 88.1: Insufficiency fracture of the lateral tibial plateau (arrowheads) is suspected in the frontal projection **(A)** and confirmed by subchondral cortical disruption (arrowheads in the externally rotated oblique projection **(B)**). (Reprinted with permission from Harris JH, Harris WH. *The Radiology of Emergency Medicine,* 4th ed. Philadelphia: Lippincott Williams & Wilkins, 2000.)

- Knee extension at the time of injury typically results in an anterior fracture, whereas flexion leads to a posterior fracture.
- Twenty to twenty-five percent of tibial plateau fractures involve capsuloligamentous structures, usually the anterior cruciate ligament/medial cruciate ligament (ACL/MCL), and are typically seen with local or split compression fractures (Fig. 88.2).

Diagnosis

- Clinical signs
  - Inability to bear weight
  - Severe joint line tenderness
  - Ecchymosis
  - Localized soft tissue swelling

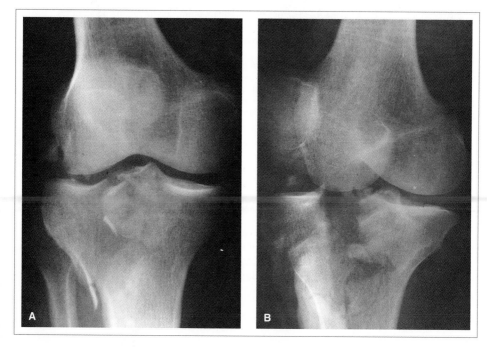

FIGURE 88.2: Comminuted fracture of the proximal tibia. In the frontal projection **(A)**, the comminuted fragments appear to be only slightly displaced. The true magnitude of the degree of displacement is more accurately portrayed in the oblique projection **(B)**. (Reprinted with permission from Harris JH, Harris WH. *The Radiology of Emergency Medicine,* 4th ed. Philadelphia: Lippincott Williams & Wilkins, 2000.)

- Plain film
  - Fracture lines may be subtle!
  - X-ray film will typically show the fracture in the anteroposterior (AP) view
  - Cross table lateral view may show a fat fluid level
  - Oblique films may show more subtle fractures and can provide more complete visualization of an obvious fracture due to the contour of the tibial plateau.
- Computed tomographic imaging
  - Very beneficial in localizing subtle fractures and confirmation when plain film only suggests fracture.
  - CT scan can evaluate the degree of depression in displaced fractures and quantify the amount of articular surface involved in a comminuted fracture.

Evaluation
- Initial assessment should focus on concomitant life-threatening injury.
- Assess the ankle and hip joints.
- A complete neurovascular examination should be performed and documented.
- Examine the knee joint for laxity to evaluate for ligamentous injury.
- Look for any signs of open fractures around the joint. A search for associated fractures on x-ray film should be performed.
- When evaluating plain films, follow the line of the tibial plateau, carefully looking for any subtle cortical disruptions.

TABLE 88.1: Factors that predict need for operative management

Degree of articular depression

Extent and separation of condylar fracture lines

Diaphyseal-metaphyseal comminution and dissociation

Integrity of surrounding soft tissue

Management
- Stable nondisplaced and bicondylar fractures with minimal displacement and no significant disruption of the articular surface can be treated with a long-leg cast or knee immobilizer for 6–8 weeks.
- Operative management considerations (Table 88.1)
  - Severe depression or displacement
    - ▶ 4–10 mm is usually acceptable for depressed fractures.
    - ▶ >10 mm depression/displacement is significant and operative management is likely.
  - Unstable joints
  - Significant ligamentous injury
  - Open fractures
  - Compartment syndrome
  - Age is another factor. Young and active patients should be treated operatively, whereas elderly patients who are not active are generally managed nonoperatively.
- Early complications are from infection, loss of reduction, development of compartment syndrome, and DVTs. The most common long-term complication is osteoarthritis.

Special Considerations
- Observe for delayed vascular compromise which may be a result of improper reduction or soft tissue swelling.
- Vascular complications, while uncommon, do occur with tibial plateau fractures. If there are clinical signs of popliteal artery injury (decreased peripheral pulses, mottling of skin, delayed capillary refill, etc.) an arteriogram should be ordered and a vascular consult obtained.
- Peroneal nerve injury may occur.
- A Segond fracture is a bony avulsion of the lateral tibial plateau that occurs where the lateral capsular ligament attaches.
  - Look for an oval-shaped fragment adjacent to the lateral tibial plateau.
  - It is an important sign for disruption of the ACL and anterolateral rotary instability.
  - It typically occurs in sports from knee flexion with an excessive internal rotation and varus stress.

Current Practices

If a patient with blunt knee injury and a benign x-ray film is unable to walk or bear weight in the emergency department, could there still be a fracture? How sensitive is the x-ray for tibial plateau fracture?

There are no published sensitivities for the use of plain film radiography to diagnose tibial plateau fractures. Most texts suggest that plain films are sufficient and adequate for the evaluation of most knee injuries. Further evaluation with computed tomography or magnetic resonance imaging is generally indicated only for those with high suspicion for fracture (i.e., "unable to walk"), equivocal plain film reading, or if there is a need to characterize the degree of displacement for a clear fracture (plain film is not good at defining this).

Do all patients with blunt knee injury need an x-ray?
No. The Ottawa Knee Rule has shown that a knee radiograph is required only for the patient with blunt knee trauma who has any one of the following:

(1) Age older than 55 years
(2) Tenderness at the head of the fibula
(3) Isolated tenderness of the patella
(4) Inability to flex to 90 degrees
(5) Inability to bear weight immediately and in the emergency department (four steps)

The Ottawa Knee Rule has demonstrated a sensitivity of 100% for identifying clinically important fractures in the original derivation and has subsequently been validated at other sites with similar sensitivities.

Suggested Readings
Emparanza J, Aginaga J. Validation of the Ottawa Knee Rules. *Ann Emerg Med.* 2001;38(4):364–368.
Everett L, Pallin D, Antosia RE. Knee and lower leg. In: Marx JA, Hockberger RS, Walls RM, Adams JQ, eds. *Marx: Rosen's Emergency Medicine: Concepts and Clinical Practice,* 6th ed. St. Louis: Elsevier, 2006.
Stiell IG, Wells GA, McDowell I, et al. Use of radiography in acute knee injuries: need for clinical decision rules. *Acad Emerg Med.* 1995;(2):966–973.

89

Ankle Fracture

Michael Rosselli

Definition

- The ankle is formed by:
  - the tibia which forms the medial malleolus, posterior malleolus, and the plafond (ceiling)
  - the fibula which forms the lateral malleolus
  - the talus
- The ankle is held together by:
  - medial ligaments (collectively termed deltoid ligament)
  - lateral ligaments (anterior talofibular ligament, the calcaneofibular ligament, and the posterior talofibular ligament)
  - syndesmosis between the distal tibia and the fibula.
- It is important to understand the anatomy because ligamentous injuries resulting in joint instability often occur with ankle fractures (Fig. 89.1).

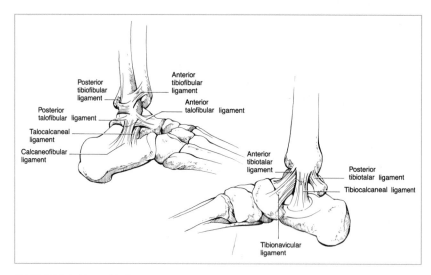

FIGURE 89.1: The ankle ligaments: **(A)** lateral view; **(B)** medial view. (Reprinted with permission from Wolfson AB, Hendey GW, Ling LJ, et al. *Harwood-Nuss' Clinical Practice of Emergency Medicine,* 5th ed. Philadelphia: Lippincott Williams & Wilkins, 2009.)

Pathophysiology

- The majority of ankle fractures are caused by abnormal motion of the talus within the mortise.
- The primary mechanisms of injury in ankle fractures are external rotation, abduction, adduction, and vertical compression.
- Typically, fractures caused by ligamentous avulsion are transverse, whereas fractures caused by talar impaction are oblique.

TABLE 89.1: Weber classification

Weber A	Fibular avulsion fracture below the tibiotalar joint line
Weber B	Fibular fracture at the joint line
Weber C	Fractures above the joint line disrupting the syndesmosis ligament

Diagnosis

- The decision to order a radiograph should be based on physical findings. Standard views include anteroposterior, lateral, and mortise views. The diagnosis is usually clear on the plain films.
- *The Ottawa Ankle Rule* is a well-established and validated clinical decision tool designed to identify the low-risk patient with ankle injury who does not require imaging. The rule has a sensitivity of 99%. An x-ray is needed if any of the following are present:
  - Bony tenderness along the distal 6 cm of the medial malleolus, posterior edge.
  - Bony tenderness along the distal 6 cm of the lateral malleolus, posterior edge.
  - Inability to bear weight for four steps both immediately postinjury and in the emergency department.

Evaluation

- Look at the ankle and the lower extremity for signs of swelling, ecchymosis, deformity, or any asymmetry from the uninjured side.
- Palpate the bones of the ankle, specifically the malleoli, the entire tibia and fibula, and the bones of the midfoot. The foot and knee should be evaluated for associated injury.
- Assess for range of motion: flexion, extension, inversion, and eversion.
- Assess neurovascular status: palpate the dorsalis pedis pulse, assess capillary refills, and check distal sensation and motor function.
- The Danis-Weber classification system for ankle fractures is commonly used and is based on the location of the fibular fracture (Table 89.1) (Fig. 89.2).

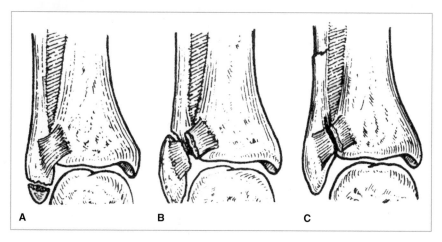

A   B   C

FIGURE 89.2: The Weber classification. (From Ankel F. The Ankle. In: Hart RG, Rittenberry TJ, Uehara DT, eds. *Handbook of orthopedic emergencies*. Philadelphia: Lippincott Raven, 1999, with permission.)

Management

Lateral Malleolar Fracture

- This is the most common fracture of the ankle, typically from an inversion injury.
- **Weber A** fractures are generally stable.
  - They may be placed in a short-leg splint, treated with RICE (rest, ice, compression ACE bandage, elevation), and advised to be non–weight bearing for one week until they follow up with an orthopedic surgeon.
  - Alternatively, isolated small avulsion fractures can be made weight bearing if the patient tolerates walking.
- **Weber B** fractures are usually stable but can be unstable.
  - The patient with a stable joint should be placed in a short-leg splint, made non–weight bearing, and given orthopedic follow-up.
  - Instability may be appreciated on examination but is more easily identified with stress views of the ankle; widening of the tibiofibular joint and disruption of the medial mortise suggest an unstable ankle. Immobilization in a long-leg posterior splint and urgent orthopedic consultation are needed. These injuries usually require operative management for improved long-term outcome.
- **Weber C** fractures are usually unstable and usually require operative care.
- Lateral malleolus fractures may not fit neatly into one category; in general, the ankle should be splinted, made non–weight bearing, and referred for orthopedic consultation. The greater the degree of fracture/joint instability, the more urgent follow-up should be.

Medial Malleolar Fracture

- Often associated with lateral or posterior malleolar fractures.
- Isolated medial fractures can occur with inversion, eversion, or direct blows.
- Isolated fractures involving the medial articulation generally warrant consultation with an orthopedist.
- With no evidence of joint instability, treatment includes a bulky short-leg splint, RICE, analgesia, and keeping the patient non–weight bearing until seen by an orthopedist (Fig. 89.3).

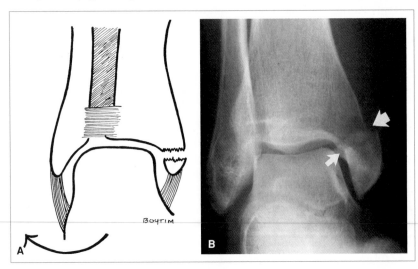

FIGURE 89.3: A, B: Eversion injury with an avulsion fracture of the medial malleolus (arrows). The avulsion fracture line is characteristically horizontal. Its presence indicates that the deltoid ligament is intact. (Reprinted with permission from Harris JH, Harris WH. *The Radiology of Emergency Medicine,* 4th ed. Philadelphia: Lippincott Williams & Wilkins, 2000.)

Bi- and Trimalleolar Fractures
- Involve the medial, lateral, and posterior malleoli (Fig. 89.4).
- In the case of fracture/dislocation, the obviously deformed joint should be reduced expeditiously in the emergency department.
- Closed fractures are rarely associated with vascular compromise, whereas open fractures are commonly associated with vascular compromise.
- If an open fracture/dislocation is present, orthopedic operative irrigation and reduction is preferred.
- For both open and closed fracture/dislocations, a long-leg posterior splint is placed followed by postreduction radiographs and vascular checks.

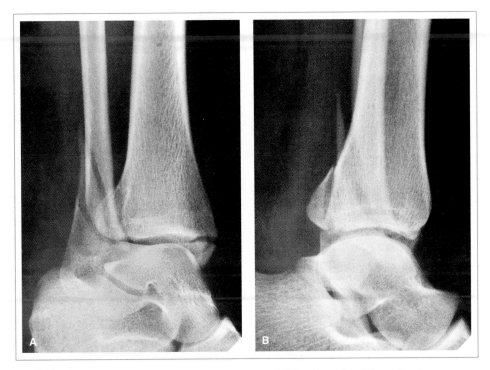

FIGURE 89.4: Trimalleolar fracture. Oblique **(A)** and lateral **(B)** radiographs of the ankle show a trimalleolar fracture affecting both malleoli and the posterior lip of the distal tibia. The latter feature is better seen on the lateral view. (Reprinted with permission from Greenspan A. *Orthopedic Imaging: A Practical Approach,* 4th ed. Philadelphia: Lippincott Williams & Wilkins, 2004.)

Posterior Marginal Fractures
- Rare
- Occur by ligamentous avulsion or by axial loading.
- Nondisplaced fractures involving <25% of the articular surface can be treated with a non–weight bearing short-leg cast for 4 weeks.
- Displaced fractures or those involving >25% often require open reduction and internal fixation.

Plafond Fractures (Anterior Marginal Tibial Fractures)
- Usually occur when the talus hits the distal tibia due to a high-energy dorsiflexion force.
- This injury requires orthopedic consultation because operative intervention is often necessary.

Pilon Fracture
- Results from axial compression that directs force vertically into the tibial plafond causing severe comminution of the distal tibia and fibula (Fig. 89.5).
- Computed tomography may be necessary to differentiate a pilon fracture from a trimalleolar fracture.
- Place the patient in a long-leg posterior splint to provide adequate stabilization and arrange for orthopedic consultation. This injury requires operative repair.

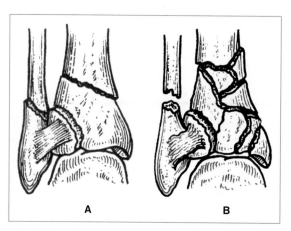

FIGURE 89.5: Pilon fracture. (From Ankel F. The Ankle. In: Hart RG, Rittenberry TJ, Uehara DT (eds). *Handbook of orthopaedic emergencies.* Philadelphia: Lippincott Raven, 1999, with permission.)

Tillaux Fracture
- Is an avulsion fracture of the anterolateral aspect of the distal tibia.
- The fracture line starts at the joint line and extends vertically, exiting at or distal to the fused physis (Fig. 89.6).
- The mechanism of this injury is external rotation and abduction, leading to avulsion of the bone element by the anterior talofibular ligament.
- Treatment is RICE, analgesics, and prompt orthopedic follow-up.

Talar Dome Fractures
- The most common sites involved are the superolateral and superomedial margins of the dome.
- Patients may present describing persistent ankle pain. Prolonged pain, swelling, and crepitus should raise suspicion for this injury. Palpating the dome of the talus with the foot plantar flexed may localize the tenderness.
- Nondisplaced fractures are treated conservatively.
- Displaced fractures should undergo operative management for the debridement and removal of any loose body.

Maisonneuve Fractures
- Are oblique fracture of the proximal fibula with either disruption of the deltoid ligament or fracture of the medial malleolus (Fig. 89.7).
- The mechanism of injury is external rotation upon an inverted or adducted foot. The force of injury is transmitted up the lower leg via the syndesmosis fracturing the relatively weak proximal fibula.
- Treatment is based on the integrity of the ankle joint and presence of a medial malleolar fracture.

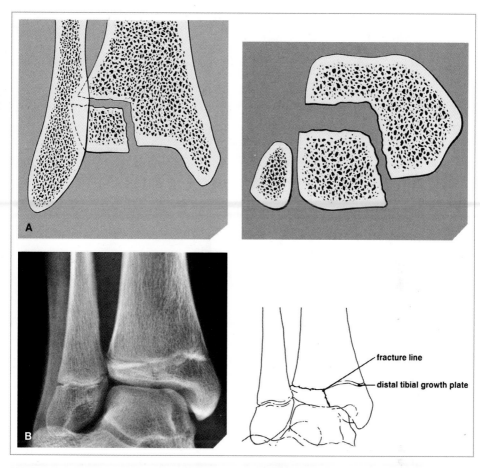

FIGURE 89.6: Tillaux fracture shown as **(A)** schematic and **(B)** oblique view of the ankle. (Reprinted with permission from Greenspan A. *Orthopedic Imaging: A Practical Approach,* 4th ed. Philadelphia: Lippincott Williams & Wilkins, 2004.)

- If the mortise joint is disrupted or there is a fracture of the medial malleolus, operative fixation is necessary.
- If the joint is not disrupted and there is no malleolar fracture, the patient can be treated in a long-leg cast for 6–12 weeks.

Special Considerations

- Isolated medial malleolus fractures are less common because the injury requires more force than lateral malleolus fractures; therefore, other associated fractures and joint instability should be suspected.
- Always palpate the proximal fibula to avoid missing a Maisonneuve fracture.
- Isolated ankle dislocation is rare, and most ankle dislocations are associated with fractures involving the malleoli.

Current Concepts/Evidence

I am familiar with the Ottawa Ankle Rule, but it does not seem like many physicians use it. Does it really work? Is it applicable to children?

This decision rule has been extensively studied and validated in both adults and children. A meta-analysis of 27 studies and 15,581 patients showed pooled sensitivities

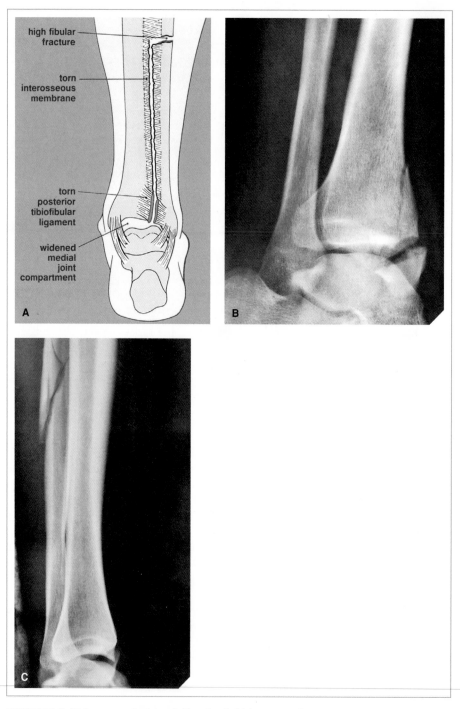

FIGURE 89.7: Maisonneuve fracture. **A:** The classic Maisonneuve fracture commonly occurs at the junction of the middle and distal thirs of the fibula. The tibiofibular syndesmosis is disrupted, and the interosseous membrane is turn up to the level of the fracture. The tibiotalar (medial) joint compartment is widened because of lateral subluxation of the talus. **B:** Oblique view of the ankle shows a communited fracture of the medial malleolus with extension into the anterior lip of the tibia. **C:** On the lateral view, a comminuted fracture of the fibula is apparent. (Reprinted with permission from Greenspan A. *Orthopedic Imaging: A Practical Approach,* 4th ed. Philadelphia: Lippincott Williams & Wilkins, 2004.)

of 97% in adults and 99% in children. Despite good data showing physician awareness of the rule and the fact that most patients with ankle sprains (85%) do not have fractures, the rule is not widely applied in practice. Patient expectations, legal pressures to diagnose all injuries, and ease of radiographs probably lead most physicians to lean on imaging despite negligible indications. Informing patients about the low yield and letting them help make the decision may be one way to avoid the time, radiation, and cost of this frequently ordered and often unnecessary test.

Suggested Readings
Bachman LM, Kolb E, Koller M, et al. Accuracy of Ottawa ankle rules to exclude fractures of the ankle and mid-foot: systematic review. *BMJ.* 2003;326(7386):417.
Hart R, Rittenberry T, Uehara D. *Handbook of Orthopedic Emergencies.* Philadelphia: Lippincott-Raven, 1999: 341–356.
Rockwood C, Green D. *Fractures in Adults,* 3rd ed. Philadelphia: Lippincott, 1991.
Shah K. Ankle and foot injuries. In: Wolfson A, ed. *Clinical Practice of Emergency Medicine,* 4th ed. Philadelphia: Lippincott Williams & Wilkins, 2005:1092–1100.

90

Ankle Dislocation

Fahad Khan

Definition

- Ankle dislocations are described by the relation of the talus to the tibia.
- Dislocations occur in every direction: anterior, posterior, superior, lateral, and medial.
- Posterior dislocations are the most common; superior dislocations are rare.

Pathophysiology

- The ankle joint is a modified saddle joint that consists of the distal fibula, tibia, and the talus bone of the foot.
- A pure dislocation (without fracture) is extremely rare. Because the ankle joint has extremely strong ligamentous support, most dislocations have associated fractures as they require forces of great magnitude.

Posterior Dislocations

- Usually result from a fall on a plantar-flexed foot.
- They are associated with isolated fractures of the posterior lip of the tibia and can include malleoli fractures and are usually associated with rupture of the tibiofibular ligaments.

Anterior Dislocations

- Result from forced dorsiflexion or a blow directed posteriorly to the distal tibia while the foot is fixed.
- The most common cause is deceleration injury seen in motor vehicle collisions.
- They are associated with malleolar fractures or a fracture of the anterior lip of the tibia.

Superior Dislocations

- Result from significant axial force, commonly from a patient landing on his or her feet from a fall of significant height.
- Cause diastasis of the tibiofibular joint, with the talus driven upward, disrupting the mortise.
- They can be associated with fractures of the talar dome.

Lateral Dislocations

- Usually occurs from a marked inversion/eversion of the foot.
- This injury is less commonly associated with rupture of the deltoid ligament and always associated with malleoli and distal fibula fractures.

Diagnosis

- Ankle dislocations have an obvious clinical presentation of significant deformity and disability.

- Plain radiographs should be obtained before reduction if there are no signs of vascular compromise or skin tenting. Anteroposterior (AP) and lateral views obtained at the bedside are adequate to assess the nature of the dislocation and associated fractures. Additional views may be obtained after reduction to determine the exact extent and severity of the associated fractures (Fig. 90.1).

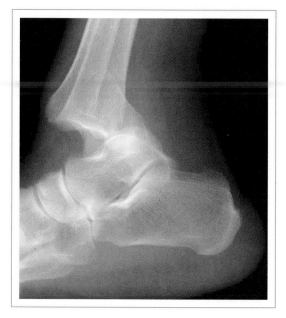

FIGURE 90.1: Ankle dislocation with "tenting"of the skin. Courtesy of Mark Silverberg, MD. (Reprinted with permission from Greenberg MI, Hendrickson RG, Silverberg M, et al. *Greenberg's Text-Atlas of Emergency Medicine*. Philadelphia: Lippincott Williams & Wilkins, 2005.)

Evaluation

Posterior

- Posterior ankle dislocations are locked in plantarflexion with the anterior tibia easily palpable.
- The foot has a shortened appearance with resistance to dorsiflexion.

Anterior

- Anterior dislocations present with a dorsiflexed foot that appears elongated.
- The talus is prominent anteriorly, and the dorsalis pedis pulse may be diminished or absent secondary to pressure from the displaced talus.

Superior

- Superior dislocations may cause the affected leg to look shortened compared with the unaffected leg, with widening and shortening of the affected ankle area.

Lateral

- Lateral dislocations present with the foot entirely displaced laterally and the skin taut over the medial aspect of the ankle joint.

Management

- Immediate reduction should be performed if there is vascular compromise or skin tenting.
- After one or two unsuccessful attempts at closed reduction, orthopedic consultation should be obtained.
- If the fracture/dislocation has an associated laceration, consider that the joint is contaminated. Open fracture/dislocations need immediate orthopedic consultation for intraoperative irrigation and reduction.

Posterior Reduction

- The patient is placed in the supine position with the knee flexed to relax the Achilles tendon. This can be accomplished by an assistant, if available, or the patient can be positioned such that the knee hangs over the end of the bed. The assistant can provide counter-traction over the calf.
- The foot is grasped with two hands, one over the heel and the other on the forefoot.
- The foot is then slightly plantarflexed, traction is applied distally, and the foot is pulled anteriorly.
- An assistant can provide downward pressure on the distal tibia as the talus is reduced (Fig. 90.2).

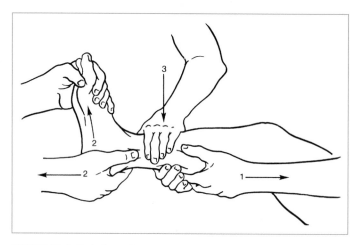

FIGURE 90.2: Technique of reduction of posterior dislocation of the ankle. (Reprinted with permission from Wolfson AB, Hendey GW, Hendry PL, et al. *Harwood-Nuss' Clinical Practice of Emergency Medicine*, 4th ed. Philadelphia: Lippincott Williams & Wilkins, 2005.)

Anterior Reduction

- Same patient positioning is used as with posterior reduction.
- An assistant provides counter-traction over the calf.
- The foot is grasped with two hands, one over the heel and the other on the forefoot.
- The foot is dorsiflexed to free the talus, traction is applied distally, and the foot is pulled posteriorly.
- An assistant can provide upward pressure on the distal tibia as the talus is reduced (Fig. 90.3).

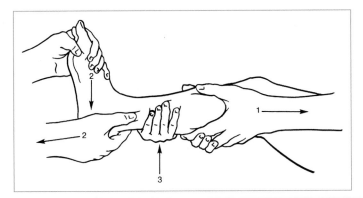

FIGURE 90.3: Technique of reduction of anterior dislocation of the ankle. (Reprinted with permission from Wolfson AB, Hendey GW, Hendry PL, et al. *Harwood-Nuss' Clinical Practice of Emergency Medicine,* 4th ed. Philadelphia: Lippincott Williams & Wilkins, 2005.)

Superior Reduction
- Evaluate carefully for a concomitant spine injury.
- Splint the joint for comfort and then obtain an emergent orthopedic consultation for an open reduction and internal fixation. If orthopedic consultation is unavailable or delayed, the foot should be reduced in the emergency department with longitudinal traction and talar manipulation.

Lateral Reduction
- An assistant provides counter-traction over the calf.
- Place one hand on the heel and the other on the forefoot.
- Longitudinal traction is applied to the foot while gently pulling it medially. Reduction usually occurs with a palpable thud.
- Orthopedic consultation is generally required for this uncommon fracture-dislocation.

Postreduction Care
- Neurovascular status should be checked before and after any reduction attempt, and after immobilization.
- After successful reduction, appropriate immobilization should be applied, including the ankle splinted at 90 degrees with a posterior leg splint and U-splint (stirrup splint) for additional support.
- Elevate the affected ankle.
- Consultation with an orthopedic surgeon for possible hospitalization and operative stabilization of the joint is recommended.

Special Considerations
- After one or two unsuccessful attempts at closed reduction, orthopedic consultation should be considered.
- Open dislocations should be managed in the operating room.
- Be aware of the rare subtalar dislocation: inferior aspect of the talus dislocates from the talocalcaneal and talonavicular joints. This more distal dislocation is more difficult to reduce and often (up to 20%) requires operative reduction.

Current Concepts/Best Evidence

Are there alternatives to procedural sedation for ankle reductions?

One small study prospectively randomized 42 consecutive patients presenting with ankle dislocation to intra-articular hematoma block with 12 cc of 1% lidocaine versus moderate sedation (medications used were left to the discretion of the treating physician) for the closed reduction procedure. Patients were asked to rate their pain improvement (0–10) both pre- and postprocedure. The average pain reduction in the hematoma block group was 4.6, the average pain reduction in the sedation group was 4.3 ($p = 0.70$, not surprising given the low numbers in each arm). The average time to reduction was 64 minutes in the hematoma block group versus 82 minutes in the sedation group. All hematoma-blocked patients were reduced in the emergency department, six required multiple attempts. Two patients in the sedation group required multiple reduction attempts and an additional patient failed closed reduction and was reduced in the operating room.

Suggested Readings

Gutman D, Savitt DL, Storrow AB. Extremity trauma. In: Knoop KJ, Stack LB, Storrow AB, eds. *Atlas of Emergency Medicine,* 2nd ed. New York: McGraw-Hill, 2002:336–337.

McNamara R, Ufberg J. Management of common dislocations. In: Hedges JR, Roberts JR, eds. *Clinical Procedures in Emergency Medicine,* 4th ed. Philadelphia: Saunders Company, 2004:983–985.

Michael JA, Stiell IG. Ankle injuries. In: Tintinalli JE, ed. *Emergency Medicine A Comprehensive Study Guide,* 6th ed. New York: McGraw-Hill, 2004:1736–1741.

Rivers CS, ed. Orthopedic emergencies. In: *Preparing for the Written Board Exam in Emergency Medicine,* 5th ed. Milford, Ohio: Emergency Medicine Educational Enterprises, Inc, 2006:456–460.

Simon RR, ed. *Emergency Procedures and Techniques,* 4th ed. Philadelphia: Lippincott Williams & Wilkins, 2002:284–285.

Wagner RB, Crawford WO Jr, Schimpf PP, et al. Quantitation and pattern of parenchymal lung injury in blunt chest trauma: diagnostic and therapeutic implications. *J Comput Tomogr.* 1988;12:270–281.

White BJ, Walsh M, Egol KA, Tejwani NC. Intra-articular block compared with conscious sedation for closed reduction of ankle fracture-dislocations. *J Bone Joint Surg.* 2008;90(4):731–734.

91

Foot Fracture

Joshua Quaas

Definition/Background
- The foot has three anatomical segments:
    - hindfoot (calcaneus and talus)
    - midfoot (navicular, cuboid, and cuneiforms)
    - forefoot (metatarsals and phalanges)
- Approximately 10% of all fractures occur in the foot (Fig. 91.1).

Pathophysiology
- Mechanisms of injury in the foot are most commonly inversions and blunt trauma.
- Falls are a less common mechanism but are associated with substantial morbidity.

Diagnosis
- The decision to order a radiograph should be based on physical findings. Standard films include anteroposterior, lateral, and oblique views.
- *The Ottawa Foot Rule* is a well-established and validated clinical decision tool designed to identify the low-risk patient with foot injury who does not require imaging. The rule has a sensitivity of 99% and is validated in both the pediatric and adult populations. An x-ray is needed if any of the following is present:
    - bony tenderness to the navicular bone
    - bony tenderness to the base of the 5th metatarsal
    - inability to bear weight for four steps both immediately postinjury and in the emergency department (ED)

Evaluation
- Look for signs of swelling, ecchymosis, deformity, and any asymmetry from the uninjured side.
- Palpate all the bones of the foot, paying special attention to the midfoot and the fifth metatarsal. The ankle (and sometimes the knee) should be evaluated for associated injury.
- Assess for range of motion: plantar and dorsiflexion, toe flexion, and extension.
- Assess neurovascular status: palpate the dorsalis pedis pulse, assess capillary refill, check distal sensation, and motor function.

Management
Calcaneal Fractures
- Usually occur from a vertical compressive force, such as a fall from height.
- Fractures are not always clearly visible; using **Bohler's angle** to measure the position of the cuboid relative to the calcaneus is helpful. Bohler's angle is

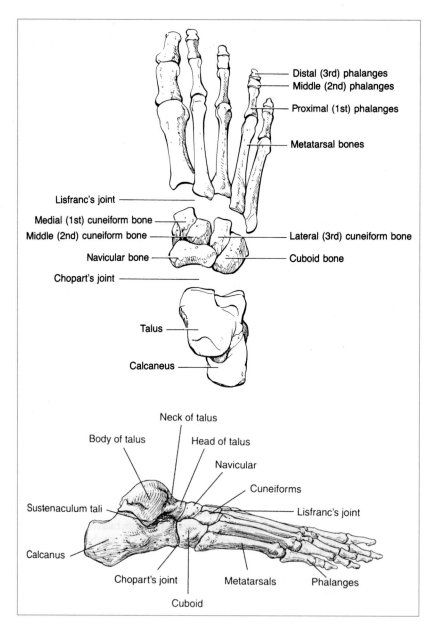

FIGURE 91.1: Bones of the foot. (Bottom from Ankel F. The Foot. In: Hart RG, Rittenberry TJ, Uehara DT, eds. *Handbook of orthopedic emergencies.* Philadelphia: Lippincott Raven, 1999, with permission.)

normally 20–40 degrees. In most cases a decrease in Bohler's angle implies a fracture (Fig. 91.2).

▪ The mechanism of force to injure this bone is significant and warrants a full body trauma evaluation. Up to 10% of patients with calcaneal fracture also have lumbar spine injuries.

▪ This fracture is associated with chronic pain and long-term decreased mobility and function.

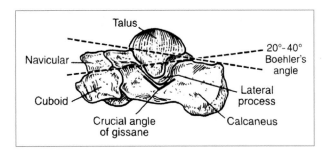

FIGURE 91.2: Boehler's angle. (From Ankel F. The Ankle. In: Hart RG, Rittenberry TJ, Uehara DT, eds. *Handbook of orthopedic emergencies.* Philadelphia: Lippincott Raven, 1999, with permission.)

- The best treatment for this fracture is controversial. It is managed both operatively and non-operatively. The patient should be placed in a short-leg posterior splint, made non–weight bearing, and should see an orthopedist within 48 hours if one is not available in the ED (Fig. 91.3).

Lisfranc Fracture-Dislocation
- This rare, oft-missed injury occurs because of direct trauma or hyperdorsiflexion of the Lisfranc joint. The dislocation is usually associated with a fracture at the base of the second metatarsal or the middle cuneiform bone.
- The foot generally presents with significant swelling and tenderness.
- This injury is generally treated with open reduction and internal fixation, and many orthopedists will keep the patient in the hospital for same or next day repair. Alternatively, the patient may be discharged in a short-leg posterior splint, made non–weight bearing, and given 24- to 48-hour orthopedic follow-up. Timing to

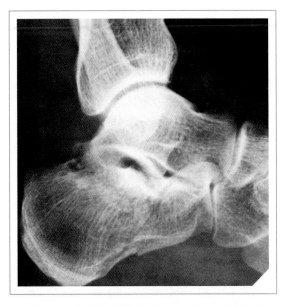

FIGURE 91.3: Fracture of the calcaneus. Lateral view shows a comminuted fracture of the calcaneus. There is a suggestion of extension of the fracture line into the subtalar joint. (Reprinted with permission from Greenspan A. *Orthopedic Imaging: A Practical Approach,* 4th ed. Philadelphia: Lippincott Williams & Wilkins, 2004.)

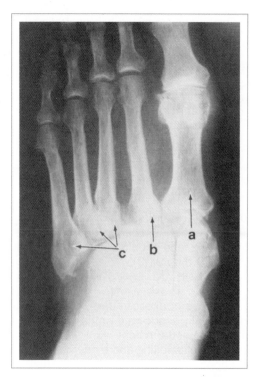

FIGURE 91.4: Radiograph of a Lisfranc dislocation: **(A)** first metatarsal; **(B)** second metatarsal; **(C)** third, fourth, and fifth metatarsals, which have been dislocated laterally. (Reprinted with permission from Wolfson AB, Hendey GW, Ling LJ, et al. *Harwood-Nuss' Clinical Practice of Emergency Medicine*, 5th ed. Philadelphia: Lippincott Williams & Wilkins, 2009.)

definitive treatment is critical for this injury to prevent long-term morbidity (Fig. 91.4).

Talus Fracture
- Talar fractures are rare and generally require high-energy trauma such as a motor vehicle accident or a fall from height.
- Talar dome fractures are difficult to identify on x-ray film. Sometimes called "osteochondritis dessicans," these patients will present later with chronic ankle pain.
- Talar body and neck fractures are usually visible on x-ray film. These injuries are treated both operatively and nonoperatively.
- Talar fractures should be placed in a short-leg, posterior splint, made non–weight bearing, and be given orthopedic follow-up.

Subtalar Dislocation
- This dislocation involves disruption of the talus from the calcaneus and navicular joints with an intact tibiotalar joint. It occurs from significant torsion stress.
- Presents with significant foot swelling and deformity (may appear to be an ankle dislocation clinically). Neurovascular compromise is uncommon.
- Diagnosis is made by plain films.
- Reduce using procedural sedation. Flex the knee. Apply longitudinal traction of the foot with initial reproduction of the injury followed by reversal of the deformity.

- If ED orthopedic consult unavailable, the patient should be put in a short-leg posterior splint and a U/sugar tong splint, made non–weight bearing, and given 24- to 48-hour outpatient orthopedic follow-up.

Midfoot Fractures
- Fractures of the cuboid, navicular, and cuneiforms are uncommon.
- The patient should be put in a short-leg posterior splint, made non–weight bearing, and given outpatient orthopedic follow-up. Definitive treatment is usually a short-leg cast for 6–8 weeks.

Fifth Metatarsal Fractures
- The proximal fifth metatarsal fractures generally occur with ankle inversion:
  - Jones fracture: transverse fracture at the proximal diaphysis.
  - Pseudo-Jones fracture (also known as Dancer's fracture): avulsion fracture by the peroneus brevis tendon at the most proximal tip of the base of the metatarsal.
- Jones fractures have a high incidence of nonunion (Fig. 91.5). These are operatively repaired in the young and active. If ED orthopedic consult unavailable, the patient should be put in a short-leg posterior splint, made non–weight bearing, and given 24- to 48-hour outpatient orthopedic follow-up.

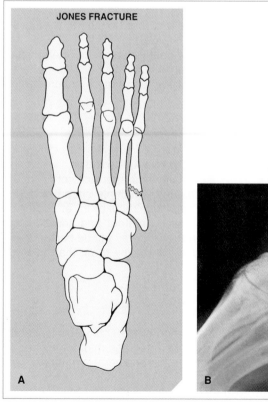
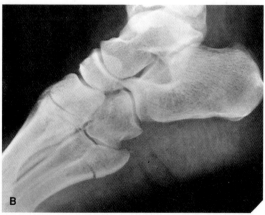

JONES FRACTURE

A

B

FIGURE 91.5: Jones fracture. **(A)** a "true" Jones fracture is located about an inch distally to the base of the fifth metatarsal. **(B)** A 43-year-old woman, while dancing, twisted her left foot and sutained a "true" Jones fracture of the fifth metatarsal. (Reprinted with permission from Greenspan A. *Orthopedic Imaging: A Practical Approach,* 4th ed. Philadelphia: Lippincott Williams & Wilkins, 2004.)

■ Pseudo-Jones fractures are stable injuries and can be treated with a hard sole shoe. If this is uncomfortable for the patient, he or she can be placed in a bulky dressing and given crutches to weight bear as tolerated.

Forefoot Injuries

■ Metatarsal and phalangeal fractures occur most commonly from direct blunt trauma.

■ Dislocations of the metatarsophalangeal joints and interphalangeal joints are caused by dorsiflexion and compression of the phalanges.

■ Plain films are adequate to evaluate for both of these injuries.

■ Metatarsophalangeal and interphalangeal dislocations are treated by longitudinal traction with gentle manipulation of the dislocated base toward the joint. A digital block is recommended for patient comfort.

■ Most foot fractures can be treated with a hard sole shoe: second, third, and fourth metatarsal fractures and almost all toe fractures. Toe fractures should be "buddy-taped" as dynamic splinting helps healing and reduces pain.

■ First metatarsal fractures and significant first toe fractures (>25% of articular surface involved, comminuted) should be placed in a short-leg splint, made non–weight-bearing, and given orthopedic follow-up. These bones are central to balance and gait and generally require casting for definitive treatment.

Special Considerations

■ With significant torsion injuries to the ankle and foot be sure to evaluate for a Maisonneuve fracture.

■ Lisfranc injuries and Jones fractures do not heal well and are often missed; this results in patient morbidity and medicolegal liability.

■ Give adequate outpatient analgesia for foot fractures; often patients will need a short course of oral narcotics.

Current Concepts/Evidence

Is the Ottawa Foot Rule just as good as the Ottawa Ankle Rule?

It is. The Ottawa Foot Rules have ~99% sensitivity and specificity of ~ 38%. This outstanding sensitivity has been externally validated by multiple sites that found comparable sensitivities. Application of the Ottawa predictive rules by ED attending physicians would have resulted in a 19% reduction in use of midfoot and ankle radiographs at one site. Many patients have the expectation that an x-ray will be part of their ED visit; spending time educating patients is the key to convincing them that an x-ray may not be necessary.

Suggested Readings

Pigman EC, Klug RK, Sanford S, Jolly BT. Evaluation of the Ottawa clinical decision rules for the use of radiography in acute ankle and midfoot injuries in the emergency department: an independent site assessment. *Ann Emerg Med.* 1994;24:41–45.

Shah K. Ankle and foot injuries. In: Wolfson AW, ed. *Clinical Practice of Emergency Medicine.* Philadelphia: Lippincott Williams & Wilkins, 2005:1092–1100.

Simon S, Sherman S, Koenigsknecht S. *Emergency Orthopedics of the Extremities,* 5th ed. New York: McGraw-Hill, 2007:472–490.

92

Thermal Burns

Kathleen A. Wittels

Definition

- Thermal burns are injuries to the skin and adjacent tissues from exposure to a heat source. These include flame, scald, steam, and contact burns. Burns are categorized as first, second, third, or fourth degree (Table 92.1).

Pathophysiology

- Five factors influence the extent of burn injury: the temperature of the agent, the heat capacity of the agent, the duration of contact with the skin, the heat and conductivity of the local tissues, and the heat transfer coefficient.
- Injury occurs both from direct cellular damage as well as by the release of local mediators.
- In patients with extensive burns, increased vascular permeability leads to significant fluid losses and results in hypovolemic shock.
- There is an initial decrease in cardiac output and increase in peripheral vascular resistance after severe burn injury.
- **Infection is the leading cause of death in patients with severe burn injuries.**

Diagnosis

- Assessment of burns requires careful examination of the skin to determine the extent and classification of the burn.
- Both first- and second-degree burns are painful. First-degree burns appear red, whereas second-degree burns will also have blisters (thin-walled for superficial

TABLE 92.1: Burn Categories

Burn degree	Burn thickness	Description
First degree	Superficial	Minor epithelial damage to the epidermis
Second degree	Superficial partial thickness	Involves the epidermis and superficial (papillary) dermis; blisters likely
	Deep partial thickness	Extends into the deep (reticular) dermis
Third degree	Full thickness	Destroy both the epidermis and the dermis
Fourth degree		Involve the fascia, muscle, or bone

and thick-walled for deep). Third-degree burns appear white and leathery and are less painful due to damage to nerve endings.

- The *Rule of 9s* is a tool to estimate the total burn surface area. It assigns 9% to the head and each arm; 18% to the chest, back, and each leg; and 1% to the perineum and genitalia. Pediatric patients have different percentages given the relatively larger head and shorter legs in children (Fig. 92.1).

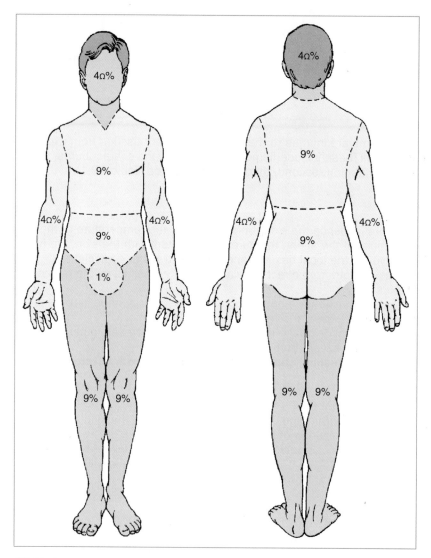

FIGURE 92.1: Rule of Nines: In "rule of nines," the adult body is divided in to surface areas of fraction or multiples of 9%, which may give a quick estimation of the burn size. (Reprinted with permission from Flint L, Meredith JW, Schwab CW, et al. *Trauma: Contemporary Principles and Therapy*. Philadelphia: Lippincott Williams & Wilkins, 2008.)

Evaluation

- Remove all clothing to allow for complete skin examination and evaluation of associated injuries.

- Assess for any **signs of airway compromise (singed nasal hairs, stridor, dysphonia).** Fiberoptic laryngoscopy is helpful to identify laryngeal edema or other airway injury. **Intubate early in this setting as edema will worsen over the first several hours and may make delayed intubation impossible.**

Management

- Oxygen should be applied immediately as smoke inhalation is commonly associated with burn injuries.
- Pain management and intravenous fluid resuscitation are the mainstays of early burn treatment.
- The *Parkland formula* estimates the fluid requirement in milliliters for the first 24 hours for adults.
  - 4 mL × %BSA burned × patient weight (kg)
  - Half of this amount (usually lactated ringers) should be given over the first 8 hours and the other half over the next 16 hours.
- Follow urine output to maintain at least 0.5 mL/kg/hr in adults and 1 mL/kg/hr in children.
- Skin should be cleansed with normal saline and dressed with antibiotic ointment. Deeper burns may require debridement.
- Prophylactic antibiotics are not necessary, but tetanus vaccination should be updated as necessary.
- Escharotomies are performed on the extremities when there is neurovascular compromise from circumferential burns. Incisions should be made medially and laterally to the level of the fascia in order to restore perfusion.
  - With severe burns to the thorax, ventilation may be impaired from constriction necessitating emergent escharotomy.
- First- and superficial second-degree burns will usually heal over a period of days to weeks as the skin reepithelializes, but deep-second degree burns have increased risk of hypertrophic scar formation and contraction.
- Third- and fourth-degree burns require skin grafting and may require extensive reconstruction and cause prolonged disability.

Special Considerations

- Transfer to a burn center is recommended by the American Burn Association under the following circumstances:
  - BSA >10%
  - Burns involving the hands, feet, perineum/genitalia, face, or major joint
  - Inhalational burns
  - All third-degree burns
- Abuse should be suspected when the burn pattern is inconsistent with the history.
  - Particularly worrisome situations include burns involving the perineum, circular burns, and burns on the lower extremities without involvement of the soles of the feet.
  - Elderly patients and children are at higher risk for abuse.

Best Evidence/Clinical Decision Rules

Should colloid solutions be used in burn resuscitation?

After burn injury, intravascular protein leaks occur through endothelial damage. Five percent of albumin has been suggested as an adjunct to crystalloid resuscitation (Fodor et al, 2006) but has not been proven to reduce organ dysfunction (Cooper et al, 2006). Currently, there is no clear consensus on its use in burn patients.

Suggested Readings

Cooper AB, Cohn SM, Zhang HS, et al. Five percent albumin for adult burn shock resuscitation: lack of effect on daily multiple organ dysfunction score. *Transfusion*. 2006;46:80–89.

Fodor L, Fodor A, Ramon Y, et al. Controversies in fluid resuscitation for burn management: literature review and our experience. *Injury*. 2006;37(5):374–379.

Greenhajgh DG. Burn resuscitation. *J Burn Care Res*. 2007;28:555–565.

93

Pediatric Trauma

Anupam Kharbanda and Jonathan St. George

Preparation

- Prior to notification: review the trauma bay and familiarize yourself with the location of essential items.
- After notification: assign management roles (airway, monitor, access, etc.).
- Team leader's responsibility is to maintain a calm atmosphere on arrival of patient.
- Ask emergency medical services, family, and witnesses to remain available for more details of the event.

Pediatric Pearls

- Calming the family member(s) and enlisting them as an ally to sooth an awake and scared child is essential to running a smooth trauma resuscitation.
- Cell phone cameras are now ubiquitous—ask for any pictures of the event.

Primary Survey

- Designed to rapidly assess and treat life-threatening pulmonary conditions.
- Follow ABCDE (Airway, Breathing, Circulation, Disability, Exposure) described below.

Pediatric Pearls

- The Broselow tape is a color-coded system that aids physicians in determining pediatric dosing and equipment for pediatric trauma and resuscitation available in most emergency departments
- Most cardiac arrests in pediatric trauma are due to airway compromise and hypoxia, not hypovolemia. Therefore, emphasis should be placed on early/aggressive airway and breathing management.

A. Airway goals: remove obstructions, maintain patency, and protect the airway

- Maintain C-spine stabilization.
- Assess the airway for patency/obstruction and structural instability (fractures).
- Open airway (jaw thrust, nasal trumpet, oral airway).
- Suction blood, secretions, and vomitus from oropharynx.
- Rapidly assess the need for a definitive airway (severe agitation, depressed mental status, facial/oropharyngeal trauma, neck trauma, multisystem trauma requiring the operating room).

Pediatric Pearls

- Large occiput causes increased forward flexion and airway obstruction. Place support under cervical spine to keep the head in a neutral position or "sniffing" position.
- A cuffed endotracheal tube is now preferred in children older than 1 year.

B. Breathing goals: optimize ventilation and oxygenation, identify/reverse specific injuries

- Give oxygen via 100% nonrebreather.
- Look and listen for good chest rise and clear breath sounds bilaterally.
- Look for signs of inadequate ventilation: **grunting, nasal flaring,** tachypnea, **retractions**, stridor, or wheezing.
- Signs of inadequate oxygenation: agitation, cyanosis, **poor capillary refill, bradycardia**, and desaturation on pulse oximetry.
- Start positive pressure ventilation (PPV) if inadequate oxygenation/ventilation does not rapidly improve.
- Identify signs of tension pneumothorax (deviated trachea, absent breath sounds, tympany, hypotension). Perform catheter/chest tube decompression.
- Identify massive hemothorax (absent breath sounds, dullness to percussion, poor chest wall motion with ventilation, and hypotension).
- Order portable chest film (CXR). Do not delay the tube thoracostomy for a CXR if the patient is unstable.
- Rapid transfer to the operating room if the initial drainage is >15 mL/kg or the chest tube output is >4 mL/kg/hr.

C. Circulation goals: identify and reverse hemodynamic compromise/shock

- Look for signs of shock (tachycardia, cool extremities, altered mental status (AMS), weak distal pulses, delayed capillary refill).
- Rapid vascular access (two large peripheral IVs). If peripheral access is delayed (>3 attempts or >1 minute), move quickly to intraosseous (IO) access.
- For shock, administer normal saline or lactated ringers solution at 20 mL/kg and rapidly infuse up to 60 mL/kg within 15–60 minutes if vitals signs do not improve. Consider early conversion to packed red blood cells (pRBCs) for clear signs of hemorrhagic shock.
- Administer 10 mL/kg of packed red blood cells if perfusion does not improve after crystalloid bolus infusions.
- Resuscitative thoracotomy is indicated if vital signs were recently lost, and a trauma surgeon is immediately available.

Pediatric Pearl: hypotension is a **late** finding. Children with hypotension can deteriorate rapidly.

- **Ultrasound: now an essential part of all trauma evaluation**
  - Perform FAST (Focused Abdominal Sonography in Trauma) examination.
  - Primarily to evaluate for pericardial effusion and intra-abdominal hemorrhage.
    - Penetrating trauma to the chest with sonographic evidence of pericardial tamponade should go directly to the operating room.
  - May look above the diaphragm for pneumothorax or hemothorax.

D. Disability goals: early identification of intracranial/spinal cord injury

- Maintain immobilization for suspected cervical spine injury.

- Determine level of consciousness: Pediatric Glasgow Coma Scale (PGCS) or the alert, voice, pain, unresponsive (AVPU) system.
- Rapid optimization of intracranial pressure is required for patients with severe head injury.
- **PGCS score of less than eight** = secure airway with an endotracheal tube
  - The head of the bed should be elevated to 20 degrees to 30 degrees.
  - Optimize hemodynamic status with fluids and blood to correct shock.
  - If cerebral herniation present, consider:
    - Hyperventilate (goal $PaCO_2$ 30–34 mm Hg).
    - Intravenous mannitol 0.5–1.0 g/kg for impending cerebral herniation.
- **For alert patients with a PGCS of greater than 9**
  - Look for signs of external head injury (infants with a scalp hematoma are at increased risk for intracranial injury).
  - Evaluate pupillary size and responsiveness.
  - Test gross motor strength.

E. Exposure goals: identify all life-threatening wounds and detect/correct hypothermia

- Identify actively bleeding or penetrating wounds.
- Apply direct pressure to bleeding wounds.
- Obtain rectal temperature to assess for hypothermia, rapidly correct core temperature of <35° C with warm blankets or Bair Hugger, and warm intravenous fluids to 40° C if large volumes are being given.

> **Pediatric Pearl:** *children can rapidly develop hypothermia because of increased BSA to volume ratio*

Secondary survey goals: to identify all other injuries to the trauma patient

- Not performed until primary survey/life-threatening conditions have been managed.
- Complete head to toe examination includes log-roll with stabilization to examine the patient's back.
- Order appropriate, clinically driven imaging and tests.
- Give appropriate medications including analgesia, sedation, antibiotics, tetanus prophylaxis, and so forth.
- Maintain appropriate monitoring, with frequent reassessment of the patient.
- Return to ABCs if patient becomes unstable.

Decision-Making Considerations
Key distinctions in pediatric anatomy and physiology

- **Size**
  - Compared to adults, a greater force per square centimeter is applied to their bodies for the same mechanism.
  - Increased risk for multiorgan injury.
- **Proportion**
  - Relatively larger head and internal organs.
  - Increased risk of intracranial injury.
  - Increased risk of internal organ injury (spleen, liver, bladder, kidney).
- **Flexibility**
  - Increased flexibility means less skeletal protection of internal organs.
  - Increased risk for SCIWORA (spinal cord injury without radiographic abnormality).
  - Increased risk of internal trauma without evidence of skeletal trauma.

TABLE 93.1: Pediatric vital signs

Age	Wt (Kg)	Respiratory rate	Heart rate	Systolic blood pressure
Preterm	2	55–65	120–180	40–60
Term newborn	3	40–60	90–170	52–92
1 month	4	30–50	110–180	60–104
6 months to 1 year	8–10	25–35	120–140	65–125
2–4 years	12–16	20–30	100–110	80–95
5–8 years	18–26	14–20	90–100	90–100
8–12 years	26–50	12–20	60–110	100–110
>12 years	>40	12–16	60–105	100–120

- **Metabolic rate**
  - Increased metabolic rate, oxygen consumption, and compensatory reserve lead to:
    - Increased risk for secondary injury due to hypoxia and hypotension
    - More rapid decompensation
    - Increased risk of inadequate resuscitation

Essential Numbers/Formulas
- Pediatric vital signs vary with age (Table 93.1)
- Weight(kg) = (age × 3) + 7
- ETT size: (age/4) + 3
- Minimum blood pressure: 70 + [2 × age (years)] = systolic blood pressure

---

Pediatric Pearl: PGCS = combined score of best eye, verbal, and motor response

---

The PGCS is essentially the same as the GCS except for the verbal scoring:

1. No verbal response.
2. Inconsolable, agitated.
3. Inconsistently inconsolable, moaning.
4. Cries but consolable, inappropriate interactions.
5. Smiles, orientated to sounds, follows objects, interacts.

Specific Pediatric Injuries by System
- Pediatric trauma is predominantly blunt, with penetrating trauma occurring in only 10% of cases.
- Most pediatric trauma can be managed nonoperatively.
- **Head injury**
  - Most deaths from trauma in children are due to head injuries.
  - Evaluation of traumatic brain injury should be a priority in all seriously injured children.
  - Anticonvulsant prophylaxis is controversial (Table 93.2).

TABLE 93.2: Anticonvulsant[a] prophylaxis recommendations

Children with two or more seizures, or seizures lasting more than a few minutes

Children with a Glasgow Coma Scale score of <8, because of the risk of developing acute posttraumatic seizures

Those suspected of having high intracranial pressures (ICPs)

[a]Load with fosphenytoin (20 mg/kg).

- **C-spine injury**
  - Increased risk for SCIWORA.
  - 50% of children with SCIWORA will have a delayed onset of paralysis, sometimes up to 4 days.
  - Cannot clear cervical spine with plain films or computed tomography without the child being alert and cooperative.
- **Chest injury**
  - Cardiac and pulmonary contusions without overlying bone fractures are common.
  - More than two-thirds of children with significant chest injury have other organ system injuries.
- **Abdominal injury**
  - Children with severe injuries can have minimal physical findings.
  - Computed tomography and diagnostic peritoneal lavage are not completely reliable in diagnosing certain injuries.
  - Splenic injury is most common, followed by liver and bowel.
  - Delayed signs of pancreatic injury make it difficult to diagnose in the emergency department.
  - Hollow viscous injuries are also difficult to diagnose and may warrant admission for serial examinations, repeat imaging, exploratory laparotomy, or diagnostic peritoneal lavage.
  - Duodenal hematoma can cause delayed small bowel obstruction (Fig. 93.1).

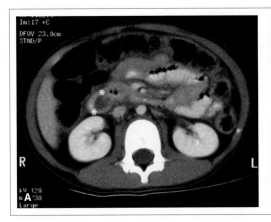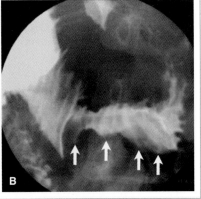

FIGURE 93.1: Rear seat passenger who sustained a lap belt injury. Axial contrast-enhanced computed tomography **(A)** and prone image from single contrast upper GI examination **(B)** demonstrate a hematoma within the duodenal wall (low attenuation region on computed tomography) (asterisks in A), with contour abnormality along the inferior portion of the duodenum (arrows) on the upper GI examination **(B)**. This is a not an uncommon type of injury with lap-belt-type injuries in which children also sustain Chance-type fractures. (Reprinted with permission from Schwartz ED, Flanders AE. *Spinal Trauma: Imaging, Diagnosis, and Management.* Philadelphia: Lippincott Williams & Wilkins, 2007.)

- **Suspect seat belt syndrome**
  - ▸ Seat belt use and characteristic abdominal wall contusions.
  - ▸ Suggestive of hollow viscous or mesenteric lacerations (other internal organ injuries also possible).
  - ▸ Caused by significant shearing and compressive forces.
- Associated lumbar or chance fractures mandate admission for observation and a complete evaluation (50% incidence of associated intra-abdominal injury).

- **Genitourinary injury**
  - Uncommon in children.
  - Associated with pelvic fractures.
  - Gross hematuria or microscopic hematuria >25 red blood cells/HPF (high power field) warrants a computed tomographic scan.
  - Asymptomatic microscopic hematuria in the stable patient does not need intervention or imaging.

- **Extremity injuries**
  - Initial management is similar to adult trauma, with the additional concern for growth plate injuries.
  - Evidence of vascular compromise requires emergent reduction and vascular evaluation.
  - Splinting in a severely injured trauma patient is usually sufficient.
  - An isolated long-bone fracture should not cause hemodynamic instability in children. Search for alternate sources of blood loss in the patient with an isolated femur fracture and signs of hemodynamic instability.
  - **Child abuse** should always be considered in pediatric trauma.
    - ▸ The most common manifestations include bruises, burns, fractures, head trauma, and abdominal injuries.
    - ▸ Death from injury in the first year of life is usually attributable to abuse (Table 93.3).

TABLE 93.3: Red flags suggesting abuse

A discrepancy between caregiver stories and clinical findings
Delayed presentation to the emergency department from the time of injury
Multiple subdural hematomas (particularly without evidence of external trauma)
Retinal hemorrhages
Perioral injuries
Ruptured viscera without history of trauma
Genital or perianal trauma
Evidence of frequent injuries (old scars or fractures on x-ray film)
Fractures of long bones in children younger than 3 years
Bizarre injuries (burns, bites, marks from objects such as belts, ropes, shoes, etc)
Sharply demarcated burns (stocking-glove injury patterns), burns in unusual locations, branding-type burns

TABLE 93.4: Specific reasons for transfer to a pediatric trauma center

Serious mechanism (ejected from vehicle, prolonged extrication, fall from significant height)

Penetrating head, chest, or abdominal trauma

Multisystem trauma

Multiple long-bone fractures

Severe head or facial trauma

Spinal fractures or spinal cord injury

Amputations

Transfer to a Pediatric Trauma Center
- Predicated primarily on physician judgment and common sense.
- Any patient who is stable after initial resuscitation that requires care beyond your facility's ability to manage, or patients who have a high likelihood of delayed complications from their injuries should be transferred for further care.
- Specific trauma scores may aid in your assessment (pediatric trauma score or revised trauma score).
- Specific reasons for transfer are listed in Table 93.4.

Suggested Readings
Holmes JF, Gladman A, et al. Performance of abdominal ultrasonography in pediatric blunt trauma patients: a meta-analysis. *J Pediatr Surg*. 2007;42:1588–594.

Hutchings L, Willett K. Cervical spine clearance in pediatric trauma: a review of current literature. *J Trauma*. 2009;67:687–691.

Kuppermann N, Holmes JF, et al. Identification of children at very low risk of clinically-important brain injuries after head trauma: a prospective cohort study. *Lancet*. 2009;374:1160–1170.

94

Geriatric Trauma

Ula Hwang

Definition
- For this chapter, we define geriatric trauma as injury to **adults ≥65 years of age** (the most commonly used definition).
- Lower and upper age parameters for "geriatric" include cutoffs of ≥45 or ≥55 years of age, with "very old" as ≥80 years age.

Background
- Epidemiology
  - By 2012, it is projected that adults ≥65 years age will account for 20% of the US population and the rate of emergency department utilization by individuals 65–74 years age will potentially double.
  - Injury-related diagnoses are the third most common reason (following heart disease and chest pain) for emergency department visits by this group.
- Mechanism of injury
  - Falls are the most common mechanism of injury to geriatric patients and are the leading cause of injury death.
  - More than one-third of adults ≥65 years fall each year and this rate has been increasing over the last decade.
- Advanced age, coupled with multiple comorbidities and decreased physiologic reserve are associated with poorer outcomes secondary to rapid decompensation.
- **The American College of Surgeons recommends that all significant trauma patients >55 years of age be transported to and cared for a designated trauma center.**
- Emergency physicians should have a lower threshold for trauma team activation and consider older age alone (≥75 years) as a criterion. Early activation of trauma teams, intensive monitoring, evaluation, and resuscitation of geriatric trauma patients improve survival.
- Emergency physicians should have a lower threshold for hospital admission and observation.
- As with pediatric patients, geriatric patient with trauma or injury should be assessed for potential abuse or neglect.

Pathophysiology—Evaluation—Management
- Loss of physiologic reserve may result in atypical or blunted response to trauma-related shock or resuscitation efforts.
- Guidelines for trauma management in geriatric patients remain the same as with younger adult patients. What differentiates trauma management for older adults from younger adults are:
  - **Greater suspicion** of occult trauma.
  - **Judicious and aggressive** evaluation and management.
  - **Physiologic changes (Table 94.1).**

TABLE 94.1: Physiologic changes with aging that impact geriatric trauma care

Changes with aging	Implication on trauma care	Management
Airway ↓ Gag/cough reflex	Increased risk for aspiration and obstruction Intubation may be more difficult secondary to degenerative changes, presence of dentures, and cervical arthritis	Consider orotracheal intubation using anesthetics, neuromuscular blockade, and in-line cervical alignment To avoid hypotension with use of rapid sequence intubation medications, doses of etomidate, barbiturates, and benzodiazepines should be reduced (doses for neuromuscular blockers are unchanged)
Breathing ↓ Respiratory muscle strength ↓ Tidal volume and lung capacity ↓ Ciliary function	Decreased ability to compensate for hypoxia Increased risk for respiratory failure; complications may develop (e.g., pulmonary edema, atelectasis, pneumonia)	Consider early intubation with significant injuries, chest wall trauma, or rising PCO_2
Circulation ↓ Force and rate of cardiac contraction ↓ Cardiac output ↓ Response to circulating catecholamines ↑ Calcification and decreased elasticity of vessels ↓ Oxygen delivery and consumption	Blunted response to shock (no compensatory tachycardia); vital signs may not reflect hemodynamic instability Overly aggressive fluid resuscitation may quickly result in volume overload Increased risk for vessel injury, hematoma formation	Hypertensive patients with normotensive pressures are hemodynamically unstable Use serial arterial blood gas analysis with lactate and base deficit levels to gauge respiratory function, reserve and need for intensive resuscitation efforts. Repeat testing 30–45 minutes postarrival with persistently high levels are indicators of inadequate resuscitation or hemorrhage Early fluid resuscitation with multiple small fluid boluses of crystalloid If no change in vital signs with crystalloid, consider early and liberal use of packed red blood cell transfusion to enhance oxygen-carrying capacity and reduce tissue ischemia
Disability (neurologic) ↓ Brain mass/cerebral atrophy Dura more adherent to skull ↓ Cerebral perfusion/blood flow Cognitive and memory impairment more common	Greater risk for traumatic brain injury (especially subdural hematomas) Intracranial hemorrhage may have minimal clinical findings Greater mortality associated with severe head injury and hypotension	Determine baseline cognitive function; cognitive impairment may not be secondary to aging Perform frequent neurologic checks
Environmental control ↓ Fat; ↓ thermoregulatory ability ↓ Basal metabolic rate	Increased risk for hypothermia (which can lead to acidosis and coagulopathy after trauma)	Consider early warming measures

(continued)

TABLE 94.1: Physiologic changes with aging that impact geriatric trauma care *(Continued)*

Changes with aging	Implication on trauma care	Management
Pain ↓ Pain perception	Blunted pain response may not reflect extent of injury, poor localization of pain Underreporting or minimizing of pain Undertreatment may exacerbate respiratory deterioration	Use alternative pain assessment methods (behavioral clues, nonnumeric scales) as needed Provide analgesia starting with low doses and titrating as needed and appropriate
Musculoskeletal system ↓ Muscle strength ↑ Bone loss/degenerative changes	Increases risk for fracture Accurate secondary survey may be challenging because of preexisting conditions	
Communication ↓ Hearing and vision	Decreased hearing and vision	Speak in a lower tone; avoid compound questions; limit background noise when possible; obtaining history may take longer Use other sources for history (medical records, family, etc.)
Psychosocial Response varies by individual; depression more common; fear common after trauma	Assess coping and support systems; provide guidance and repeat information as needed; anticipate unique discharge needs (functional impairment, fear of falling, loss of independence) Goals of care and end-of-life concerns	Ascertain advanced directives via medical records, primary physician, family, friends
Comorbidities Chronic disease is common (e.g. COPD, cardiovascular disease, diabetes, hypertension, renal failure)	Multiple comorbidities increase patient vulnerability and may exacerbate injury Cardiovascular disease and diabetes are associated with worse outcomes	Accurate medical history is critical
Medications Polypharmacy common; Medications may alter normal response to shock or resuscitation efforts	Cardiac medications: β-blockers blunt tachycardia Warfarin, clopidogrel, aspirin: increase risk of bleeding Psychotropic medications may affect cognitive function	Reverse warfarin effects with vitamin K (10 mg slow intravenous infusion for emergency reversal, 1–2.5 mg oral for nonemergency reversal), prothrombin complex concentrate, fresh frozen plasma

Diagnosis

- Knowing the patient's baseline cognitive and functional abilities is critical to determine whether changes present are acute.
- Gathering information about the mechanism of injury, past medical history, and medications is critical in geriatric patients as these may impact physiologic response to shock and resuscitation efforts.

- Imaging considerations.
  - Follow routine trauma protocols with radiographic imaging for adult patients.
  - Lower threshold for computed tomographic imaging with head injury. Strongly consider head computed tomography in all patients ≥65 years age presenting with traumatic brain injury.
  - Complaints of neck pain warrant immediate cervical immobilization. Persistent neck pain with normal radiographs should be followed by computed tomography of the neck.
  - While prior studies indicate that National Emergency X-radiography Utilization Study (NEXUS) criteria may be used in older adults to rule out the need for radiographic imaging, geriatric trauma patients are at increased risk for C1 and C2 cervical fractures (especially falls from a standing height) and fractures at multiple levels that may be unstable. As head computed tomography is often used for geriatric trauma patients, the addition of a C1–C2 computed tomography is recommended.

Special Considerations

Determine advanced directives and end-of-life care decisions for the patient. Patients may not need to be transferred to an intensive care unit setting following these principles:

- Communication with the patient, family, and professional colleagues.
- Framing the discussion within the individual and familial cultural context.
- All patients deserve a precise diagnosis.
- Decisions are based on a risk-benefit analysis for the patient.
- Patient autonomy is paramount.
- Due deliberation is made.
- Consensus before a final decision is made.

Best Evidence/Clinical Decision Rules

A study using data from the prospective NEXUS found that the NEXUS decision instrument may be safely applied to neurologically intact and cognitively functioning geriatric patients (≥65 years) with blunt trauma.

Use of the Injury Severity Score in geriatric patients thus far has had mixed outcomes in predicting survival.

Suggested Readings

Champion H, Copes W, Buyer D, et al. Major trauma in geriatric patients. *Am J Public Health.* 1989;79:1278–1282.

Demetriades D, Karaiskakis M, Velmahos G, et al. Effect on outcome of early intensive management of geriatric trauma patients. *Br J Surg.* 2002;89:1319–1322.

Demetriades D, Sava J, Alo K, et al. Old age as a criterion for trauma team activation. *J Trauma.* 2001;51:754–757, 756–758.

Finelli F, Jonsson J, Champion H, et al. A case control study for major trauma in geriatric patients. *J Trauma.* 1989;29:541–548.

Jacobs D. Special considerations in geriatric injury. *Curr Opin Crit Care.* 2003;9:535–539.

Lomoschitz F, Blackmore C, Mirza S, et al. Cervical spine injuries in patients 65 years old and older: epidemiologic analysis regarding the effects of age and injury mechanism on distribution, type, and stability of injuries. *AJR Am J Roentgenol.* 2002;178:573–577.

Mack L, Chan S, Silva J, et al. The use of head computed tomography in elderly patients sustaining minor head trauma. *J Emerg Med.* 2003;24:157–162.

Oreskovich M, Howard J, Copass H, et al. Geriatric trauma: injury patterns and outcome. *J Trauma.* 1984;24:565–572.

Scalea T, Simon H, Duncan A, et al. Geriatric blunt multiple trauma: improved survival with early invasive monitoring. *J Trauma.* 1992;30:129–134.

Touger M, Gennis P, Nathanson N, et al. Validity of a decision rule to reduce cervical spine radiography in elderly patients with blunt trauma. *Ann Emerg Med.* 2002;40:287–293.

95 Trauma During Pregnancy

Resa Lewiss

Introduction

- Trauma is the cause of most nonobstetric morbidity and mortality during pregnancy.
- Blunt injury, falls, and direct assault account for the majority of traumas.
- Trauma is associated with increased risk of preterm labor, placental abruption, maternal-fetal hemorrhage, and miscarriage.
- Sufficient fetal resuscitation is possible only with sufficient maternal resuscitation.

First 15 Minutes (Fig. 95.1)

- Mandatory supplemental oxygen
- Large-bore intravenous line (IV)
- Normal vital signs do not rule out significant hemorrhage
  - Because of the physiologic changes in pregnancy (see below), vital signs demonstrating maternal shock occur after 30–35% volume loss.
  - Resuscitate with intravenous fluids and blood products if necessary.
  - Vasopressors compromise uterine blood flow.
- Laboratory profile
  - Trauma laboratories
  - Rh status: if Rh negative, will likely need Rh immune globulin (RhoGAM)
    - If <12 weeks, standard RhoGAM dose adequate (50 μg IM)
    - If >12 weeks gestation, obtain Kleihauer-Betke assay to determine degree of maternal-fetal hemorrhage and then give appropriate RhoGAM dose (300 μg IM typically sufficient)
      - The Kleihauer-Betke assay quantifies the degree of fetal-maternal hemorrhage in the Rh negative patient using maternal blood sample.
      - 300 μg dose of RhoGAM for each 30 mL of fetal blood.
  - DIC screen
    - Complete blood counts (including platelets), coagulation profile (including PT, aPTT), d-dimer, and fibrinogen.
- Left lateral decubitus position or right hip/wedged up 15 degrees to prevent supine hypotension secondary to IVC compression by gravid uterus >20 weeks' gestation.
- Earlier intubation and gastric decompression.

Physical Examination

- Physical examination of the abdomen is less reliable due to decreased sensitivity of abdominal wall and peritoneum.
- Bony pelvis protects fetus <12 weeks.
- General physical examination of the gravid patient:
  - Abdomen/pelvis
    - Less reliable in the gravid patient
    - Visually inspect for ecchymosis, contractions, abdominal contour

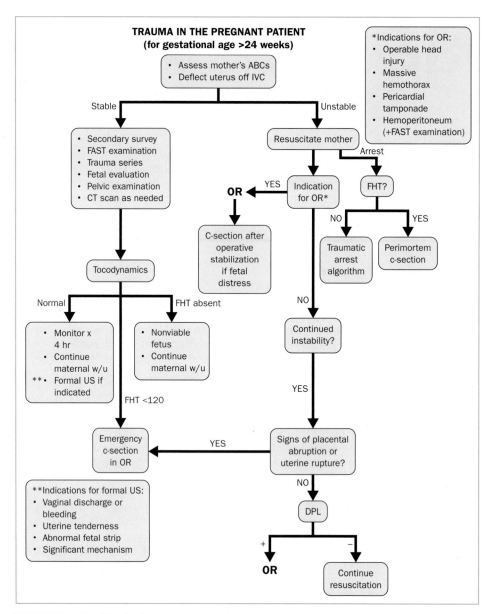

FIGURE 95.1: Algorithm for the management of the pregnant trauma patient. IVC, inferior vena cava; OR, operating room; FAST, focused assessment with sonography for trauma; CT, computed tomographic; FHT, fetal heart tones; US, ultrasound; DPL, diagnostic peritoneal lavage. (Redrawn with permission from Bisanzo M, Bhatia K, Filbin MR. *Emergency Management of the Trauma Patient: Cases, Algorithms, Evidence*. Philadelphia: Lippincott Williams & Wilkins, 2006.)

▷ Auscultate bowel sounds and fetal heart sounds
▷ Palpate for tenderness, guarding, uterine contour, contractions, fetal parts
▷ Measure fundal height
  ◆ Height in centimeters estimates gestational age in weeks (after 24 weeks).
  ◆ Repeat examination during resuscitation.

- Sterile pelvic examination
  - If <20 weeks and suspicious for injury, evaluate genital tract for injury (tears, bone fragments), vaginal bleeding, and secretions.
  - If >20 weeks and vaginal bleeding present, do not examine/manipulate cervix; consult obstetrician/gynecologist.
  - Premature rupture of membranes.
    - pH 7 amniotic fluid; pH 5 vaginal secretions.
    - Ferning–dried vaginal secretions form branching pattern on microscopy.
    - Nitrazine test–turns purple with alkaline amniotic fluid (risk of false positive with blood or urine contamination).

Emergency Interventions
- Standard ATLS algorithm applies
- Tetanus prophylaxis when indicated
- Uterine irritability/preterm labor
- Frequent contractions common after trauma
- Mandatory external fetal monitoring >20 weeks for at least 4 hours
  - Cardiotocographic monitoring is standard for evaluating fetal distress.
    - Normal heart beat 120–160/min
    - Uterine contractions
    - Decreased beat to beat variability concerning
    - Late decelerations concerning
  - Emergency department or labor and delivery unit is appropriate based upon maternal stability and workup.
- Tocolytics should be given only with obstetric consultation.
- X-ray and computed tomographic scan.
  - Should NOT be withheld if necessary for maternal evaluation
  - Risk negligible if <10 rad and individual trauma films each <1 rad
    - Greatest risk to fetal viability: 2 weeks postconception
    - Greatest risk to embryogenic organogenesis: 2–8 weeks postconception
    - Negligible risk after 20 weeks
  - Standard x-rays deliver minimal radiation
    - Shield abdomen and pelvis when possible
    - Collimate the x-ray beam when possible
  - Computed tomographic scan
    - Minimal exposure with shielded abdomen with head computed tomography (CT) or chest CT
    - <20 weeks, shield uterus and scan upper abdomen for CT
    - >20 weeks, minimal risk to fetus
    - Intravenous contrast not contraindicated
- Ultrasound
  - Trauma ultrasound [focused assessment with sonography for trauma (FAST)]
    - Splenic injury most common cause of intraperitoneal hemorrhage
  - Pelvic ultrasound
    - Fetal heart tones, fetal movement, location of placenta
    - Difficult to detect uterine rupture or fetal-placental injury
    - Does NOT rule out placental abruption
- Diagnostic peritoneal lavage
  - If necessary, should be performed with an open supraumbilical approach.

Physiology of Pregnancy
- Maternal circulating blood volume is increased
  - Up to 50% from baseline by 28 weeks gestation

- Physiologic anemia
  - Red blood cell mass does not increase at the same rate as the whole blood volume
- Cardiac output is increased
  - 1.0–1.5 L/min at 10 weeks' gestation
- Heart rate is increased
  - 10–20 beat/min increase in the second trimester
- Blood pressure is decreased
  - 10–15 mm Hg decrease in the second trimester
    - ▶ <12 weeks, the uterus is protected by the bony pelvis.
    - ▶ >12 weeks, the uterus becomes intra-abdominal and more vulnerable to trauma.
    - ▶ Bladder moves anteriorly and is more vulnerable to trauma.
    - ▶ Gravid uterus pressing on IVC >20 weeks' gestation commonly causes supine hypotension.
    - ▶ Engorgement of pelvic and lower limb vessels.
  - Increased risk of retroperitoneal bleed
- Respiratory compensation limited
  - Diaphragm rises
  - Residual lung volume is decreased by 25%
  - Functional residual capacity decreased
  - Respiratory alkalosis due to increased respiratory rate
- Delayed gastric emptying and decreased intestinal motility
  - Gastroesophageal reflux increased frequency
  - Aspiration risk increased
- Fetal brain and skull most susceptible to blunt and penetrating trauma

Injuries Unique to Pregnancy
- Placental abruption
  - Premature separation of placenta from uterine wall.
  - Second most common cause of fetal death (after maternal death).
  - Etiologies: trauma, maternal hypertension, cocaine, vascular disease, fibroids, diabetes, smoking, fetal anomalies.
  - Relatively inelastic placenta shears off plastic uterus.
  - Signs and symptoms: abdominal pain, vaginal bleeding, and frequent uterine contractions.
  - Cardiotocographic monitoring may show fetal distress.
  - Ultrasound is specific but not sensitive.
- Uterine rupture
  - Rare (more likely later in pregnancy)
  - Etiology: blunt trauma especially to the uterus
  - Signs and symptoms: Abdominal pain, loss of uterine contour, and unexpected palpation of fetal parts through gravid abdomen
  - X-ray or ultrasound demonstrate fetus in abnormal location

Emergency Interventions
- Consultations
  - Emergent
    - ▶ Trauma service
    - ▶ Obstetrics-gynecology service for >20 weeks' gestation

- Urgent
  - Social services
  - Domestic violence advocate
- Perimortem cesarean delivery
  - Fetal survival with good neurological outcome directly correlated to time of maternal death (<5 minutes is best).
  - Attempt if >23 weeks' gestation
    - Continue maternal resuscitation
    - Emergent consultations: obstetrics-gynecology and neonatology
    - Procedure (performed by the most experienced physician present)—see Chapter 102 "Perimortem C-Section" for details
      - First: Single vertical incision into peritoneum epigastrium to pubic symphysis.
      - Second: Single vertical incision into uterus from fundus to bladder reflection.
      - Third: Deliver child.
      - Fourth: Clamp umbilical cord.

Special Considerations

- Shock manifests later and after more significant volume loss than in a nonpregnant patient.
- Vasopressor use may compromise uterine perfusion, so use caution when initiating therapy.
- Penetrating trauma to the abdomen.
  - Gunshot
    - Gravid uterus protects maternal abdominal viscera.
    - Mandatory exploratory laparotomy is controversial and depends upon maternal and fetal status.
  - Stab
    - Observation versus exploratory laparotomy is controversial.
- Electrical injuries
  - Fetus affected most when current passes through uterus.
  - Examine for fetal heart beat.
- Thermal burns
  - Larger burn area correlates with greater risk to fetus.
    - Burn formulas not applicable
  - Increased risk of third spacing, CO toxicity.
    - Hyperbaric therapy if symptomatic or CO >15 mm Hg

Suggested Readings

Bhatia K, Cranmer H. Trauma in Pregnancy. In: Marx JA, Hockberger RS, Walls RM, eds. *Rosen's Emergency Medicine: Concepts and Clinical Practic*, 7th ed. Philadelphia: Mosby, 2010:252–261.

Goldman SM, Wagner LK. Radiologic management of abdominal trauma in pregnancy. *Am J Roentgenol.* 1996;166(4):763–767.

Ma OJ, Mateer JR, DeBahnke DJ. Use of ultrasonography for the evaluation of pregnant trauma patients. *J Trauma.* 1996;40:665–667.

Section Editor: Kaushal Shah

96

Rapid Sequence Intubation and Gum-Elastic Bougie

Todd A. Seigel and Leon D. Sanchez

General

Management of the airway is the most critical intervention in the care of the trauma patient. While the general approach to emergency airway management serves as the framework for airway management of the trauma patient, these patients merit several other specific considerations. Early intubation improves outcome in severely injured patients, and early airway management should be considered. Traumatic injuries to the airway, head, and neck impact both the method of intubation and the pharmacologic agents chosen for induction. Acute hemorrhage from chest, abdominal, or extremity trauma may also result in hemodynamic compromise. Finally, the increased potential for a difficult or failed airway must be considered and prepared for. Similar to the emergent management of any airway, **rapid sequence intubation (RSI) is the preferred method of airway management of the trauma patient.**

Indications

- Glasgow Coma Scale (GCS) score of ≤8
- Decreased mental status with impending failure of airway protection
- Failure to maintain the airway
- Failure of ventilation
- Failure of oxygenation
- Protect the combative trauma patient from additional harm
- Other therapeutic indication such as need for paralysis or hyperventilation

Contraindications

- Absolute
  - Total upper airway obstruction
  - Total loss of facial landmarks
- Relative
  - Anticipated difficult airway
  - Likelihood of injury from the procedure
  - Use of intubation when a less invasive technique would suffice

Nasotracheal intubation is generally inappropriate for the trauma patient, but in the absence of head or neck trauma, nasotracheal intubation can be considered with the following caveats:

- Absolute
  - Apnea
  - Basilar skull or facial fracture

- Neck trauma or cervical spine injury
- Head injury with suspected increased intracranial pressure
- Nasal or nasopharyngeal obstruction
- Combative patients or patients *in extremis*
- Patients with coagulopathy
- Pediatric patients

Landmarks

- Viewing the oropharynx from above, the tongue will be the most anterior structure.
- The pouch-like vallecula separates the tongue from the epiglottis which sits above the airway. The larynx sits anterior to the esophagus.
- The vocal cords sit as an inverted "V" within the larynx.
- Landmarks may be distorted secondary to traumatic injury or obstructed by blood or vomit (Fig. 96.1).

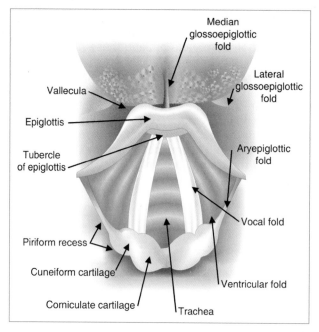

FIGURE 96.1: Larynx visualized from the oropharynx. Note the median glossoepiglottic fold. It is pressure on this structure by the tip of a curved blade that flips the epiglottis forward, exposing the glottis during laryngoscopy. Note the valleculae and the pyriform recesses are different structures, a fact often confused in the anesthesia literature. The cuneiform and corniculate cartilages are called the arytenoid cartilages. The ridge between them posteriorly is called the posterior commissure. (Reused with permission from Redden RJ. Anatomic considerations in anesthesia. In: Hagberg CA, ed. *Handbook of difficult airway management.* Philadelphia: Churchill Livingstone; 2000:9.)

Technique for Orotracheal Intubation

The approach to the technique for RSI can be summarized in 7 discrete steps, each beginning with the letter P. This approach is an appropriate framework appropriate for evaluating the trauma patient, though these patients merit some additional considerations.

- Preparation
  - Assess airway: LEMON mnemonic to predict difficulty of airway; aspects of the mnemonic may be limited or impossible secondary to cervical spine

immobilization or trauma. Therefore, *every airway in a trauma patient should be considered a difficult airway, even without overt trauma to the head or neck.*

▸   **L**ook externally: If you get the sense that an airway appears difficult, it likely is.

▸   **E**valuate anatomy: The 3-3-2 Rule (Fig. 96.2).

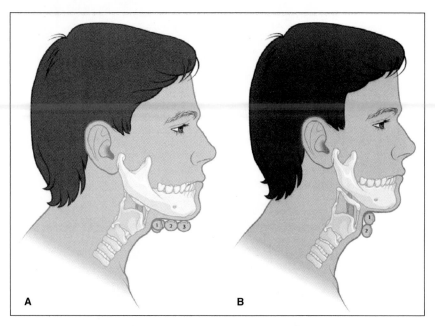

FIGURE 96.2: A: The second 3 of the 3-3-2 rule. **B:** The 2 of the 3-3-2 rule. (From Walls RM, Murphy MF, Luten RC, et al. *Manual of emergency airway management.* Philadelphia: Lippincott Williams & Wilkins; 2004:77, with permission.)

◆   Mouth opening: If the patient's open mouth can fit less than 3 of the patient's own fingers, it is predictive of a difficult airway.

◆   Thyromental distance: A distance less than 3 of the patient's finger widths is predictive of difficult airway. This can be assessed in the trauma patient once cervical spine collar is opened prior to intubation.

◆   Hyomental distance: A distance of less than 2 of the patient's finger widths is predictive of a difficult airway.

▸   **M**allampati Score: Roughly correlates the size of internal oropharyngeal structures with successful intubation attempts. Graded as class I-IV. Will likely be difficult or impossible to attempt in the trauma patient (Fig. 96.3).

▸   **O**bstruction: Any evidence of upper airway obstruction heralds a difficult airway; total upper airway obstruction is an absolute contraindication to orotracheal intubation.

▸   **N**eck mobility: Neck mobility is crucial to obtaining the optimum view of the larynx. Hindrance to neck extension, including cervical spine immobilization, predicts difficulty in intubation.

•   Equipment

▸   Endotracheal tube (ETT): Prepare two ETTs, 8.0 and 7.0. The larger tube is suitable for most adult men and the smaller for most adult women. If

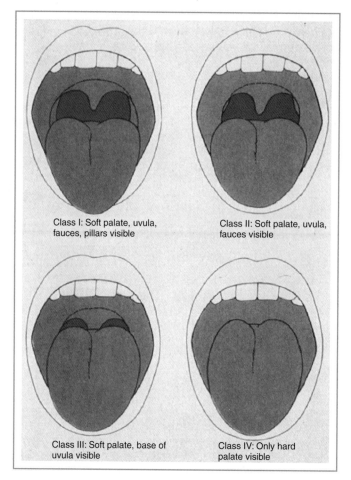

Class I: Soft palate, uvula, fauces, pillars visible

Class II: Soft palate, uvula, fauces visible

Class III: Soft palate, base of uvula visible

Class IV: Only hard palate visible

FIGURE 96.3: The Mallampati Scale. (From Walls RM, Murphy MF, Luten RC, et al. *Manual of emergency airway management*. Philadelphia: Lippincott Williams & Wilkins; 2004:78, with permission.)

difficulty is encountered using a larger tube, the smaller tube is readily available. Check the integrity of the cuff prior to use. Place the stylet in the tube.

▶ Laryngoscope and blades: Ensure that the light source works in two laryngoscopes and prepare blades (Macintosh 3 and 4, Miller 3 and 4). Use a blade you feel comfortable with.

- Rescue airway devices at the bedside, including an oral airway, a gum-elastic bougie, and a laryngeal mask airway.
- Surgical intervention prepared if needed.
- Ensure that patient is monitored with a functional intravenous line
- Position patient and adjust bed height
- Have pharmacologic agents drawn and ready to push
- Assign roles to the other members of the team in the room

- **Preoxygenation**
  - Ideally, deliver 100% oxygen for 3 minutes; non-rebreather mask delivers approximately 70%. Note that oxygen saturation may never reach 100%, despite preoxygenation, particularly in patients with significant or airway trauma.

- This replaces nitrogen in functional residual capacity with oxygen.
- When time is critical or patient is following commands, preoxygenation is achieved in eight vital capacity breaths.
- This allows approximately 8 minutes of apnea in 70 kg adult; this time varies on the basis of patient body habitus and medical history. Trauma patients with significant chest injury may desaturate quickly.

■ **Pretreatment**

This refers to the administration of medications to attenuate the potential adverse effect of intubation, that is, increased intracranial pressure. Although not every patient requires pretreatment, it should be considered for any trauma patient with potential intracranial injury. Pretreatment may mitigate the rise in intracranial pressure as well as the sympathetic response to intubation. Although data exist suggesting varied efficacy of each individual agent, the "five-drug cocktail" should be considered for pretreatment of head injured patients.

- **Lidocaine** 1.5 mg/kg 3 minutes prior to airway manipulation—mitigates physiologic response to intubation that may increase intracranial pressure (ICP).
- **Vecuronium** 0.01 mg/kg—as a defasciculating agent prior to administration of succinylcholine as fasciculations may increase ICP. Theoretically should be given 1–3 minutes prior to succinylcholine for adequate effect. It is no longer recommended in the third edition of Ron Wall's Manual of Emergency Airway Management.
- **Fentanyl** 3 mcg/kg, which also mitigates physiologic response to intubation but may be limited by patient's hemodynamic status as it can cause hypotension.
- **Succinylcholine** 1.2 mg/kg and **etomidate** 0.3 mg/kg remain the standard induction and paralytic agents. Ketamine potentially raises ICP and should be avoided in these patients until the evidence is clearer. Although crush injury is a known contraindication to succinylcholine, the potential danger does not exist in the acute (<6 hours) traumatic period and should still be used.

■ **Protection and Positioning**

Secondary to potential neck injury and cervical spine immobilization, approach to positioning is a pivotal difference in management of the trauma patient. Appropriate positioning to ensure cervical spine immobilization may limit the view of the airway.

- Sellick's maneuver: Firm pressure against cricoid cartilage to protect from aspiration.
- In-line stabilization: In the nontrauma patient, the "sniffing" position is typically employed. That position creates neck extension with slight flexion of lower cervical spine and optimally aligns the pharyngeal and laryngeal airway. *It should be avoided in the trauma patient.* Prior to intubation, the cervical collar should be opened but not removed. Another person in the room is assigned the dedicated task of holding the patient's neck while the airway is managed. This person kneels at the head of the bed and places his hands on the patient's shoulders. The elbows are near the patient's ears, and gentle pressure is applied such that the forearms of the person holding stabilization keep the cervical spine immobilized (Fig. 96.4).

■ **Paralysis and Induction**

The goal of the rapid sequence is to maintain the shortest amount of apnea as possible such that intermittent ventilation is not required.

- In the trauma patient with suspected head injury, the "five-drug" cocktail should be considered. Vecuronium, lidocaine, and fentanyl should be administered prior to the induction agent.
- The induction agent should then be given, as a bolus, in sufficient dose to produce immediate loss of consciousness. Common induction agents are

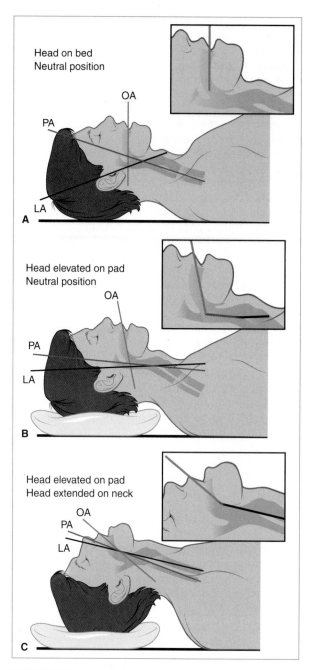

FIGURE 96.4: A: Anatomic neutral position. The oral axis (*OA*), pharyngeal axis (PA), and laryngeal axis (*LA*) are at greater angles to one another. **B:** Head, still in neutral position, has been lifted by a pillow flexing the lower cervical spine and aligning the *PA* and *LA* axes. **C:** The head has been extended on the cervical spine, aligning the *OA* with the *PA* and *LA* axes, creating the optimum sniffing position for intubation. (From Walls RM, Murphy MF, Luten RC, et al. *Manual of emergency airway management*. Philadelphia: Lippincott Williams & Wilkins; 2004:56, with permission.)

propofol (1.5–3 mg/kg) and etomidate (0.3 mg/kg), though etomidate is the induction agent of choice for the trauma patient. Etomidate is not vasoactive and will preserve blood pressure. It should be used in the hypotensive trauma patient or a patient with suspected occult hemorrhage.

- The paralytic should then be administered. Succinylcholine (1.5–2 mg/kg) is the paralytic of choice in RSI due to its rapid onset.
- Fasciculations will occur approximately 20–30 seconds after the administration of succinylcholine
- Apnea will occur almost uniformly by 1 minute.

- **Placement of the Tube and Proof of Placement**
  - Open patient's mouth.
  - Holding the handle in the left hand, insert the blade of choice starting from the right side of the mouth with the goal of sweeping the tongue fully to the left.
  - Apply gentle upward and forward pressure (approximately 45 degrees) to visualize the airway; avoid the temptation to use the laryngoscope as a lever.
  - If cords are not immediately visible, try slowly withdrawing laryngoscope to allow the cords to drop into view.
  - Keep the cords under direct visualization; ask someone to hand you the ETT.
  - Pass the tube through the vocal cords and stop when the cuff is just past the cords.
  - Remove stylet and inflate balloon.

- **Proof of Tube Placement**
  There are several ways to confirm tube placement:
  - Direct visualization of the tube passing through the cords is paramount.
  - Auscultate over the stomach and then over the lungs to confirm placement.
  - Confirm placement in trachea with color change on end-tidal carbon dioxide detector.
  - Obtain postintubation chest x-ray film.

- **Postintubation Management**
  - Maintain proper ventilator settings.
  - Administer appropriate amounts of sedation to keep the patient comfortable.
  - Nasogastric tube should be inserted to decompress the stomach.
  - Obtain arterial blood gas to determine adequate oxygenation and ventilation.

Technique for Gum-Elastic Bougie Insertion

Specific limitations in the trauma patient may compromise the view of the airway. Preparation for a difficult or failed airway should be undertaken prior to direct laryngoscopy. The bougie is a long, semirigid device, much like a stylet, with a bent/angled tip that can be used to guide the placement of the ETT when the view of the vocal cords is obscured.

Preparation

- Preoxygenation, pretreatment, paralysis, and positioning are executed as described above, in preparation for laryngoscopy.
- If the view of the vocal cords is inadequate for confident placement of the ETT, the bougie can be used.
- The ETT must be a size $\geq$ 6.0.
- Bougie may be lubricated with sterile water or KY jelly.

Placing the Bougie (Fig 96.5)

- The bougie should be oriented such that the angled tip is directed anteriorly.

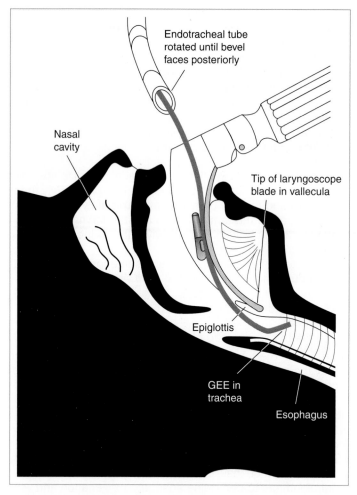

FIGURE 96.5: Proper placement of the gum-elastic bougie entails navigating the angled tip anteriorly into the trachea followed by sliding the endotracheal tube over the bougie. It is best to keep the laryngoscope blade in place throughout the procedure.

- The bougie should be carefully advanced through the partial view of the vocal cords. If the cords are completely obscured, the bougie may be placed blindly as anteriorly as possible.
- Check for **"palpable clicks"**: the perceptible snaps of the bougie as it passes along the rings of cartilage in the trachea.
- Check for **"hold-up"**: the resistance encountered during insertion of a bougie; it occurs as a result of the tip reaching the carina/small bronchi.
- If "palpable clicks" and/or "hold up" are present, slide the ETT over the bougie. If "clicks" and "hold-up" are absent, bougie is likely in the esophagus and should be removed.
- When passing the ETT over the bougie, rotate the ETT 90 degrees counter-clockwise before passing thru cords to prevent bevel tip from catching on arytenoids or cords.

- Once the ETT is in place, pull out the bougie.
- Confirm tracheal ETT placement using conventional methods.

Complications
- Incorrect tube placement: esophageal airway or mainstem intubation.
- Prolonged hypoxia.
- Witnessed aspiration.
- Broken teeth, excessive bleeding secondary to mucosal damage.
- Pneumothorax and pneumomediastinum.
- Cardiac dysrhythmia.
- Complications or side effects from pharmacologic therapy, including hypotension.

Precautions
- Failure to confirm IV access and patency prior to initiation of RSI.
- Not allowing onset of action of sedation and paralysis medications prior to attempting intubation.
- Failure to consider concomitant injuries when selecting pharmacologic agents.
- Failure to maintain adequate stabilization of the cervical spine.
- Failure to maintain visualization of cords when passing the ETT.
- Using the laryngoscope as a lever.

Pearls
- In the trauma patient, aggressive airway management should be considered early, especially in the combative or hemodynamically unstable patient.
- Even in trauma, RSI is the airway management strategy of choice.
- Every patient with trauma should be assumed to have a cervical spine injury, and for this reason, is considered a "difficult airway."
- Concomitant injuries, such as head trauma and chest trauma, impact the physiology and mechanics of airway management, as well as choices of pharmacologic agents used in intubation.
- If an esophageal intubation is detected, the tube should be removed and the patient should be ventilated.
- If direct laryngoscopy is difficult, placement of an ETT over a bougie should be considered.

Suggested Readings
Shah KH, Kwong BM, Hazan A, Newman DH, Wiener D. Success of the gum elastic bougie as a rescue airway in the emergency department [published online ahead of print November 8, 2008]. *J Emerg Med.*

Vissers RJ. Advanced airway support. *Emergency Medicine Manual.* New York: McGraw-Hill, 2004.

Walls RM, Murphy MF, Luten RC, Schneider RE. *Manual of Emergency Airway Management*, 2nd ed. Philadelphia: Lippincott Williams & Wilkins, 2004.

Wolfson AB, Reichman EF. Resuscitation. *Harwood Nuss' Clinical Practice of Emergency Medicine.* Philadelphia: Lippincott Williams & Wilkins, 2004.

97

Cricothyroidotomy—Standard and Needle

Alden Landry and Jason Imperato

Indications

- Used to provide emergent airway access if a safer, less invasive airway (oral or nasotracheal intubation) cannot be established or is contraindicated, such as:
  - Major midface and jaw injuries
  - Massive oropharyngeal bleeding
  - Burns around the mouth
  - Possible spinal trauma preventing adequate ventilation
  - Inability to open a patient's mouth
- Needle cricothyroidotomy should be performed in children younger than 12 years.

Contraindications

- Absolute
  - An oral or nasal airway can be established
  - Significant injury or fracture of the cricoid cartilage
  - Partial or complete transection of the airway
  - Patients younger than 12 years (Needle cricothyroidotomy is the procedure of choice for this age group)
- Relative
  - Neck mass, swelling, or cellulitis
  - Neck hematoma
  - Coagulopathy

Landmarks

The cricothyroid membrane is best identified by palpating the laryngeal prominence, which is the palpable protuberance at the anterior superior aspect of the larynx. Approximately one of the patient's finger breadths inferior to the laryngeal prominence is a small depression which is the cricothyroid membrane and below it is the cricothyroid cartilage (Fig. 97.1).

Technique—Standard

- Identify the landmarks—see above landmarks section
- Prepare the neck
  - If time permits, apply appropriate antiseptic solution.
  - If time permits and patient is conscious, infiltrate skin of anterior neck with 1% lidocaine solution.
- Immobilize the larynx
  - This is done by placing the thumb and long finger on opposite sides of the superior laryngeal horns, allowing the physician to relocate and reidentify the cricothyroid membrane at any time during the procedure (Fig. 97.2).

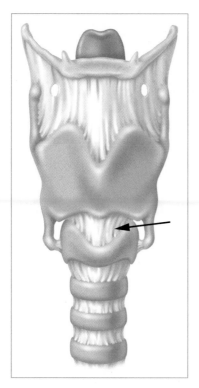

FIGURE 97.1: Anatomy of the larynx. The cricothyroid membrane (arrow) is bordered above by the thyroid carilage and below by the cricoid cartilage. (From Walls RM, Murphy MF, Luten RC, et al. *Manual of Emergency Airway Management*, 2nd ed. Philadelphia: Lippincott Williams & Wilkins; 2004:162, with permission.)

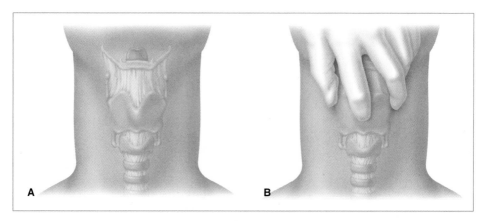

FIGURE 97.2: A: Surface anatomy of the airway. **B:** The thumb and long finger immobilize the superior cornua of the larynx; the index finger palpates the cricothyroid membrane. (From Walls RM, Murphy MF, Luten RC et al. *Manual of Emergency Airway Management*, 2nd ed. Philadelphia: Lippincott Williams & Wilkins; 2004:162, with permission.)

- Incise the skin
  - Using a #11 blade, make a vertical midline incision approximately 2 cm in length.
  - Care should be made to extend the incision down to but not through any of the deep structures of the neck.
- Reidentify the membrane
  - Use your index finger to palpate the anterior larynx, with your thumb and long finger maintaining immobilization of the larynx.
  - Leave your index finger on the cricothyroid membrane.
- Incise the membrane
  - Removing index finger.
  - Incise the cricothyroid membrane at least 1 cm in length in a horizontal direction.
- Insert the tracheal hook
  - Insert and turn the tracheal hook so that it is oriented in a cephalad direction.
  - Light upward and anterior traction is applied to bring the airway immediately out of the skin incision (Fig. 97.3).

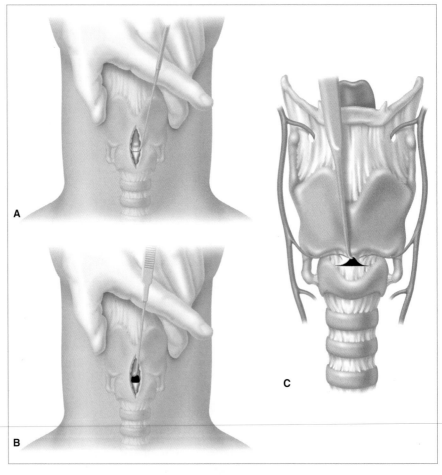

FIGURE 97.3: A: The tracheal hook is oriented transversely during insertion. **B** and **C:** After insertion cephalad traction is applied to the inferior margin of the thyroid cartilage. (From Walls RM, Murphy MF, Luten RC et al. *Manual of Emergency Airway Management*, 2nd ed. Philadelphia: Lippincott Williams & Wilkins; 2004:162, with permission.)

- Insert the Trousseau dilator
  - Insert minimally into the wound with the blades oriented superiorly and inferiorly, allowing the dilator to open and enlarge the wound vertically.
- Insert the tracheostomy tube
  - With its inner cannula in place, gently insert the tracheostomy tube through the incision between the blades of the Trousseau dilator.
  - Rotate the Trousseau dilator to allow advancement of the tube.
  - Remove the Trousseau dilator once the tube is firmly seated against the anterior neck.
- Inflate the cuff and confirm tube position
  - Ventilate patient and auscultate both lungs for equal breath sounds.
  - Confirm color change of carbon dioxide detector.

Technique—Needle
- Find landmarks in the same way as for standard cricothyroidotomy.
- Attach a large-bore needle (12- or 14-gauge) with a catheter to a 3-mL syringe.
- Partially fill the syringe with saline.
- Immobilize the trachea.
- Insert the needle into the cricothyroid membrane at a 90-degree angle.
- Attempt to withdraw air through the needle.
  - If air bubbles are seen in the syringe, proper placement is confirmed.
- Change the angle to 45 degrees and advance the catheter over the needle into the larynx and then withdraw the needle and syringe.
- Attach an endotracheal tube connector to the catheter.
- Stabilize the tube.
- Ventilate the patient and check for proper tube placement.

Complications
- Hemorrhage
- Pneumomediastinum
- Infection
- Voice change
- Subglottic stenosis
- Laryngeal/tracheal injury

Common Pitfalls
- Malposition
- Poor identification of anatomical landmarks
- Failure to stabilize trachea

Pearls
- Numerous commercial cricothyrotomy devices are available. Several use a modified Seldinger technique which is similar to the method used for placement of central venous catheters.
- Cricothyroidotomy is the surgical airway of choice in an emergency.

Suggested Readings

Vissers RJ. Advanced airway support. *Emergency Medicine Manual*. New York: McGraw-Hill, 2004:3–8.

Walls RM, Murphy MF, Luten RC, Schneider RE. *Manual of Emergency Airway Management*, 2nd ed. Philadelphia: Lippincott Williams & Wilkins, 2004.

Wolfson AB, Reichman EF. Resuscitation. *Harwood Nuss' Clinical Practice of Emergency Medicine*. Philadelphia: Lippincott Williams & Wilkins, 2004.

98

Lateral Canthotomy

Dean Straff

Indications

Retrobulbar hemorrhage is an ocular emergency that is most commonly a result of direct trauma to the eye, recent retrobulbar anesthesia, or eyelid surgery. If untreated, orbital compartment syndrome develops with resultant optic nerve ischemia and irreversible vision loss in as little as 90–120 minutes. See also Chapter 26 (Retrobulbar Hemorrhage).

- Primary indications
  - Retrobulbar hemorrhage with
    - acute loss of visual acuity
    - increased intraocular pressure
    - severe proptosis
    - diffuse subconjunctival hemorrhage
    - marked periorbital edema
  - An unconscious or uncooperative patient with an intraocular pressure >40 mm Hg.
- Secondary indications
  - Suspected retrobulbar hemorrhage with
    - associated afferent pupillary defect
    - ophthalmoplegia
    - resistance to retropulsion
    - cherry-red macula
    - optic nerve head pallor
    - severe eye pain

Contraindications

- Suspected ruptured globe

Landmarks

- The lateral canthal tendon is a combined tendon-ligament that provides structural fixation of the lids (tarsal plates) and orbicularis oculi muscle to the inner aspect of the bony lateral orbital wall (zygoma) just posterior to the orbital rim.
- The tendon has an inferior and superior crux.
- The point at which the tendon attaches is entitled Whitnall tubercle.
- Eisler's pocket, a small pocket of orbital fat, lies anterior to the lateral canthal tendon.
- Upon cutting the inferior crux of the lateral canthal tendon, the lower lid loses its structural fixation to the lateral orbital wall and becomes lax, releasing the increased intraocular pressure from the eye.

Technique

- Positioning is critical. The patient must be in the supine position and has to be able to cooperate throughout the procedure. Unexpected head movement may

lead to iatrogenic globe injury. Depending on the clinical scenario, the patient may
need to be restrained, undergo conscious sedation, or even be intubated and
paralyzed.

- The lateral canthus should be prepped and draped in a sterile fashion.
- Irrigate the eye with normal saline to remove surrounding debris.
- **Anesthetize** the lateral canthus with approximately 1 mL of 1% or 2% lidocaine
  with epinephrine to obtain both local anesthesia and hemostasis.
- A **straight clamp** is placed horizontally across the lateral canthus (the skin of
  the lateral corner of the eye) for 1–2 minutes to compress tissues and achieve
  hemostasis.
- Release the clamp, leaving an impression for where the incision is to be made.
- Use a pair of forceps to pick up the skin around the lateral orbit.
- **Use scissors and cut** a 1–2 cm horizontal incision in the tissue starting at the
  lateral corner of the eye and extending laterally. This will open skin, orbicularis
  muscle, orbital septum, palpebral conjunctiva, and expose Eisler's fat pocket
  (Fig. 98.1).

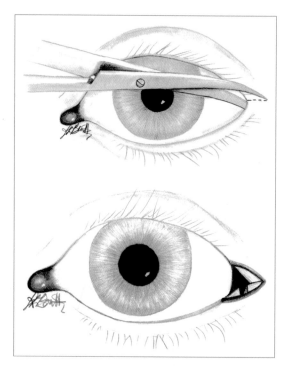

FIGURE 98.1: Lateral canthotomy and cantholysis. The inferior arm of the lateral canthal tendon
has been incised to release the globe. (From Knoop KJ, Dennis WR. Eye trauma. In: Wolfson AB, ed.
Harwood-Nuss' Clinical Practice of Emergency Medicine, 4th ed. Philadelphia: Lippincott Williams &
Wilkins; 2005:952, with permission.)

- **Retract the lid down** and away from the lateral orbit separating the conjunctiva
  and the skin.
- Palpate the inferior portion of the lateral canthal tendon by using your finger or the
  tip of the scissors.
- With the scissors pointed inferoposteriorly toward the lateral orbital rim (pointing
  away from the globe), dissect and **cut the inferior crux of the lateral canthal
  tendon.** This critical incision is approximately 1–2 cm in depth and length.

- If this procedure is insufficient, dissect superiorly and cut the superior crux of the lateral canthal tendon.
- Releasing the pressure of the hematoma will help prevent further visual loss or restore vision to the effected eye.

Complications

- Iatrogenic globe injury.
- Excessive bleeding.
- Local infection or abscess formation.
- Fibrosis may develop limiting extraocular motility.
- Improper direction of scissors superiorly may lead to injury to the levator aponeurosis, resulting in ptosis.
- The lacrimal gland and lacrimal artery also lie superiorly; care must be taken to avoid these structures.
- Loss of adequate lower lid suspension and ectropion (can be repaired at a later date by ophthalmologist).

Common Pitfalls

- Failure to adequately position, sedate, and anesthetize the patient.
- It is extremely important to immediately test visual acuity post-procedure. If vision fails to improve, operative orbital decompression or hematoma evacuation is required.

Pearls

- Despite high intraorbital pressures, only a small amount of blood is usually expressed from the hematoma upon completion of the emergent orbital decompression.
- Almost immediately after a successful procedure, there will be a noticeable improvement of extraocular muscle movements and visual acuity, resolution of afferent pupillary defect, decrease in intraocular pressure, and resolution of the severe eye pain.
- Formal intraocular pressure testing with instruments such as a Tono-pen is contraindicated in patient with suspected ruptured globe injury.
- If it is unclear whether there is retrobulbar hemorrhage or another ocular process occurring, an emergent computed tomographic scan of the orbits may be helpful to clarify the diagnosis. However, imaging may delay treatment and result in permanent vision loss.
- Always call an emergent ophthalmology consult when this procedure is performed.
- Retrobulbar hemorrhage can also occur spontaneously. It has been reported to occur in people with hemophilia, von Willebrand disease, disseminated intravascular coagulation, leukemia, hypertension, atherosclerosis, straining, venous anomalies, and intraorbital aneurysm of the ophthalmic artery.

Suggested Readings

McInnes G, Howes DW. Lateral canthotomy and cantholysis: a simple, vision-saving procedure. *CJEM.* 2002;4(1):49–52.

Roberts JR, Hedges JR, eds. *Clinical Procedures in Emergency Medicine.* 4th ed. Portland, Ore: WB Saunders Co, 2004:1275.

Rosen P, Barkin R. *Emergency Medicine: Concepts and Clinical Practice*. St Louis: Mosby, 2002:910.

Titinalli JE, Kelen GD, Strapczynski JS. *Emergency Medicine: A comprehensive Study Guide*. 6th ed. New York: American College of Emergency Physicians, McGraw-Hill Co, 2004:1458.

Vassallo S, Hartstein M, Howard D, Stetz J. Traumatic retrobulbar hemorrhage: emergent decompression by lateral canthotomy and cantholysis. *J Emerg Med*. 2002;22(3):251–256.

99

Tube Thoracostomy

Chilembwe Mason

Indications

"Chest tube" is used to evacuate abnormal collections of air or fluid from the pleural space in the following conditions:

- Pneumothorax
- Hemothorax
- Chylothorax
- Empyema
- Drainage of recurrent pleural effusion
- Prevention of hydrothorax after cardiothoracic surgery

Contraindications

- None for unstable injured patients
- **Relative contraindications**
  - Anatomic abnormalities—pleural adhesions, emphysematous blebs, or scarring
  - Coagulopathy

Landmarks

- Chest tube placement preferred at the fourth or fifth intercostal space at the mid to anterior axillary line but multiple sites are possible (see Fig. 99.1).
- Intercostal nerve and vessels are located along the inferior margin of each rib; therefore, the tube should pass immediately over the superior surface of the lower rib.

Supplies

There exist several commercially packaged thoracostomy kits. However, the surgeon should be familiar with the required equipment should these kits not be available. Standard equipment includes:

- Antiseptic solution, drapes, and towel clips
- One percent lidocaine, 20 mL
- 25-gauge needle, 22-gauge needle, 10-mL syringe
- No. 10 scalpel blade with handle, Kelly clamps (two), and forceps
- Thoracostomy tube selection
  - Trauma: No. 36–40 French
  - Nontraumatic: No. 24–32 French
  - Children: No. 20–24 French
  - Infants: No. 18 French
- Pleurovac (collection bottle, underwater seal, suction control)
- Connecting tubing

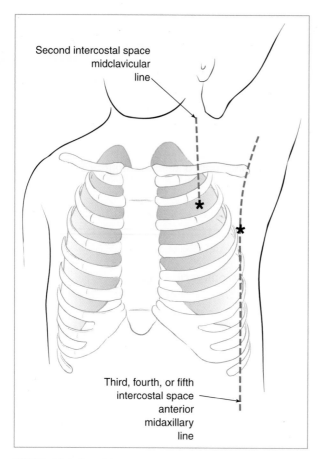

Second intercostal space
midclavicular
line

Third, fourth, or fifth
intercostal space
anterior
midaxillary
line

FIGURE 99.1: Possible sites for chest tube placement. (From Connors KM, Terndrup TE. Tube thoracostomy and needle decompression of the chest. In: Henretig FM, King C, eds. *Textbook of Pediatric Emergency Procedures*. Philadelphia: Lippincott Williams & Wilkins, 1997:399.)

- Gauze pads, adhesive tape, 4 × 4-in. pads, petroleum gauze or Xeroform gauze dressing, antibiotic ointment
- 2, 1, or 0 suture (not 2-0 or 1-0), needle driver, and suture scissors

Technique

Preparation

- Nasal oxygen and continuous pulse oximetry monitoring should be arranged for.
- If patient is stable, parenteral analgesics or conscious sedation should be used.
- Elevate the head of the bed to 30–60 degrees.
- Patient's arm on the affected side is placed over the patient's head.
- Sterilize the area where the tube will be inserted with povidone-iodine or chlorhexidine solution.
- Drape the area with sterile towels.

Assemble the suction-drain system according to manufacturer's recommendations; adjust the suction until a steady stream of bubbles is produced in the water column.

General Basic Steps

Analgesia
Incision
Blunt dissection
Verification
Insertion
Securing the tube
Confirmation

Analgesia
- Produce local anesthesia using up to 5 mg/kg of 1% lidocaine with epinephrine (1:100,000).
- Inject the subcutaneous area with a small-bore (25-gauge) needle.
- Generously infiltrate the muscle, periosteum, and parietal pleura in the area of the tube's eventual passage using a larger bore needle.

Incision
- Using a no. 10 scalpel blade make at least a 3–4 cm transverse incision through the skin and subcutaneous tissue.
- One method is to make the incision at an intercostal space lower than the thoracic wall entry site, so the tube may be "tunneled" up over the next rib.

Blunt Dissection
- Use a large Kelly clamp or scissor (this often takes considerable force) (Fig. 99.2).

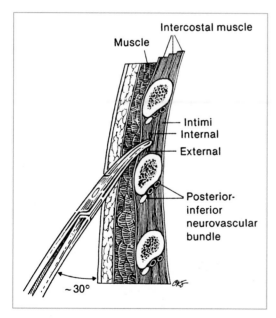

FIGURE 99.2: Perform blunt dissection through the subcutaneous tissues and intercostal muscles with a Kelly clamp. (From Feliciano DV. Tube thoracostomy. In: Benumof JL, ed. *Clinical Procedures in Anesthesia and Intensive Care*. Philadelphia: JB Lippincott Co, 1992, with permission.)

- Track is created over the rib by pushing forward with the closed points and then spreading and pulling back with the points spread.
- Push through the muscle and parietal pleura with the closed points of the clamp until the pleural cavity is entered.

- A palpable pop is felt when the pleura is penetrated, and a rush of air or fluid should occur at this point.

Verification
- Once the pleura is penetrated, insert a gloved finger into the chest wall track to verify that the pleura has been entered and that no solid organs are present (Fig. 99.3).

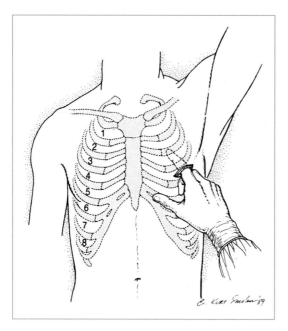

FIGURE 99.3: Perform finger thoracotomy before insertion of the thoracostomy tube. (From Feliciano DV. Tube thoracostomy. In: Benumof JL, ed. *Clinical Procedures in Anesthesia and Intensive Care.* Philadelphia: JB Lippincott Co, 1992, with permission.)

- The finger can be left in place to serve as a guide for tube insertion.

Insertion
- It is recommended that the tube be held in a large curved clamp with the tip of the tube protruding from the jaws.
- Pass the tube over, under, or beside the finger into the pleural space.
- The tube is advanced superiorly, medially, and posteriorly until pain is felt or resistance is met; then pulled back 2–3 cm (Fig. 99.4).
- Ensure that all the holes in the chest tube are within the pleural space.

Securing the Tube (Numerous Methods Are Acceptable)
- Close the remainder of the incision using a large 0 or 1 silk or nylon suture keeping the ends long.
- Suture ends are wrapped and tied repeatedly around the chest tube, then knotted securely. The sutures are tied tightly enough to indent the chest tube slightly to avoid slippage.
- A horizontal mattress (or Purse-string) suture is placed approximately 1 cm across the incision on either side of the tube, essentially encircling the tube. This suture helps secure the tube and eventually facilitates closing the incision when the chest tube is removed.

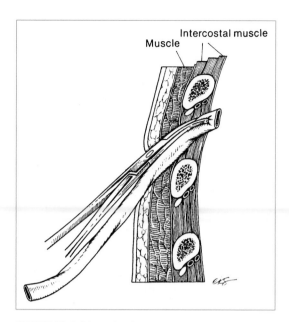

Muscle

Intercostal muscle

FIGURE 99.4: Direct the thoracostomy tube posteriorly and superiorly in patients with pleural effusions including hemothoraces. (From Feliciano DV. Tube thoracostomy. In: Benumof JL, ed. *Clinical Procedures in Anesthesia and Intensive Care.* Philadelphia: JB Lippincott Co, 1992, with permission.)

- Place occlusive dressing of petroleum-impregnated gauze where the tube enters the skin; then cover with two or more gauze pads.
- Wide cloth adhesive tape can be used to hold the tube more securely in place.

Confirmation

Indicators for correct placement are as follows:

- Condensation on the inside of the tube
- Audible air movement with respirations
- Free flow of blood or fluid
- Ability to rotate the tube freely after insertion

Attach tube to previously assembled water seal or suction.

- Observing bubbles in the water seal chamber when the patient coughs is a good way to check for system patency.

Obtain chest radiograph.

Complications

- Hemothorax
- Pulmonary edema
- Bronchopleural fistula
- Empyema
- Subcutaneous emphysema
- Infection
- Contralateral pneumothorax
- Subdiaphragmatic placement of the tube
- Localized hemorrhage

Common Pitfalls

- Use of inadequate local anesthesia
- Making the initial skin incision too small
- Failure to advance the chest tube far enough into the pleural space
- Directing the tube toward the mediastinum can cause a contralateral pneumothorax

Pearls

- For a pneumothorax, direct the tube superiorly and anteriorly. For a hemothorax, direct the tube posteriorly.
- Clamp both ends of the tube during insertion to avoid being contaminated by fluid.
- If there is no lung re-expansion after chest tube placement consider that the tube may not be in the pleural cavity, that the most proximal hole is outside the chest cavity, or that there is a large air leak from the tracheobronchial tree.
- Immediate drainage of more than 20 mL/kg (approximately 1,000–1,500 mL in an adult) of blood from the pleural cavity or a continued output of at least 200 mL/hr for 4 hours is an indication for a thoracotomy.

Suggested Readings

Kirsch TD, Mulligan JP. Tube thoracostomy. In: Roberts JR, Hedges JR, eds. *Clinical Procedures in Emergency Medicine*, 4th ed. Philadelphia: WB Saunders, 2004:187–209.

Simon RR, Brenner BE. *Emergency Procedures and Techniques*, 4th ed. Philadelphia: Lippincott Williams & Wilkins, 2002:172–179.

100

Thoracotomy

Oscar Rago and Barbara Kilian

Indications

- Penetrating chest trauma
  - Loss of pulses at any time with initial vital signs in the field
  - Systolic blood pressure <70 mm Hg after aggressive fluid resuscitation
- Blunt trauma
  - Witnessed loss of pulses or systolic blood pressure <70 mm Hg after aggressive fluid resuscitation AND
  - Initial chest tube output >20 mL/kg of blood, OR
  - Confirmed or highly suspected pericardial effusion, OR
  - Confirmed or highly suspected ongoing intra-abdominal hemorrhage (controversial)
- Goals
  - Relief of cardiac tamponade
  - Support of cardiac function with open massage, aortic cross-clamping, and/or internal cardiac defibrillation
  - Control of cardiac, pulmonary, or great vessel hemorrhage

Contraindications

- Injuries with no witnessed vital signs
- Multisystem blunt trauma
- Severe head injury

Risks/Consent Issues

- This is an emergent procedure and does not require written consent.

Landmarks

- Left-sided supine anterolateral approach over the fifth rib, fourth intercostal space (Fig. 100.1).
- In males incise below the nipple, in females below the inframammary fold.

Technique

- Patient preparation
  - Patient should be intubated and a nasogastric tube should be placed.
  - Order intravenous fluids, epinephrine 1 mg intravenous, and stat blood.
  - Place towels under the left chest and the left arm above the head.
  - Sterilize the incision area with copious povidone-iodine solution.
  - In patients with signs of life, consider induction, sedation, and paralysis.
- Incision and dissection
  - Using a no. 20 blade, incise from the sternal border to the posterior axillary line. Cut firmly through subcutaneous tissue to the intercostal muscle.
  - Using scissors cut the intercostal muscles.

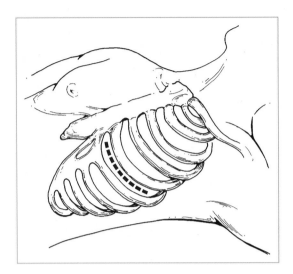

FIGURE 100.1: Thoracotomy landmark.

- Temporarily stop ventilations just before exposing the pleura to avoid lacerating the lung.
- Insert rib spreader (handle down) once the intercostal muscles are separated.
- Use a Gigli saw or trauma shears to cut the sternum for right-sided exposure.

■ Pericardiotomy
  - Hold the pericardium with forceps and use scissors to cut from the cardiac apex to the aortic root (Fig. 100.2).

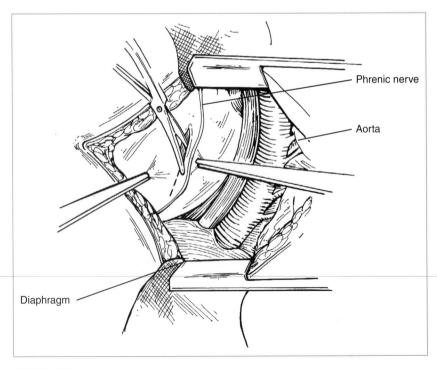

Phrenic nerve

Aorta

Diaphragm

FIGURE 100.2: Pericardium.

- The incision should be made anterior and lateral, avoiding the left phrenic nerve.
- Evacuate fresh blood and clots from the pericardial cavity.
■ Cardiac massage
- Direct, two-handed cardiac massage should be started as soon as possible (see Fig. 100.3); the left hand is placed over the right ventricle, whereas the right hand supports the surface of the left ventricle.

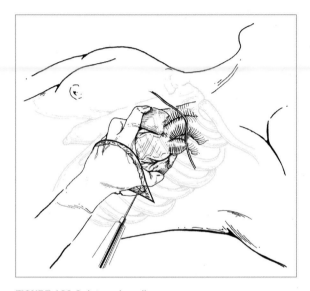

FIGURE 100.3: Internal cardiac massage.

- Avoid fingertip pressure and apply the compression force perpendicular to the septum.
- Avoid direct pressure on coronary arteries and allow for relaxation in diastole.
- To defibrillate, apply paddles perpendicular to the ventricles; use 20–60 J.
■ Control of hemorrhagic wounds
- Ventricular cardiac wounds.
- Initially, apply direct finger pressure.
- Use staples to repair large ventricular wounds.
- Nonabsorbable 2-0 silk sutures can also be used.
- The use of Teflon pledgets may help prevent tearing of the myocardium (see Fig. 100.4).
- For atrial wounds, use occlusion clamps (digital pressure may not work) or Foley catheter (see Fig. 100.5) for temporary control of bleeding.
■ Great vessel wounds
- Hemorrhage can generally be controlled using clamps or digital pressure (see Fig. 100.6).
- Both subclavian arteries can be cross-clamped as needed.
- Laparotomy pads can be used to tamponade hemorrhage.
■ Aortic cross-clamping
- Indicated if the systolic blood pressure cannot be maintained above 70 mm Hg.
- The aorta can be found posterior and lateral to the esophagus by running the fingers from the incision posteriorly toward the vertebral column, identifying

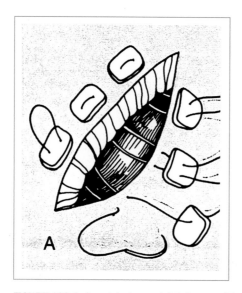

FIGURE 100.4: A ventricular septal defect resulting from a penetrating injury. Penetrating communications can often be closed by simple pledgeted mattress sutures. (From Simon RR, Brenner BE. *Emergency Procedures and Techniques,* 4th ed. Philadelphia: Lippincott Williams & Wilkins, 2002:166, with permission.)

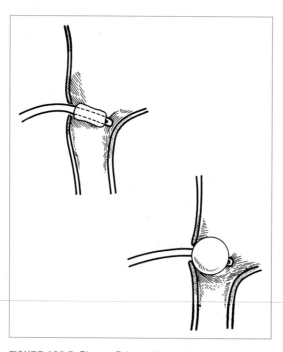

FIGURE 100.5: Place a Foley catheter tip into the wound. Inflate the balloon and pull back the catheter to control bleeding. Then proceed with more definitive repair. (From Simon RR, Brenner BE. *Emergency Procedures and Techniques,* 4th ed. Philadelphia: Lippincott Williams & Wilkins; 2002:167, with permission.)

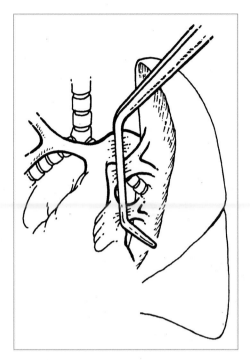

FIGURE 100.6: Occlusion of the pulmonary hilum with a Satinsky clamp. (From Simon RR, Brenner BE. *Emergency Procedures and Techniques,* 4th ed. Philadelphia: Lippincott Williams & Wilkins, 2002:170, with permission.)

the esophagus by palpation of the nasogastric tube, and dissecting away the anterior pleura.

- Once aorta is isolated, a vascular clamp is applied to the aorta by using the left index finger to secure the clamp (see Fig. 100.7).
- Check the brachial artery pressure and if it is >120 mm Hg the clamp should be released and adjusted to maintain a blood pressure below 120 mm Hg.

Complications

- Aortic or esophageal injuries due to cross-clamping
- Myocardial injury secondary to open cardiac massage
- Phrenic nerve transaction
- Fractured ribs
  - Wound infection and/or sepsis (rare)

Common Pitfalls

- Incision too small: It is acceptable to incise past the posterior axillary line.
- Rib spreader handle up: Does not allow for extension of incision to right chest.
- Pericardium not opened: Myocardial injuries cannot be excluded without direct visualization.
- Phrenic nerve injury: The nerve runs vertically on the anterior pericardial surface.

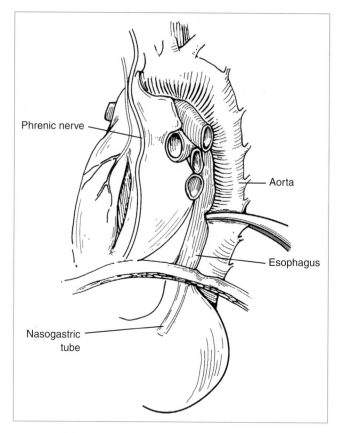

FIGURE 100.7: Aortic clamp.

Pearls

- The most important predictors of survival include injury mechanism (stab wounds carry the most favorable prognosis), injury location, and the presence of pulses.
- Always perform tube thoracotomy to identify potential right-sided injuries, if not extending the thoracotomy to the right side.
- A patient with an organized cardiac rhythm is a good candidate for a thoracotomy.
- Make the incision on top of the fifth rib to avoid the intercostal arteries.
- Start the incision 2 cm lateral to the sternal edge to avoid the internal mammary arteries.
- When cutting the pericardium diligently avoid myocardial laceration. Ribs may be broken while deploying the spreader; avoid getting cut by sharp bone edges.
- Health care needle-stick exposures have been reported at a high rate during emergency department thoracotomy. Be careful to take universal precautions and avoid needle injuries!

Suggested Readings

Cothren CC, Moore EE. Emergency department thoracotomy for the critically injured patient: objectives, indications, and outcomes. *World J Emerg Surg*. 2006;1:4.

Roberts J, Hedges J. *Clinical Procedures in Emergency Medicine*, 4th ed. Philadelphia: WB Saunders, 2004.

http://www.trauma.org/index.php/main/article/361/. Accessed June 2007.

101

Diagnostic Peritoneal Lavage

Laura Withers and Raymond Wedderburn

General

Diagnostic peritoneal lavage (DPL) is a sensitive (~95%) means to rapidly evaluate for intra-abdominal injury in the trauma patient.

Indications

- In blunt trauma
  - Unexplained hypotension
  - Patient with an equivocal examination, altered sensorium, or who is otherwise difficult to assess (especially if computed tomography [CT] is unavailable).
  - Patient taken emergently to the operating room for extra-abdominal procedure, who requires further abdominal assessment or who will not be a candidate for serial examinations because of anesthesia.
- In penetrating trauma
  - A hemodynamically stable, asymptomatic patient with an anterior abdominal wall stab wound and evidence of fascial penetration but no obvious indication for laparotomy.

Contraindications

- Absolute contraindications
  - Meets indications for exploratory laparotomy
- Relative contraindications
  - Prior abdominal surgery—consider open technique
  - Pregnancy—consider open technique with supraumbilical approach
  - Morbid obesity
  - Ascites or advanced cirrhosis
  - Coagulopathy

Risks/Consent Issues

- In patients who require DPL because of altered sensorium, consent is implied. Discussion with the patient and/or family should be held when possible.
- The incidence of complications may be lower for open diagnostic peritoneal lavage compared with the percutaneous technique; however, the percutaneous technique is somewhat faster.

Landmarks

The incision or puncture site is in the midline, one-third of the distance from the umbilicus to the symphysis pubis (Fig. 101.1). In the pregnant patient or the patient with a pelvic fracture, the incision should be made just above the umbilicus.

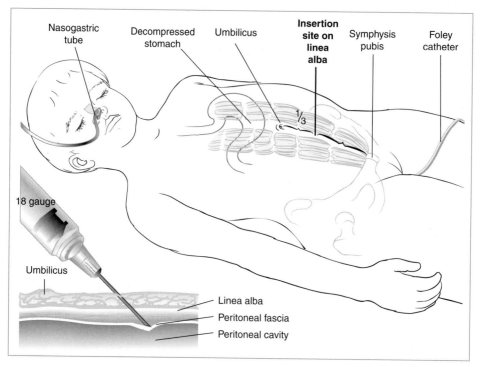

FIGURE 101.1: Anatomical landmarks for diagnostic peritoneal lavage. (From VanDevander PL, Wagner DK. Diagnostic peritoneal lavage. In: Henretig FM, King C, eds. *Textbook of Pediatric Emergency Procedures.* Philadelphia: Williams & Wilkins, 1997:358, with permission.)

Technique

- ▪ Patient preparation
  - • Place a urinary catheter to empty the bladder (if not contraindicated).
  - • Place a nasogastric tube (if not contraindicated) and keep it connected to suction to decompress the stomach.
  - • Gather instruments, sterile supplies, and appropriate sterile gown.
  - • Prepare the abdomen from costal margin to pubis and from flank to flank with povidone/iodine solution (Betadine) or chlorhexidine and create a sterile field with towels or drapes.
  - • Inject local anesthesia (1% lidocaine with epinephrine is preferred) in the skin area where the incision will be made.
- ▪ Open technique
  - • Using a no. 10, 11, or 15 blade scalpel make a 2- to 4-cm incision in the vertical direction at a site one-third of the distance from the umbilicus to the pubis.
  - • Divide the subcutaneous tissue down to the level of the fascia.
  - • Grasp the fascia with clamps and elevate it. Incise it sharply.
  - • Grasp the peritoneum with two clamps, release one and regrasp so that the bowel that may be caught can fall away. Repeat with the second clamp. Incise peritoneum sharply (Fig. 101.2).
  - • Insert a peritoneal dialysis catheter into the abdomen directing it gently toward the pelvis (Fig. 101.3).
  - • Follow directions under "Common Technique for Aspiration and Lavage" section.

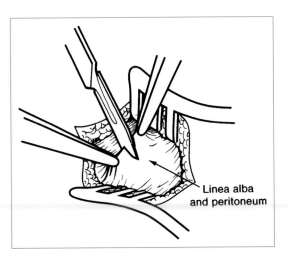

FIGURE 101.2: Make an incision between two hemostats that pick up the peritoneum and fascia as shown. (From Simon RR, Brenner BE. *Emergency Procedures and Techniques*. Philadelphia: Lippincott Williams & Wilkins, 2002:17, with permission.)

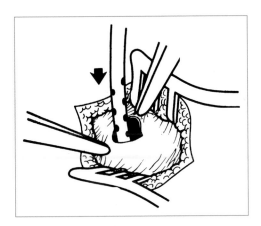

FIGURE 101.3: Pass a catheter through a 2-cm incision and direct it toward the pelvis. (From Simon RR, Brenner BE. *Emergency Procedures and Techniques*. Philadelphia: Lippincott Williams & Wilkins; 2002:17, with permission.)

- At the conclusion of the procedure (after the catheter is removed), the fascial incision should be closed with no. 0 or no. 1 PDS or nylon suture. Skin can be closed with staples.
- Percutaneous technique
  - Elevate the skin on either side of the needle insertion site, between clamps.
  - Insert an 18-gauge beveled needle in a syringe through the skin and soft tissue. The fascia will cause resistance, which will be felt to release when the needle enters the abdomen. Advance the needle 0.5–1 cm into the abdomen. Draw back on the needle. Easy aspiration confirms abdominal location.
  - The J-shaped or flexible side of a guide-wire is threaded through the needle. STOP if resistance is met or when approximately 5 cm of wire remains outside the abdomen (Fig. 101.4).
  - Leaving the wire in place, remove the needle.
  - Make a 0.5- to 1-cm incision at the insertion site.

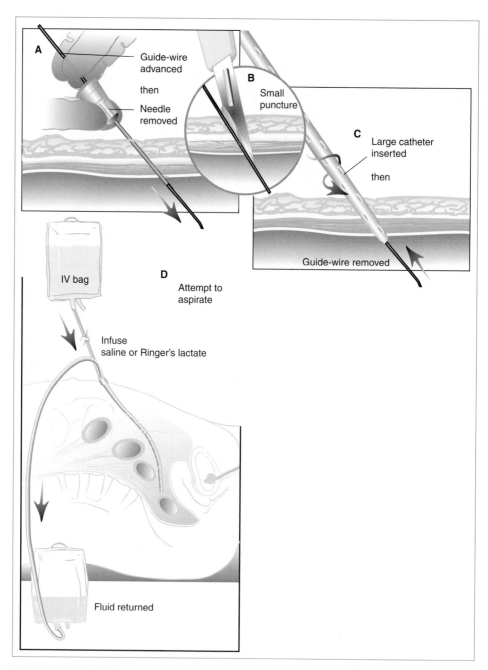

FIGURE 101.4: A: Guide-wire advanced through needle. **B:** Small puncture with scalpel. **C:** Lavage catheter advanced into the peritoneal cavity over the guide-wire. **D:** An initial attempt is made to aspirate blood from the peritoneal cavity; 10–15 mL/kg normal saline or Ringer's lactate is infused via the lavage catheter; the bag is dropped to a level below the abdomen and the fluid is recovered by gravity. (From VanDevander PL, Wagner DK. Diagnostic peritoneal lavage. In: Henretig FM, King C, eds. *Textbook of Pediatric Emergency Procedures*. Philadelphia: Williams & Wilkins, 1997:362, with permission.)

TABLE 101.1: Interpretation and appropriate action based on lavage findings

Findings	Interpretation	Action
>100,000 RBCs	Positive for **blunt** trauma	Laparotomy
20,000–100,000 RBCs	Indeterminate for **blunt** trauma	Consider further imaging: correlate clinically
>10,000 RBCs	Positive for **penetrating** trauma	Laparotomy
<10,000 RBCs	<2% chance of missed injury	May still need to evaluate for diaphragmatic injury in penetrating trauma
>500 WBCs	Positive	Laparotomy

RBCs, red blood cells; WBCs, white blood cells.

- Insert a dialysis catheter over the wire into the abdomen in the direction of the pelvis (dilatation with a dilator may be required as a separate step before catheter insertion).
  - Remove the wire.
- Common technique for aspiration and lavage
  - Connect the dialysis catheter to a syringe and aspirate.

Interpretation of Results (Table 101.1)
- If 10 mL of gross blood is aspirated, the DPL is positive and the patient should undergo immediate laparotomy.
- If bile, enteric contents, or food particles are aspirated, the DPL is positive and the patient should undergo immediate laparotomy.
- If aspiration yields <10 mL of blood, instill 10 mL/kg (up to 1 L) of warm normal saline into the abdomen. Shift the abdomen gently (i.e., place in Trendelenburg, then reverse Trendelenburg positions) and allow the fluid to remain for 5–10 minutes.
- Place the empty infusion bag or container on the floor below the patient to allow the fluid to drain. The container should be vented to promote drainage of the fluid. Drain at least half of the infused fluid.
- Send a sample of 20 mL to the laboratory for red blood cell and white blood cell counts.

Complications
- Local wound complications such as infection, dehiscence, and hematoma may be higher with open technique.
- Intraperitoneal injury to solid organs, bowel, bladder, and vasculature may be more common with the percutaneous technique.
- Procedure can cause pain.

Common Pitfalls
- False-positives may occur in the presence of pelvic fractures.
- If resistance is encountered when placing the catheter or infusing fluid, stop and check the catheter position. If the catheter is preperitoneal, DPL can be reattempted.
- If adequate fluid cannot be siphoned, the catheter may be obstructed and can be gently manipulated. Gently changing the patient's position or shifting the abdomen may release compartmentalized fluid.

Pearls

- DPL does not evaluate the retroperitoneum. It should be evaluated by computed tomographic scan in the stable patient.
- DPL may be falsely positive, particularly in the presence of pelvic fractures. A positive DPL does not mandate laparotomy. Stable patients with positive DPL may be candidates for nonoperative management.
- DPL, CT, and FAST (focused abdominal sonogram for trauma) can substitute or augment each other. The particular clinical situation, capacity of the particular institution, and skills of the providers are important considerations.
- Infusion of fluid can confound future CT and ultrasound findings.

Suggested Reading

Marx JA. Peritoneal procedures. In: Roberts JR, Hedges J, eds. *Clinical Procedures in Emergency Medicine*, 4th ed. Philadelphia: WB Saunders, 2004:841–851.

102 Perimortem C-Section

Penelope Chun Lema and Armin Perham Poordabbagh

Indications
- Gravid patient with a potentially viable fetus of ≥24 weeks' gestational age and imminent maternal death or unresponsive to cardiopulmonary resuscitation (CPR) for 5 minutes.
- **Survival of mother and infant is greatest when procedure is performed within 5 minutes of maternal arrest.**

Contraindications
- Patient with fetus <24 weeks' gestational age.
- Lower limit of fetal viability varies depending on institution and available resources.

Risk/Consent Issues
- Verbal consent from family when possible.

Technique
- Patient preparation
  - Procedure should be performed by the most experienced person available.
  - Contact all essential personnel (i.e., neonatology/pediatrics, obstetrics).
  - Continue CPR on maternal patient throughout entire procedure.
  - Estimate fetal age/maturity (if unknown from history).
  - Height of uterine fundus reaches the umbilicus at 20 weeks' gestational age and increases approximately 1 cm for each additional week.
  - Four finger breadths above the umbilicus is approximately 24 weeks' gestational age.
- Incision
  - Use a scalpel with a no. 10 blade.
  - Make a midline vertical incision on the abdomen from just above the symphysis pubis extending to the umbilicus along the linea nigra/linea alba.
  - Incise through all layers of the abdominal wall to the peritoneal cavity (Fig. 102.1).
  - Use retractors (if available) to retract abdominal wall and expose the uterus.
- Reflect bladder inferiorly
  - If a full bladder obstructs view of the uterus, decompress bladder with a puncture incision and deflate with either pressure or suction.
  - Bladder repair may be done later (if mother survives).
  - Make a small vertical incision (2–5 cm) along the lower uterine segment until amniotic fluid is encountered.
  - Be careful not to cause inadvertent injury to the underlying fetus.
  - Insert index finger into incision and lift the uterus away from the fetus.
  - Use bandage (blunt-ended) scissors to extend the incision either transversely or vertically.

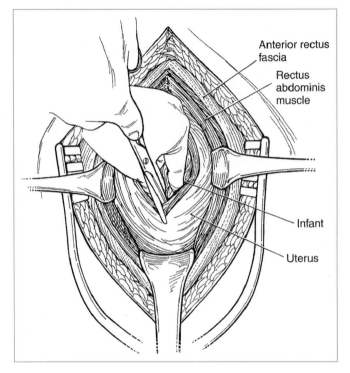

FIGURE 102.1: Anatomical landmarks.

- Avoid tearing the uterine vessels located along the lateral margins of the uterus when making a transverse incision.
- Incision should be large enough for delivery of the fetal head and body.
- Deliver baby (Fig. 102.2).
  - Place hand into the uterus and gently deliver the infant's head. Check for nuchal cord.
  - If the infant's feet are first encountered, continue as a breech delivery.
  - Suction the mouth and nares with bulb suction.
  - Complete delivery of the infant's shoulders and thorax.
  - Clamp and cut the umbilical cord.
  - Continue neonatal resuscitation as necessary.
  - Check maternal pulses and continue CPR.
  - Relief of aortocaval compression by the uterus improves maternal hemodynamics.
  - Cases of maternal survival have been reported.

Complications
- Bladder injury
- Bowel injury
- Fetal lacerations and injury
- Neonate with neurologic deficits and/or demise
- Maternal bleeding and infection
- Maternal morbidity

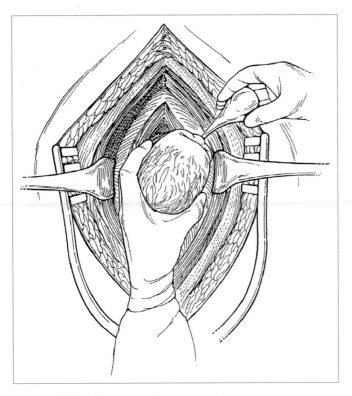

FIGURE 102.2: Delivery through cesarean section.

Common Pitfalls

- Use of fetal Doppler or ultrasonography—not practical before procedure and creates unnecessary time delay!

Pearls

- Fetal survival is dependent on time from maternal cardiac arrest to fetal delivery.
- Begin cesarean delivery within 4 minutes of cardiopulmonary arrest and complete delivery of infant within 5 minutes of arrest.
- Prognosis of fetal survival is greater with the sudden death of a previously healthy mother or in those fetuses with later gestational age.
- Continue CPR throughout procedure and reassess maternal vital signs after delivery. Maternal survival after relief of aortocaval compression has been reported.
- Neonatologist/pediatrician and obstetrician should be present when possible.

Suggested Readings

Benrubi GI. *Handbook of Obstetric and Gynecologic Emergencies*, 3rd ed. Philadelphia: Lippincott Williams & Wilkins, 2005.

Roberts JR, Hedges JR. *Clinical Procedures in Emergency Medicine*, 4th ed. Philadelphia: WB Saunders, 2004:1137–1139.

Wolfson AB, Hendey GW, Hendry PL, et al. *Harwood-Nuss' Clinical Practice of Emergency Medicine*, 4th ed. Philadelphia: Lippincott Williams & Wilkins, 2005:521.

103

Retrorograde Urethrogram

Michael Rosselli

Introduction

- For injury identification purposes, the genitourinary system is best divided into the upper urinary tract (kidneys, ureters), the lower urinary tract (bladder, urethra) and external genitalia (penis, scrotum, testes or vagina, labia minora, labia majora).
- Trauma to the urinary tract accounts for about 10% of all injuries seen in the emergency department.
- Early clinical suspicion, appropriate and reliable radiologic studies, and prompt surgical intervention, when indicated, are the keys to successful diagnosis and management.

Indications

- Blood at the urethral meatus
- Abnormal position of the prostate on rectal examination
- Perineal ecchymosis
- Scrotal ecchymosis
- Blood from the introitus/vaginal vault

Contraindications

- No absolute contraindications exist.

Landmarks

- The dome of the bladder is covered by peritoneum, and the bladder neck is fixed to neighboring structures by reflections of the pelvic fascia and by true ligaments of the pelvis.
- In males, the bladder neck is contiguous with the prostate, which is attached to the pubis by puboprostatic ligaments.
- In females, pubourethral ligaments support the bladder neck and urethra.
- The body of the bladder receives support from the urogenital diaphragm inferiorly and the obturator internus muscles laterally.

Technique

- Dilute stock contrast solution with saline 1:10 (10% solution).
- Lay patient supine.
- Acquire a plain film (KUB) of reference prior to injecting contrast.
- In males, secure the penis with a folded 4 × 4 gauze with your long finger and ring finger of your nondominant hand (be sure to stretch the penis perpendicularly across the patient's thigh to prevent urethral folding).
- After sterile preparation, a catheter-tipped Toomey irrigating syringe or a regular 60 cc piston syringe is gently placed inside the urethral meatus until a snug fit is ensured.

- Inject approximately 50–60 cc of dilute contrast material slowly under constant pressure for more than 30–60 seconds. During the injection of the last 10 cc of contrast material, the x-ray film (urethrogram) is taken.
- *Alternative technique* (Fig. 103.1):
  - Insert a Foley catheter just inside the urethral meatus.
  - Inflate the balloon with 2 cc of sterile water for a snug fit within the fossa navicularis.
  - Inject contrast at a constant rate similar to the technique defined above.

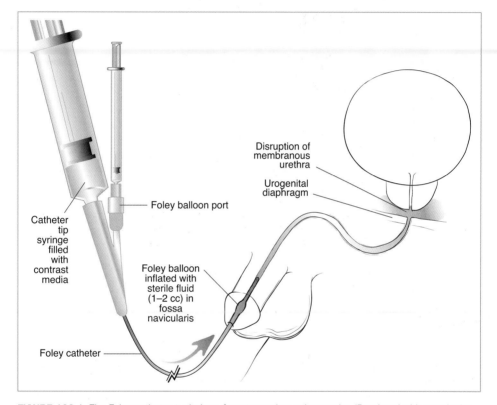

FIGURE 103.1: The Foley catheter technique for retrograde urethrography. (Reprinted with permission from King C, Henretig FM et al. *Textbook of Pediatric Emergency Procedures* 2nd ed. Philadelphia: Lippincott Williams & Wilkins, 2008.)

Complications

- Insertion of a Foley catheter may extend a partial urethral tear into a complete urethral tear.

Findings

- Urethral injury is indicated by
  - Extravasation of contrast material (Fig. 103.2)
    - Anterior tears will demonstrate extravasation below the urogenital diaphragm.
    - Posterior tears will demonstrate extravasation above the urogenital diaphragm.
  - Failure of contrast material to reach bladder

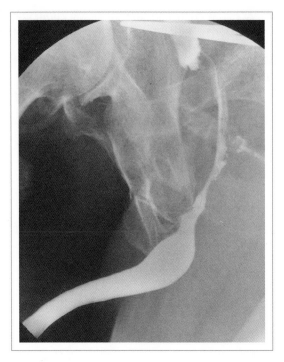

FIGURE 103.2: Retrograde urethrogram with partial tear of membranous urethra. (Reprinted with permission from Wolfson AB, Hendey GW, Ling LJ, et al. *Harwood-Nuss' Clinical Practice of Emergency Medicine*, 5th ed. Philadelphia: Lippincott Williams & Wilkins, 2009.)

- If retrograde urethrogram is positive for injury
  - Do not pass urethral catheter
  - Obtain urology consultation

Suggested Readings

Carroll PR, McAninch JW. Major bladder trauma: mechanisms of injury and a unified method of diagnosis and repair. *J Urol*. 1984;132(2):254–257.

Corriere JN Jr, Sandler CM. Bladder rupture from external trauma: diagnosis and management. *World J Urol*. 1999;17(2):84–89.

Hoecker C, Ruddy R. Emergent radiologic evaluation of renal and genitourinary trauma. In: Henretig F, King C, eds. *Pediatric Emergency Procedures*. Philadelphia: Lippincott Williams & Wilkins, 1997:429–434.

Schneider R. Urologic procedures. In: Roberts JR, Hedges JR, eds. *Clinical Procedures in Emergency Medicine*, 4th ed. Philadelphia: Saunders, 2004:1107–1112.

104

Escharotomy

Steven Shuchat and Jeffrey P. Green

Indications
- Used to decompress accumulated edema under tight, unyielding eschar following full-thickness burn.
- Circumferential extremity burn with evidence of neurovascular compromise:
  - Cyanosis
  - Deep tissue pain
  - Progressive paresthesia
  - Decreased or absent pulses
  - Elevated compartment pressure
  - Decreased arterial flow on Doppler ultrasound
  - Pulse oximetry <95% of effected extremity (without systemic hypoxia)
- Thoracic burn with evidence of respiratory compromise from eschar
- Circumferential neck burn
- Abdominal burn with evidence of increased intra-abdominal pressure (usually estimated by bladder pressure)
- Circumferential penile burn

Contraindications
- No evidence of tissue hypoperfusion by physical examination
- Normal arterial Doppler ultrasound
- Adequate respiration despite eschar
- No evidence of increased intra-abdominal pressure

Risk/Consent Issues
- Often difficult to obtain consent from major burn victims; escharotomy is a lifesaving procedure and should be performed even if informed consent from the patient cannot be obtained.
- Procedure can cause pain (local and systemic analgesia will be provided).
- Risk of bleeding (minimized with proper technique).
- Whenever the skin is broken, there is potential for introducing infection (sterile technique will be utilized).

Landmarks
Escharotomy sites are depicted in Figure 104.1.

Technique
- Do not delay procedure for transfer to burn center.
- Incision to subcutaneous level so that eschar is released, preferably with bovie cautery device to minimize bleeding.

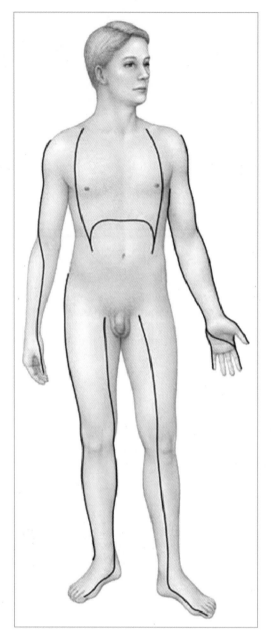

FIGURE 104.1: Escharotomy sites. (From Haro LH, Miller S, Decker WW. Burns. In: Wolfson AB, ed. *Harwood-Nuss' clinical practice of emergency medicine*, 4th ed. Philadelphia: Lippincott Williams & Wilkins; 2005:1106, with permission.)

- Thoracic escharotomy.
  - Longitudinal incisions along each midclavicular line from 2 cm below the clavicle to the tenth rib; connect with two transverse incisions across the chest, forming a square.
- Extremity eschar
  - Incision to subcutaneous layer only.
  - Cut through the entire length of the burn eschar.

Complications of Escharotomy
- Hemorrhage from superficial veins
- Infection
- Damage to underlying structures
- Complications of poorly done procedure
- Muscle necrosis
- Nerve injury, that is, foot drop

Common Pitfalls
- Underestimating the extent of the burn; often burns will not fully declare their penetration for 24–72 hours
- Failure to frequently reevaluate airway patency
- Failure to consider concomitant carbon monoxide or cyanide exposure
- Failure to use bovie cautery for escharotomy

Pearls
- More than 1 million thermal burns occur annually.
- Obtain carboxyhemoglobin level to evaluate for carbon monoxide poisoning for closed space burns.
- Suspect cyanide poisoning for burns involving wool, silk, nylon, and polyurethane found in furniture or paper.
- Never apply silver sulfadiazine to the face because it can cause skin discoloration.
- Always give tetanus prophylaxis.
- Individually wrap toes and fingers.
- For sulfa allergic patients, bacitracin is appropriate for initial burn infection prophylaxis.
- Escharotomy should not be delayed for transfer to burn center.

Suggested Readings
Chapter 14. *Resources for Optimal Care of the Injured Patient*. Committee on Trauma, American College of Surgeons, 1999.

Simon RR, Brenner BE. *Emergency Procedures and Techniques*, 4th ed. Philadelphia: Lippincott Williams & Wilkins, 2002:395–397.

Wolfson AB. *Harwood-Nuss' Clinical Practice of Emergency Medicine*, 4th ed. Philadelphia: Lippincott Williams & Wilkins, 2005:1101–1107.

Indications

- Emergency venous access for fluid resuscitation and drug infusion
- Central venous pressure and O_2 monitoring
- Infusions requiring central venous administration (vasopressors, hyperosmolar solutions, hyperalimentation)
- Routine venous access due to inadequate peripheral intravenous sites
- Introduction of pulmonary artery catheter
- Introduction of transvenous pacing wire

Contraindications

- No absolute contraindications
- Relative contraindications
  - Coagulopathic patients
  - Overlying infection, burn, or skin damage at puncture site
  - Distorted anatomy or trauma at the cannulation site
  - Combative or uncooperative patients
  - Penetrating trauma with suspected proximal vascular injury
  - Pneumothorax on contralateral side (risk of bilateral pneumothoraces)
  - Chronic obstructive pulmonary disease

Risks/Consent Issues

- Pain (local anesthesia will be given)
- Local bleeding and hematoma
- Infection (sterile technique will be utilized)
- Pneumothorax or hemothorax and need for potential chest tube

Landmarks

- The right side is often preferred because of the lower pleural dome on the right and also because the thoracic duct is on the left.
- **Infraclavicular approach** (most commonly used) (Fig. 105.1).
  - Make needle entry at bisection of middle and medial thirds of the clavicle.
  - Aim toward suprasternal notch.
  - Orient bevel inferomedially to facilitate wire entry.
- **Supraclavicular Approach** (Fig. 105.2).
  - Make needle entry just above clavicle, 1 cm lateral to insertion of clavicular head of sternocleidomastoid (SCM).
  - Aim to bisect angle between SCM and clavicle (or toward contralateral nipple).
  - Orient bevel upward.

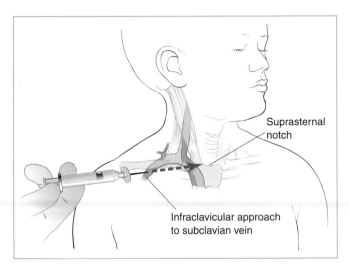

FIGURE 105.1: Infraclavicular approach for subclavian vein cannulation. (From Lavelle J, Costarino A, Jr. Central venous access and central venous pressure monitoring. In: Henretig FM, King C, eds. *Textbook of Pediatric Emergency Procedures*. Philadelphia: Williams & Wilkins, 1997:273, with permission.)

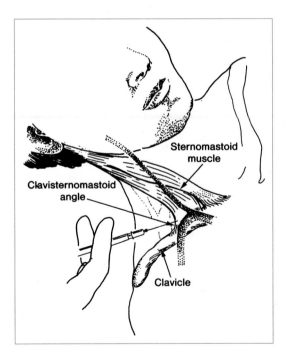

FIGURE 105.2: Supraclavicular subclavian approach. The site of entry is at the junction of the lateral aspect of the clavicular head of the sternocleidomastoid muscle with the superior border of the clavicle, called the clavisternomastoid angle. Direct the needle at a 5-degree angle from the coronal plane, at 50 degrees from the sagittal plane, and at 40 degrees from the transverse plane. (From Simon RR, Brenner BE. *Emergency Procedures and Techniques*, 4th ed. Philadelphia: Lippincott Williams & Wilkins; 2002:463, with permission.)

Technique

- **Patient reparation**
  - Place patient in 15-degree Trendelenburg position.
  - Ensure continuous pulse oximetry, electrocardiogram, and blood pressure.
  - Prepare the clavicular area with povidone-iodine solution, including the neck in case subclavian vein access fails and internal jugular vein access is necessary.
  - Apply sterile drapes.

Note: Unless immediate emergent access is warranted, the physician attempting, the procedure must wear cap, eye shields, and mask with sterile gown and gloves.

- **Locate the subclavian vein**
  - Analgesia: Use 25- or 27-gauge needle to anesthetize skin and subcutaneous tissue with 1% lidocaine.
  - Insert introducer needle (see "Landmarks" section).
  - Infraclavicular: At a shallow angle to the skin, advance the needle just posterior to the clavicle at the junction of medial and middle thirds. Apply posterior pressure on needle to direct it under the clavicle, aiming toward suprasternal notch.
  - Supraclavicular: Insert the needle 1 cm superior to clavicle and 1 cm lateral to SCM clavicular head. Direct the needle 10–15 degrees upward from the horizontal plane, just posterior to the clavicle aiming toward the contralateral nipple or bisection of angle between SCM and clavicle.
  - Aspirate continuously with the dominant hand while advancing the needle.
  - If redirecting needle, always withdraw to the level of skin first.
  - Once the vessel is located, free-flowing venous blood is aspirated.
- **Seldinger technique**
  - Stabilize and hold needle in place with nondominant hand. Remove the syringe from the needle and cap the hub with your thumb to minimize risk of air embolism.
  - Advance guide-wire through introducer needle. The wire should pass easily and not be forced. **Never let go of the guide-wire!**
  - If resistance is met, withdraw the wire and rotate it, adjust location or angle of needle entry, or remove wire and reaspirate with syringe to ensure that needle is still in vessel.
  - Remove the needle, always holding wire in place.
  - Make a superficial skin incision with the sharp scalpel bevel angled away from wire to allow easy passage of the dilator.
  - Pass the dilator over the guide-wire, always holding onto wire.
  - Advance the dilator through the skin and into the vessel with a slow, firm, twisting motion.
  - Remove dilator, leaving the guide-wire in place.
  - Pass the catheter over the wire until it emerges from the catheter's proximal end. **While holding the guide-wire,** advance catheter through the skin and into the vessel with a similar slow, firm, twisting motion.
  - Withdraw the guide-wire through the catheter.
  - Attach syringe to catheter hub and aspirate blood to confirm placement in the vein.
  - Flush and saline lock catheter lumen.
- **Final steps**
  - If inserting multilumen central line, always aspirate, flush, and heplock all lumen.
  - Suture the catheter to the skin using silk or nylon sutures.
  - Cover skin insertion site with sterile dressing.

- **Confirmation**
  - Obtain chest x-ray film to verify correct line placement and to rule out complications. The line tip should be in the superior vena cava, just superior to the right atrium.

Complications
- Arterial puncture or cannulation
- Vessel laceration or dissection
- Pneumothorax or hemothorax
- Air embolism
- Catheter tip embolism
- Catheter malposition
- Dysrhythmias
- Lost guide-wire
- Tracheal puncture or endotracheal cuff perforation
- Venous thrombosis
- Insertion site cellulitis
- Line sepsis

Common Pitfalls
- Use of inadequate local anesthesia
- Inadequate incision with scalpel
- Advancing the guide-wire into the atrium and right ventricle can cause dysrhythmias, which can be corrected by retracting the guide-wire. Always have patient on cardiac monitor.

Pearls
- In cases of penetrating thoracic trauma, place subclavian line on the same side as the chest wound because of the risk of bilateral pneumothoraces, unless proximal vascular injury is suspected.
- If unsuccessful, move next to the ipsilateral internal jugular. Do not attempt the opposite side without a chest x-ray first (risk of bilateral pneumothoraces).
- Never let go of guide-wire. One end must always be held to prevent its embolism into the vessel.
- Never force the guide-wire or catheter. Applying excessive force on insertion and removal may cause vessel injury, breakage, or embolism.
- Always occlude open hub of needle to prevent air embolism.

Suggested Readings
Rosen P, Sternbach G, Chan T, et al. *Atlas of Emergency Procedures*. St. Louis, Missouri: Mosby, 2001:78–81.

Simon RR, Brenner BE. *Emergency Procedures and Techniques*. Philadelphia: Lippincott Williams & Wilkins, 2002:452–469.

106

Bedside FAST Ultrasonography: Focused Assessment with Sonography for Trauma

Andreana Kwon and David Riley

Indications

- Yes or No: Is there intra-abdominal fluid or fluid around the heart?
- The assessment of blunt thoracoabdominal trauma with significant mechanism of injury.
- The assessment of penetrating torso trauma if operative management is not immediately indicated.

Contraindications

- The FAST examination should never delay a patient's transport to the operating room when operative management is clearly indicated.

Risks/Consent Issues

- The only theoretical risk is allergy to the ultrasound gel.

Advantages

- Noninvasive and no sedation required.
- Can be performed at the bedside while resuscitative efforts are simultaneously being performed.
- Can be performed at the bedside on patients too unstable for the computed tomographic imaging suite.
- Can be repeated serially along with changes in symptoms or hemodynamic stability.

Landmarks

- Subcostal
  - Probe placed in the subxiphoid region pointed toward the heart detects fluid in pericardial sac.
- Hepatorenal
  - Probe placed in the right midaxillary line between the 8th and 11th ribs detects fluid in the hepatorenal space (Morrison's Pouch).
- Splenorenal
  - Probe placed in the left posterior axillary line between the 8th and 11th ribs detects fluid in the splenorenal recess.
- Suprapubic
  - Probe placed 2 cm superior to the symphysis pubis detects fluid in the retrovesical or retrouterine space.

Technique

- The standard four FAST views: subcostal, hepatorenal-Morrison's Pouch, splenorenal, and suprapubic (see Fig. 106.1).

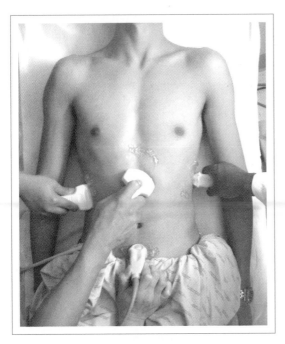

FIGURE 106.1: The four views of the FAST examination. (Reprinted with permission from Shah K, Mason C. *Essential Emergency Procedures*. Philadelphia: Lippincott Williams & Wilkins, 2007.)

- Subcostal/subxiphoid view (Fig. 106.2).
  - With the probe in the transverse plane, place it in the subxiphoid area and aim toward the patient's left shoulder to see a four-chambered view of the heart.

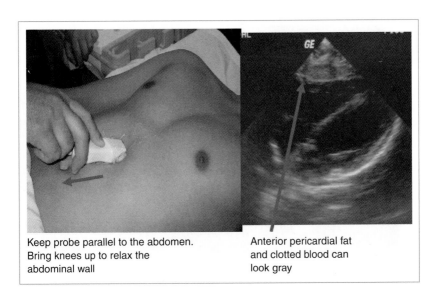

Keep probe parallel to the abdomen.
Bring knees up to relax the
abdominal wall

Anterior pericardial fat
and clotted blood can
look gray

FIGURE 106.2: Subcostal view. (Reprinted with permission from Shah K, Mason C. *Essential Emergency Procedures*. Philadelphia: Lippincott Williams & Wilkins, 2007.)

- Sweep the probe anteriorly and posteriorly to view the entire pericardium.
- Unclotted blood will appear as an anechoic black "stripe" within the hyperechoic pericardial sac (Fig. 106.3).

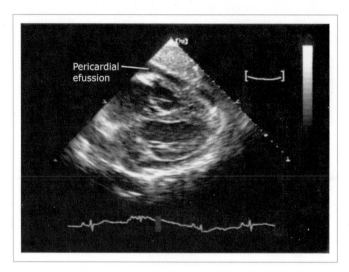

FIGURE 106.3: Ultrasound image taken from the subxiphoid transducer position demonstrating fluid in the pericardial space. (Reprinted with permission from Cosby KS, Kendall JL. *Practical Guide to Emergency Ultrasound*. Philadelphia: Lippincott Williams & Wilkins, 2005.)

- Hepatorenal-Morrison's Pouch view (Fig. 106.4).
  - With the indicator pointed toward the patient's right axilla, place probe in the midaxillary line between 8th and 11th ribs.
  - Hold the probe in a longitudinal or an oblique plane to aid visualization through rib spaces.

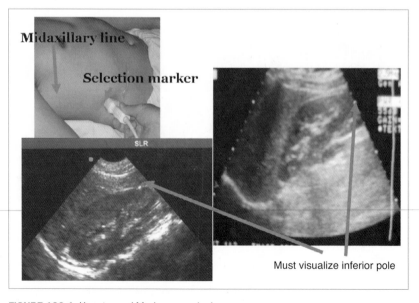

FIGURE 106.4: Hepatorenal-Morison pouch view.

- Unclotted blood or fluid will appear as an anechoic black "stripe" in the space between the liver and right kidney (Fig. 106.5).

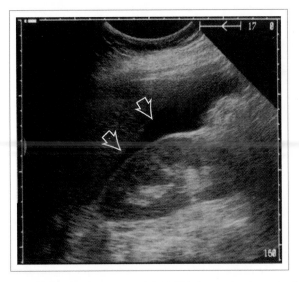

FIGURE 106.5: Intraperitoneal fluid. This image demonstrates free fluid within the peritoneal cavity. Fluid is seen as a black anechoic stripe in Morison's pouch (arrows), which is the potential space between the liver and the kidney. (Reprinted with permission from Harwood-Nuss A, Wolfson AB, et al. *The Clinical Practice of Emergency Medicine*, 3rd ed. Philadelphia: Lippincott Williams & Wilkins, 2001.)

- Splenorenal view (Fig. 106.6).
  - With the indicator pointed toward the patient's left axilla, place the probe in the left posterior axillary line between the 8th and 11th ribs, also at an oblique plane.

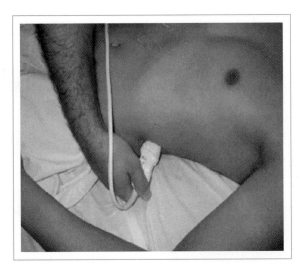

FIGURE 106.6: Location of probe for splenorenal view. (Reprinted with permission from Shah K, Mason C. *Essential Emergency Procedures*. Philadelphia: Lippincott Williams & Wilkins, 2007.)

- Turn the probe longitudinally to enhance your view.
- Unclotted blood or fluid will appear as an anechoic black "stripe" in the space between the spleen and left kidney (Fig. 106.7).

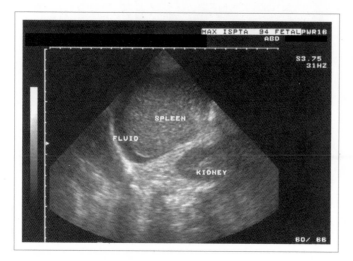

FIGURE 106.7: Peritoneal fluid detected in the left subdiaphragmatic space. (Reprinted with permission from Cosby KS, Kendall JL. *Practical Guide to Emergency Ultrasound*. Philadelphia: Lippincott Williams & Wilkins, 2005.)

- Suprapubic view (Fig. 106.8).
  - This view is facilitated by a full bladder.
  - With the indicator pointing toward the patient's head, place the probe 2 cm superior to the symphysis pubis along the midline.
  - Aim the probe caudally into the pelvis.
  - Rotate the probe 90 degrees counterclockwise for transverse images.

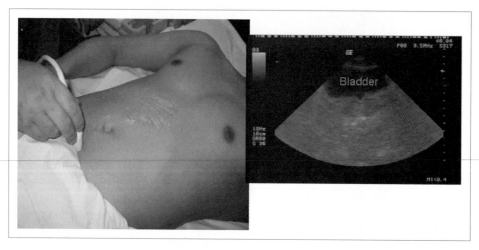

FIGURE 106.8: Suprapubic view.

- Look for anechoic blood adjacent to the bladder and anterior peritoneum (Figs. 106.9 and 106.10).

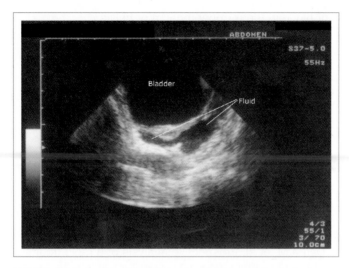

FIGURE 106.9: Sonographic appearance of fluid collecting posterior to the bladder in male patients with the transducer in the transverse orientation. (Reprinted with permission from Cosby KS, Kendall JL. *Practical Guide to Emergency Ultrasound*. Philadelphia: Lippincott Williams & Wilkins, 2005.)

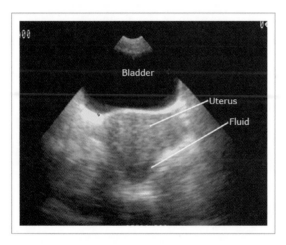

FIGURE 106.10: Ultrasound image of free fluid located posterior to the uterus with the transducer in the transverse orientation. (Reprinted with permission from Cosby KS, Kendall JL. *Practical Guide to Emergency Ultrasound*. Philadelphia: Lippincott Williams & Wilkins, 2005.)

Precautions

- Sensitivity of the examination may be dependent on several factors including the experience of the sonographer, position of patient, equipment used, and the number of serial examinations performed.
- Examination may be obscured by obese body habitus, subcutaneous air, pregnancy, preexisting peritoneal fluid, or increased bowel gas.
- Inferior pole of both kidneys must be visualized to avoid missing early fluid/blood accumulation.

- The FAST examination should *not* be used for the following:
    - Detecting contained solid organ injuries
    - Detecting bowel injuries
    - Detection of blood in the retroperitoneum or pelvis

Pearls

- Placing the patient in Trendelenburg position makes the examination of the RUQ and LUQ more sensitive.
- Remember that fresh unclotted blood will appear anechoic, but fibrin formation during the clotting process can produce variable echoes.
- The sensitivity of the examination will be increased with increasing volume of fluid in the peritoneum.

Suggested Readings

Kimura A, Otsuka T. Emergency center ultrasonography in the evaluation of hemoperitoneum: a prospective study. *J Trauma*. 1991;31:20–23.

Ma OJ, Mateer JR. *Emergency Ultrasound*. New York: McGraw-Hill, 2003.

Ma OJ, Mateer JR, Ogata M, et al. Prospective analysis of a rapid trauma ultrasound examination performed by emergency physicians. *J Trauma*. 1995;38:879–885.

Indications

- Yes or No: Is there a pneumothorax? Is there pleural fluid?
- The assessment of blunt thoracoabdominal trauma or unexplained hypotension.
- The assessment of penetrating torso trauma if operative management is not immediately indicated.

Contraindications

- The E-FAST examination should never delay a patient's transport to the operating room when operative management is clearly indicated.

Risks/Consent Issues

- The only theoretical risk is allergy to the ultrasound gel.

Advantages

- Noninvasive and no sedation required.
- Can be performed at the bedside while resuscitative efforts are simultaneously being performed.
- Can be performed at the bedside on patients too unstable for the computed tomographic imaging suite.
- Can be repeated serially along with changes in symptoms or hemodynamic stability.

Landmarks

- Anterior thorax
  - Probe placed in the mid-clavicular line in the sagittal plane; probe marker positioned cephalad.
- Right pleural-hepatorenal
  - Probe placed in the right mid-axillary line in the coronal plane at the level of the 8–11th ribs with the diaphragm as a landmark; probe marker positioned towards the axilla.
- Left pleural-splenorenal
  - Probe placed in the left posterior axillary line in the coronal plane at the level of the 8–11th ribs with the diaphragm as a landmark; probe marker positioned towards the axilla.

Technique

- The E-FAST standard views in addition to the basic FAST examination: **Bilateral Anterior Thorax, Right Pleural-Hepatorenal, and Left Pleural-Splenorenal**
- Anterior thorax
  - With the indicator pointed toward the patient's head, place the probe in the second or third intercostal space in the midclavicular line.
  - Slide the probe caudally for evaluation of a pneumothorax.

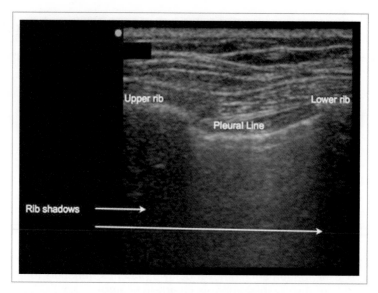

FIGURE 107.1: The bat sign (rib shadow, pleura, rib shadow).

- The upper rib-pleural line-lower rib profile is referred to as the **bat sign** (Fig. 107.1).
- Normal lung findings
  - ▸ visible sliding at the level of the pleura in B-mode
  - ▸ **comet tails**—vertical reverberation artifacts arising from the pleural line (Fig. 107.2)
  - ▸ **seashore sign** in M-mode (Fig. 107.3)
- Lung findings suggestive of a pneumothorax
  - ▸ loss of pleural sliding, as there is loss of contact between the visceral and the parietal pleura
  - ▸ absence of comet tails
  - ▸ **stratosphere sign** or **bar code sign** in M-mode (Fig. 107.4)

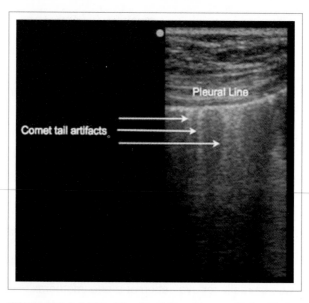

FIGURE 107.2: Bright white pleural line with comet tail artifacts.

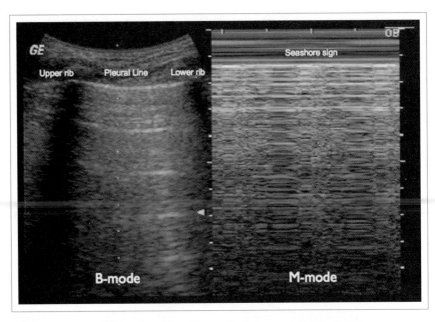

FIGURE 107.3: M-mode demonstrates the seashore sign seen in normal lung.

- Lung sliding may be absent in patients who are not spontaneously breathing, complete atelectasis, apnea, pleural scarring, or intubation on the opposite side.
- The **lung point** is the transition between collapsed and normally expanded lung. Although difficult to locate, the lung point is reportedly 100% specific for pneumothorax when identifiable.
- Table 107.1 compares the signs suggestive of normal lung versus pneumothorax.

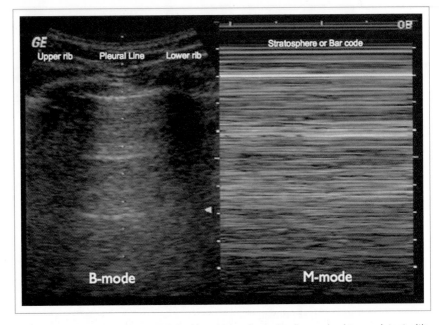

FIGURE 107.4: M-mode demonstrating the stratosphere sign/bar code sign consistent with pneumothorax. (Courtesy of Dr. Marina Del Rios.).

TABLE 107.1: Signs suggestive of normal lung versus pneumothorax using ultrasonography

Normal lung	Pneumothorax
Lung sliding	Absence of lung sliding
Comet tail artifact	Absence of comet tails
Seashore sign	Stratosphere/bar code sign Lung point

■ **Right pleural-hepatorenal view**
- With the indicator pointed toward the patient's right axilla, place probe in the midaxillary line at the level of 8th and 11th ribs.
- Slide the probe 1–2 spaces superiorly to visualize the space above the diaphragm.
- The presence of **"mirror imaging"** of the liver or spleen above the hyperechoic line representing the hemidiaphragm is evidence against pleural fluid (Fig. 107.5).
- Unclotted blood or fluid will appear as an anechoic black "stripe" in the space above the diaphragm (Fig. 107.6).

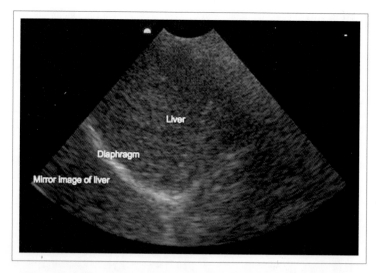

FIGURE 107.5: Right pleural-hepatorenal space. "Mirror imaging" (evidence against the presence of pleural fluid) is demonstrated.

■ **Left pleural-splenorenal view**
- With the indicator pointed toward the patient's left axilla, place the probe in the left posterior axillary line at the level of the 8th and 11th ribs, also at an oblique plane.
- If a rib shadow precludes the ability to evaluate this area, rotate the probe obliquely toward the back.
- Slide the probe 1–2 spaces superiorly to visualize the space above the diaphragm.
- Unclotted blood or fluid will appear as an anechoic black "stripe" in the space above the diaphragm.
- Rotate the probe toward the back if rib shadows prevent full evaluation.

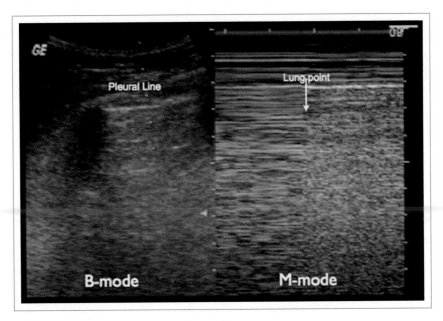

FIGURE 107.6: Right pleural-hepatorenal space with pleural fluid.

Precautions

- Sensitivity of the examination may be dependent on several factors including the experience of the sonographer, position of patient, equipment used, and the number of serial examinations performed.
- Examination may be obscured by obese body habitus, subcutaneous air, preexisting pleural fluid, or pleural disease.
- The E-FAST examination is *not* the modality of choice to detect solid organ injuries.

Pearls

- Remember that fresh unclotted blood will appear anechoic, but fibrin formation during the clotting process can produce variable echoes.
- The sensitivity of the examination will be increased with increasing volume of fluid in the thorax.

Suggested Readings

Abrams BJ, Sukumvanich P, Seibel R, et al. Ultrasound for the detection of intra-peritoneal fluid: the role of Trendelenburg positioning. *Am J Emerg Med.* 1999;17(2):117–120.

Blaivas M, Lyon M, Duggal S. A prospective comparison of supine chest radiography and bedside ultrasound for the diagnosis of traumatic pneumothorax. *Acad Emerg Med.* 2005;12(9):844–849.

Lichtenstein D, et al. The lung point: an ultrasound sign specific to pneumothorax. *Intensive Care Med.* 2000;26(10):1434–1440.

Lichtenstein DA. *Ultrasound in the Critically Ill.* New York: Springer-Verlag France, 2002:96–115.

Lichtenstein DA. Ultrasound in the management of thoracic disease. *Crit Care Med.* 2007;35(5 suppl):S250–S261.

Rothlin MA, et al. Ultrasound in blunt abdominal and thoracic trauma. *J Trauma.* 1993;34(4):488–495.

108 Wound Closures and Suture Materials

Brandon Godbout

Standard skin closure methods

Closure method	Indication	Advantages	Disadvantages	Disposition	Notes
Wound tape	Superficial wounds Linear Low tension	Fast Easy application Lowest infection rate Low cost Painless **Method of choice in:** Avulsed and friable tissue in elderly	Easily removed Greatest risk to fall off **Does not work with:** Hairy regions Moist skin Irregular wounds Moderate-high tension wounds	Generally in place for 2 weeks May vary with laceration location Keep dry for first 24 hours Gentle wash after 24–48 hours	Always dry skin before placement Apply Benzoin to edges for increased strength Cosmetically similar results in small superficial facial lacerations compared to tissue adhesives
Tissue adhesives	Superficial wounds Clean approximation Low tension Flat areas	Fastest method Easy application Antimicrobial properties No need for removal Low cost Painless **Method of choice in:** Simple facial lacerations in children	Less tensile strength Avoid placing near highly active regions (i.e., joints) Small increased risk for wound dehiscence compared with other methods	Sloughs off in 7–10 days Keep dry for first 24 hours Gentle wash after 24–48 hours No need for return or follow-up visit	Caution around eyes Apply multiple (2–3) layers Do not apply into wound Hold wound together after application for 1 minute Comparable cosmetic outcome and rate of infection compared with other wound closure methods
Staples	Superficial wounds Linear Scalp and extremities	Fast Low cost Low tissue reactivity **Method of choice in:** Simple scalp lacerations without involvement of galea aponeurotica	Least precise Removal more painful than sutures Interference with computed tomographic/magnetic resonance imaging	***Staple removal*** Scalp 10 days Extremity 7–10 days	If galea aponeurotica involved, must place deep dermal sutures before staples for effective closure Infection rates and cosmetic outcomes similar to sutures Do not use on face

(continued)

Closure method	Indication	Advantages	Disadvantages	Disposition	Notes
Sutures	Most wounds, including irregular and moderate to high tension lacerations **Suture size guide** Hand/finger **5–0** Face **5–0/6–0** Most others: **4–0**	Lowest wound dehiscence rate Greatest strength **Method of choice in:** Moderate to high-tension wounds Irregular lacerations Deep lacerations Structures requiring precise approximation Difficult hemostasis	Time-consuming Painful Must return for removal Greatest tissue reactivity Costly Operator dependent	**Suture removal** Face 3–5 days Scalp 6–8 days Extremity 10–14 days Back 10–14 days High tension 10–14 days (joints/hands)	High-tension wounds may also require deep dermal absorbable sutures No difference in cosmetic outcome, wound dehiscence, or infection rates in absorbable versus nonabsorbable sutures used during simple wound repair in pediatric patients

Suture characteristics based on location

Location	Suture type	Suture size	Removal
Scalp	Superficial: Nonabsorbable Deep: Absorbable	4–0 or 5–0 3–0 or 4–0	6–8 days
Face	Superficial: Nonabsorbable Deep: Absorbable	6–0 5–0	3–5 days followed by adhesive tape
Ear	Superficial: Nonabsorbable	6–0	10–14 days
Chest/abdomen	Superficial: Nonabsorbable Deep: Absorbable	4–0 or 5–0 3–0 or 4–0	8–10 days
Back	Superficial: Nonabsorbable Deep: Absorbable	4–0 or 5–0 3–0 or 4–0	10–14 days
Extremities	Superficial: Nonabsorbable Deep: Absorbable	4–0 or 5–0 3–0 or 4–0	10–14 days
Hand	Superficial: Nonabsorbable Deep: Absorbable[a]	5–0 5–0	10–14 days
Foot/sole	Superficial: Nonabsorbable Deep: Absorbable	3–0 or 4–0 4–0	12–14 days
Penis	Superficial: Nonabsorbable	5–0 or 6–0	8–10 days

[a]Deep sutures in the hand should generally be avoided as there is high risk for inadvertently tying important neurovascular structures.

Characteristics of absorbable sutures

Suture type	Quality	Indication	Absorption	Notes
Polyglactin (Vicryl Rapide)	Braided	Subcutaneous/intraoral closures	Day 14: 0% tensile strength retained	Faster rate of hydrolysis than plain Vicryl
Polyglactin (Vicryl)	Braided	Subcutaneous/intraoral closures	Day 28: 8% tensile strength retained	Tensile strength roughly equivalent to Dexon
Polyglycolic Acid (Dexon)	Monofilament or braided	Subcutaneous/intraoral closures	Day 28: 5% tensile strength retained	Tensile strength roughly equivalent to Vicryl
Polydioxone (PDS)	Monofilament	Subcutaneous closures	Day 28: 58% tensile strength retained	Useful in deeper wounds requiring prolonged strength or suture
Polyglyconate (Maxon)	Monofilament	Subcutaneous closures	Day 28: 59% tensile strength retained	Useful in deeper wounds requiring prolonged strength or suture
Catgut-plain	Sheep intestinal intima	Intraoral closures	Quickly absorbed in 5–7 days	Rarely used. Often breaks down before wounds have healed
Catgut-chromic	Chromic acid Treated catgut	Intraoral closures	Absorbed within several weeks	Tensile strength is twice that of plain catgut. High tissue reactivity

Characteristics of nonabsorbable sutures

Suture type	Quality	Indication	Absorption	Notes
Nylon (Ethilon)	Monofilament	Skin closures	1 year: 89% tensile strength retained	Low cost. Minimal tissue reactivity
Polypropylene (Prolene)	Monofilament	Skin/subcuticular closures	No loss of tensile strength	Colored—easy visibility in hairy areas. Slippery—may require extra knots for security
Polyester (Dacron)	Braided	Tendon repairs	No loss of tensile strength	Most elastic
Silk	Braided	Intraoral closures	Complete absorption in months	Induces strong tissue reaction. Best handling

Suggested Readings

Farion K, Osmond MH, Hartling L, et al. Tissue adhesives for traumatic lacerations in children and adults. *Cochrane Database Syst Rev.* 2002(3);CD003326.

George TK, Simpson DC. Skin wound closure with staples in the accident and emergency department. *J Roy Coll Surg Edinburg.* 1985;30:54.

Hollander JE, Giarrusso E, Cassara G, Valentine S, Singer AJ. Comparison of staples and sutures for closure of scalp lacerations. *Acad Emerg Med.* 1997;4:460.

Hsiao WC, Young KC, Wang ST, Lin PW. Incisional hernia after laparotomy: randomised comparison between early-absorbable and late-absorbable suture materials. *World J Surg.* 2000;24:747–751.

Karounis H, Gouin S, Eisman H, Chalut D, Pelletier H, Williams B. A randomized, controlled trial comparing long-term cosmetic outcomes of traumatic pediatric lacerations repaired with absorbable plain gut versus nonabsorbable nylon sutures. *Acad Emerg Med.* 2004;11:730.

Ritchie AJ, Rocke LG. Staples versus sutures in the closure of scalp wounds: a prospective, double-blind, randomized trial. *Injury.* 1989;20:217.

Roberts J, Jerris H. *Clinical Procedures in Emergency Medicine.* Philadelphia: Saunders, 2004.

Singer AJ, Hollander JE. Methods for wound closure. In: Tintinalli J, ed. *Emergency Medicine: A Comprehensive Study Guide*, 6th ed. New York: McGraw-Hill, 2004:292–298.

Singer AJ, Hollander JE, Quinn J. Evaluation and management of traumatic lacerations. *New Engl J Med.* 1997;337:1142–1148.

Singer AJ, Quinn JV, Hollander JE, Clark RE. Closure of lacerations and incisions with octyl cyanoacrylate: a multi-center randomized clinical trial. *Surgery.* 2002;131:270.

Zempsky WT, Grem C, Nichols J, Parrotti D. Prospective comparison of cosmetic outcomes of facial lacerations closed with steri-strips or dermabond. *Acad Emerg Med.* 2001;8:438.

Zempsky WT, Parrotti D, Grem C, Nichols J. Randomized controlled comparison of cosmetic outcomes of simple facial lacerations closed with Steri Strip Skin Closures or Dermabond tissue adhesive. *Pediatr Emerg Care.* 2004;20(8):519–524.

Index

Note: Italicized *t* and *f* refer to tables and figures.